Requisites in
DERMATOLOGY
Cosmetic Dermatology

For Elsevier

Commissioning Editor: Thu Nguyen
Development Editor: Claire Bonnett
Project Manager: Hemamalini Rajendrababu and Jess Thompson
Designer: Stewart Larking
Illustrator: Richard Prime

Requisites in DERMATOLOGY

Cosmetic Dermatology

Edited by

Murad Alam, MD
Chief, Section of Cutaneous and
Aesthetic Surgery
Associate Professor, Department of
Dermatology, Otolaryngology, and Surgery
Feinberg School of Medicine,
Northwestern University
Chicago, IL, USA

Hayes B. Gladstone, MD
Director, Division of Dermatologic Surgery
Associate Professor
Department of Dermatology
Department of Otolaryngology – Head and
Neck Surgery, Stanford University
Stanford, CA, USA

Rebecca C. Tung, MD
Staff Physician,
Department of Dermatology
The Cleveland Clinic
Cleveland, OH, USA

Series editor

DIRK M ELSTON

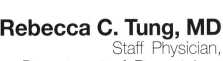

SAUNDERS

ELSEVIER

Edinburgh   London   New York   Oxford   Philadelphia   St Louis   Sydney   Toronto 2009

SAUNDERS
ELSEVIER

An imprint of Elsevier Limited

First published 2009

ISBN: 978-0-7020-3143-4

British Library Cataloguing in Publication Data
A catalogue record for this book is available from the British Library

Library of Congress Cataloging in Publication Data
A catalog record for this book is available from the Library of Congress

ELSEVIER your source for books, journals and multimedia in the health sciences
www.elsevierhealth.com

Working together to grow libraries in developing countries
www.elsevier.com | www.bookaid.org | www.sabre.org

ELSEVIER   BOOK AID International   Sabre Foundation

The Publisher's policy is to use paper manufactured from sustainable forests

Printed in China

Contents

Contributors

Murad Alam, MD
Chief, Section of Cutaneous
and Aesthetic Surgery
Associate Professor, Department of
Dermatology, Otolaryngology, and Surgery
Feinberg School of Medicine
Northwestern University
Chicago, IL, USA

R. Sonia Batra, MD
Clinical Assistant Professor of Dermatology
USC Keck School of Medicine
Los Angeles, CA, USA

Daniel Berg, MD, FRCPC
Professor of Dermatology
Department of Medicine
Director, Dermatologic Surgery
University of Washington Medical Center
Seattle, WA, USA

David Beynet, MD
Chief Resident
UCLA Division of Dermatology
David Geffen School of Medicine at UCLA
Los Angeles, CA, USA

Tina Bhutani, BSc
MD Candidate
Keck School of Medicine
University of Southern California
Los Angeles, CA, USA

Joel L. Cohen, MD
Director, DermSurgery, About Skin
Dermatology
Englewood, CO, USA

Paul C. Cotterill, BSc, MD, ABHRS
President, International Society of Hair
Restoration Surgery
Diplomate, American Board of Hair
Restoration Surgery
Toronto, ON, Canada

Paul M. Friedman, MD
Director, DermSurgery Laser Center
Clinical Assistant Professor
Department of Dermatology
University of Texas Health Science Center
Houston, TX, USA

Hayes B. Gladstone, MD
Director, Division of Mohs Micrographic
Surgery, Cutaneous Laser Surgery, and
Aesthetic Dermatologic Surgery
Department of Dermatology
Stanford University School of Medicine
Stanford, CA, USA

Joseph Greco, MD
Clinical Instructor
UCLA Division of Dermatology
David Geffen School of Medicine
at UCLA
Los Angeles, CA, USA

Jillian Havey, BSc
MD Candidate
Clinical Trials Unit
Department of Dermatology
Northwestern University
Feinberg School of Medicine
Chicago, IL, USA

Carolyn I. Jacob, MD
Chicago Cosmetic Surgery and
Dermatology
Chicago, IL, USA

Jeremy Kampp, MD
Department of Dermatology
Stanford University Medical Center
Stanford, CA, USA

Joy H. Kunishige, MD
Department of Dermatology
University of Texas Health Science Center
Houston, TX, USA

Rajeev Mallipeddi, BSc(Hons), MD, MRCP
Consultant Dermatologist and Director
Dermatological Surgery and Laser Unit
St John's Institute of Dermatology
St Thomas' Hospital
London, UK

Isaac M. Neuhaus, MD
Assistant Professor
Dermatologic Surgery & Laser Center
Department of Dermatology
University of California, San Francisco
San Francisco, CA, USA

Divya Singh-Behl, MD
Deerfield Dermatology
Deerfield, IL, USA

Brian Somoano, MD
Department of Dermatology
Stanford University Medical Center
Stanford, CA, USA

Teresa Soriano, MD
Associate Clinical Professor of Medicine
Co-director, UCLA Dermatologic
Surgery and Laser Center
UCLA Division of Dermatology
David Geffen School of Medicine
at UCLA
Los Angeles, CA, USA

Jamison E. Strahan, MD
Department of Dermatology
University of Colorado Health
Sciences Center
Aurora, CO, USA

Lily Talakoub, MD
Department of Dermatology
University of California, San Francisco
San Francisco, CA, USA

Amy Forman Taub, MD
Medical Director
Advanced Dermatology, Skinfo, SKINQRI
Assistant Clinical Professor,
Northwestern University Medical School,
Department of Dermatology
Lincolnshire, IL, USA

Rebecca Tung, MD
Staff Physician
Department of Dermatology
Cleveland Clinic Foundation
Cleveland, OH, USA

Sarah Weitzul, MD
Assistant Professor
Southwestern Medical School
Dallas, TX, USA

Siegrid S. Yu, MD
Assistant Professor
Dermatologic Surgery and Laser Center,
Department of Dermatology,
University of California, San Francisco
San Francisco, CA, USA

Dedications

Series Dedication

This series of textbooks is dedicated to my wife Kathy and my children, Carly and Nate. Thank you for your love, support and inspiration. It is also dedicated to the residents and fellows it has been my privilege to teach and to the patients who have taught me so much.

Dirk M. Elston

Cosmetic Dermatology Dedications

To my parents, Rahat and Rehana; my sister, Nigar; and B and E. With love and thanks.

Murad Alam

This book is dedicated to my parents, who provided me with the opportunity and freedom to pursue my dreams, and to my lovely fiancée, Theresa, for her support and feedback during this project.

Hayes B. Gladstone

To my parents, Eleanor and M – Thank you for your continued love, support, enthusiasm and smiles!

Rebecca Tung

Also in the series

Requisites in
DERMATOLOGY

Series Editor: Dirk M Elston

Dermatopathology
Dirk M Elston and Tammie Ferringer

Cosmetic Dermatology
Murad Alam, Hayes B Gladstone,
and Rebecca C Tung

Pediatric Dermatology
Howard B Pride, Albert C Yan, and
Andrea L Zaenglein

Dermatologic Surgery
Allison T Vidimos, Christie T Ammirati,
and Christine Poblete-Lopez

General Dermatology
Kathryn Schwarzenberger, Andrew E Werchniak,
and Christine J Ko

Series foreword

The Requisites in Dermatology series of textbooks is designed around the principle that learning and retention are best accomplished when the forest is clearly delineated from the trees. Topics are presented with an emphasis on the key points essential for residents and practicing clinicians. Each text is designed to stand alone as a reference or to be used as part of an integrated teaching curriculum. Many gifted physicians have contributed their time and energy to create the sort of texts we wish we had had during our own training and each of the texts in the series is accompanied by an innovative on-line module. Each on-line module is designed to complement the text, providing lecture material not possible in print format, including video and lectures with voice-over. These books have been a labor of love for all involved. We hope you enjoy them.

Series preface

We embarked on this series of textbooks with a simple idea: to create the type of texts we wish we had had during our own training. Each text is concise, with an attempt to focus on the essentials. We have used images, tables, and algorithms where possible to make the material accessible. Each chapter emphasizes the key points essential for practicing clinicians and those in training. We have taken advantage of online technology, creating a module to complement each text, providing material such as video that is of value to the reader, but not possible in print format. Many talented individuals have devoted countless hours to the creation of these texts. We hope you enjoy them.

Volume preface

Murad Alam, Hayes B. Gladstone, and Becki Tung set out to create a text that captures the essentials of cosmetic dermatology. The text is designed to stand alone as reference, and to function as part of an integrated curriculum. Along with the other texts in the Requisites series, it provides information essential for the physician in practice as well as for residents and fellows. Topics include the approach to the cosmetic patient, the evolving role of cosmeceuticals in dermatology, the cosmetic use of botulinum toxin, fillers, and lasers. Chapters address both ablative and nonablative light sources as well as skin tightening with radiofrequency and other emerging technologies. Specific chapters are devoted to hair transplantation, liposuction, and other advanced cosmetic surgical procedures. This book has been a labor of love for all involved. We hope you enjoy it.

Acknowledgments

We are grateful for Claire Bonnett's insightful guidance, the continuous support of the entire editorial and production team including Joanne Husovski, Karen Bowler, and Sue Hodson, and the extraordinary patience of the medical illustrators at Elsevier. Many thanks are also due to Jillian Havey for coordinating the efforts of the chapter authors. Finally, we wish to thank our teachers, patients, and the generations of dermatologic surgeons who have pioneered the advanced techniques discussed in this book.

Chapter 1

Approach to the cosmetic patient

*David Beynet, Joseph Greco,
and Teresa Soriano*

Key Points

- Proper patient selection is paramount to optimize surgical outcome and patient satisfaction.
- A complete medical and psychosocial history, and focused physical examination, should be performed prior to cosmetic procedures.

Introduction

A cosmetic patient visit has specific nuances that a regular medical visit does not have. Many of the treatments given and issues addressed are for conditions that are not pathologic, but rather are normal physiologic phenomena. This poses a potential clinical conundrum to medical physicians, who have been taught that one of the cardinal rules of medicine is, "First, do no harm." An argument can be made that any procedure with risk should not be performed for a nonpathologic condition.

However, some may contend that many cosmetic procedures can be performed safely, and that the benefits outweigh the risks. The benefits of cosmetic procedures can extend beyond the improvement of the physical appearance. Numerous studies have shown that increased attractiveness has been associated with an increased rate of employment and promotion, a higher average income and social status, and increased self-confidence and psychological well-being. Hence, enhancing an individual's physical appearance may potentially improve his or her quality of life.

The preoperative assessment is a crucial component in the selection and management of cosmetic patients. This includes an understanding of the patient's concerns for aesthetic improvement and the procedures he or she is willing to undertake. Other aspects of the preoperative visit include a thorough evaluation of the patient's medical and psychosocial history, a detailed examination of the area of concern, discussion of potential interventions, photographic documentation, and informed consent.

Rise in cosmetic procedures

With the advent of less invasive dermatologic procedures and the mainstream popularity of aesthetic procedures, it is not surprising to see the exponential increase of cosmetic procedures. According to the American Society for Aesthetic Plastic Surgery, Americans spent over $12 billion on cosmetic procedures in 2006. The total number of cosmetic procedures performed in the USA increased by 446% between 1997 and 2006. There was a 98% rise in surgical procedures and an impressive 747% increase in nonsurgical procedures. Liposuction was the most common surgical cosmetic procedure, and botulinum toxin A injection was the most commonly performed nonsurgical cosmetic procedure (Fig. 1-1).

In the USA, individuals seeking cosmetic procedures span several decades and racial ethnic backgrounds. In 2006, 72% of individuals seeking cosmetic procedures were between 35 and 64 years old (Fig. 1-2). More men and people from minority ethnic groups are seeking facial rejuvenation procedures. Although women still comprise the large majority of individuals seeking cosmetic procedures, men had nearly 1 million procedures in 2006. Racial ethnic minorities comprised 22% of individuals who had cosmetic procedures in 2006 (Fig. 1-3). Thus, contemporary cosmetic surgeons need to be knowledgeable and sensitive to varying backgrounds, expectations, and treatment modalities for men and women of different ages and skin types.

Concept of beauty

The patient's and society's concepts of beauty are important factors to be considered in the initial evaluation of a cosmetic patient. Studies have shown that a single ideal standard for beauty is difficult to ascertain. Features of beauty may vary based on gender, geographical, cultural, and historical differences. However, certain concepts of

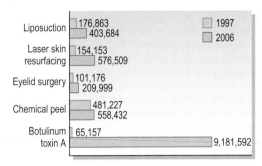

Figure 1-1 Increase in selected cosmetic procedures from 1997 to 2006. Data from the American Society for Aesthetic Plastic Surgery

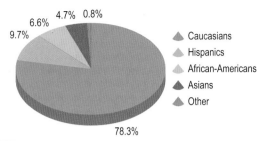

Figure 1-3 Percentage of total procedures according to race, 2006. Reprinted from the American Society for Aesthetic Plastic Surgery

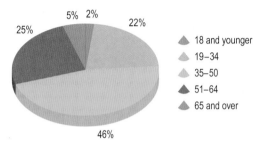

Figure 1-2 Percentage of total cosmetic procedures according to age, 2006. Data from the American Society for Aesthetic Plastic Surgery

beauty tend to remain constant across different cultures and historical time periods.

A beautiful face is thought to be the most important factor for determining overall attractiveness, particularly in the case of female beauty. Facial symmetry as a determinant of attractiveness has been addressed in several studies. From these studies, it seems that, although symmetry has a positive influence on attractiveness, overall facial averageness (of which symmetry is just one component) is more important. Evidence for this comes from a higher rating of attractiveness for facial images created through digital averaging of many faces. Attractiveness tends to increase as the faces become more average. However, although average faces are rated as attractive, they are not among the most attractive. The most attractive faces in general have extreme features as well. In summary, symmetry and averageness are important factors in establishing facial attractiveness, but unique and extreme features may lead to above-average beauty.

With growing cultural diversity and more people from minority ethnic groups seeking aesthetic procedures, it is also important to be aware of ideals of beauty specific to particular cultures. For example, a common desire of Asian patients is to have a more Western eye shape with an increased palpebral angle. They also find rounded jawlines secondary to large mandibles and hypertrophic

masseteric muscles less attractive. Korean patients often desire a near perfect complexion without lentigos, nevi, or other pigmentary abnormalities. To achieve optimal postoperative results and patient satisfaction, cosmetic surgeons need to understand the patient's psychosocial background and adjust the perioperative care and surgical management accordingly.

The initial consultation

The preoperative consultation is essential to establish a relationship between the patient and physician. This should be done in a comfortable setting where patients and physicians can have time to exchange valuable information. During this visit, the physician obtains key information to determine whether or not the patient is appropriate for the procedure.

The focus of the initial consultation should center around a discussion of the patient's concerns and the patient's expectations. When dealing with knowledgeable and experienced cosmetic patients, this task may be fairly straightforward. For example, a patient may come in specifically requesting botulinum toxin to improve prominent glabellar frown lines. However, in many instances, cosmetic patients, particularly those desiring overall facial rejuvenation, often present without one specific concern. A good starting point with these patients is to ask what they would like improved in their appearance. They commonly reply, "Everything!" or "I want to look younger." It is helpful to have a hand-held mirror and to ask the patient to point out specific concerns. They often identify multiple areas of concern, but also tend to prioritize what bothers them the most. What may seem to be a cosmetic flaw to the physician may not be what troubles the patient. If the physician wishes to suggest an area for treatment that the patient has not mentioned, care should be taken not to offend the patient or to lower his or her self-esteem.

The initial consultation should also consist of a discussion of the spectrum of levels of intervention, and patients should understand the risks and benefits at each level. For example, a 50-year-old woman with diffuse photo-aging and significant fixed rhytides can be presented with various treatment options depending on her expectations and level of risk. Retinoids, sunscreens, and good lifestyle habits may be an appropriate initial therapy for minor and subtle improvements. More significant interventions with botulinum toxin, fillers, and laser therapies may provide quicker and more significant results, but may come with increased risk. An even more aggressive approach, such as a facelift, would likely give the most dramatic and significant effect but at potentially greater risks and downtime. Prior to treatment, the physician should address the patient's specific expectations and tailor the treatment regimen accordingly.

Preoperative assessment and patient selection

A complete medical history is a key element in the preoperative evaluation. It is helpful to have the patient complete a medical history questionnaire during the initial office visit. For established patients, it is wise to review and update this information periodically, particularly before more invasive procedures. In addition to the traditional medical history, inquiry should be made regarding the patient's history of cosmetic procedures and level of satisfaction with these past procedures. This can greatly assist the physician in determining the patient's expectations and level of risk. In addition, any prior cosmetic procedure should be taken into account when performing the physical examination as the patient's baseline state may have been altered by surgical procedures, such as a browlift, or transiently improved by noninvasive procedures, such as dermal fillers.

Physicians should be aware of medical conditions that can influence wound healing such as connective tissue disorders, diabetes, and keloids. For noninvasive procedures, the focus on particular diseases will depend on the nature of the cosmetic procedure. For example, a history of herpes simplex is significant in patients considering laser resurfacing, whereas a history of venous thrombosis should be investigated in patients considering sclerotherapy and ambulatory phlebectomy. In certain instances, after thorough medical history and examination, the cosmetic surgeon can play a critical role in diagnosing underlying medical conditions. For example, a woman who desires laser hair removal for hirsutism may have an underlying hyperandrogen disorder, or an individual presenting for laser treatment of facial telangiectasias may have lupus erythematosus. Although these scenarios may be infrequent, identifying any underlying associated medical condition can dictate whether or not to proceed with the cosmetic procedure.

Special attention must also be given to the patient's psychosocial history. Caution must be taken in dealing with individuals who have sought multiple cosmetic procedures and remain dissatisfied. In addition, one should suspect a diagnosis of body dysmorphic disorder in a patient who has undergone multiple procedures without signs of obvious significant abnormality, and avoid performing any cosmetic procedure on these individuals. A formal psychiatric referral should be considered in patients with possible psychiatric disorder.

The patient's social history is an important element of the preoperative assessment. Information regarding their occupation and recreational activities can affect interventions chosen for the patient. For example, a more conservative approach should be taken in treating an actor's face as any complications may affect his or her future profession. Some lifestyles do not afford the patients the downtime necessary for certain procedures. Also included in the social history is the patient's use of tobacco. This is particularly important for patients undergoing invasive procedures, as smokers can have an increased risk of postoperative wound complications.

As with any medical procedure, it is vital to obtain an accurate list of the patient's current and recently discontinued prescriptions and over-the-counter medications. Of particular interest in performing cosmetic procedures are medications that can affect wound healing. For example, the use of topical retinoids can influence results of a chemical peel, and oral retinoids taken within months prior to a laser procedure can potentially affect wound healing. Blood thinners such as clopidogrel and warfarin can potentially lead to an increased risk of postoperative bleeding with more invasive procedures. Over-the-counter medications such as aspirin, nonsteroidal anti-inflammatory agents, vitamin E, gingko biloba, and St John's wort may also have similar effects. Furthermore, some medications can interact with local tumescent anesthesia.

Laboratory tests are indicated in the preoperative workup for invasive procedures such as rhytidectomy, eyelid surgery, and liposuction. Basic tests, such as a complete blood count, electrolytes, coagulation profiles, and a pregnancy test in women of childbearing potential, should be obtained. Electrocardiography is typically recommended for patients over 40 years of age or with a history of cardiac disease who are undergoing invasive aesthetic procedures that require general anesthesia. Occasionally, some laboratory tests may be indicated for noninvasive procedures. For example, a skin biopsy is prudent prior to laser therapy of a cutaneous lesion suspicious for malignancy. A lower-extremity duplex scan may be indicated prior to sclerotherapy in patients suspected of having larger vessel disease.

Table 1-1 Fitzpatrick's skin type classification

Skin type	Skin features	Tanning ability
I	White skin, blue eyes, blonde or red hair	Always burns, does not tan
II	White skin, blue eyes	Easily burns, tans poorly
III	Darker white skin	Mild burn, average tan
IV	Brown skin	Occasionally burns, tans easily
V	Dark brown skin	Rarely burns, tans very easily
VI	Black skin	No burns, dark tan

Table 1-2 The Glogau photo-aging classification

Type	Typical age range	Severity	Features
I	Late 20s to 30s	Mild	Minimal wrinkling, no actinic keratosis, requires little or no make-up
II	30s to 40s	Moderate	Early with facial motion, early actinic keratosis
III	50s or older	Advanced	Persistent wrinkling, visible actinic keratosis, discoloration with telangiectasias
IV	60s to 70s	Severe	Generalized wrinkling, actinic keratoses with or without malignancy

A thorough problem-focused physical examination is an essential element of the initial assessment of a cosmetic patient. The importance of having good lighting and a comfortable setting for the physician and patient cannot be over-emphasized. For example, evaluation of the aging face should be done with the patient in an upright position, with particular attention to the skin type, texture, and signs of photo-aging. The patient's Fitzpatrick skin type (Table 1-1) can assist in selecting therapeutic modalities and perioperative care, given the risk of postinflammatory hyperpigmentation in darker skin types. The degree of photo-aging can be classified using the Glogau photo-aging classification (Table 1-2). In addition to rhytides and telangiectasias, areas of dyschromia, scars, and skin laxity should be noted.

PEARLS

Ideal cosmetic surgical patient

Psychologically and medically stable

Clearly defined area of dissatisfaction

Procedure can give objective improvement

Realistic expectations

Self-motivated

Discussion of diagnosis and procedures

In order to maximize surgical outcomes and patient satisfaction, it is important to diagnose the condition accurately and then offer the best possible intervention in properly selected patients. For example, the exact nature of pigmented lesions should be identified before offering treatment options. A dermatologic surgeon may offer laser treatments to lentigos but would avoid laser therapy of a lesion suspicious for lentigo maligna; bleaching agents and a tincture of time would likely be offered to treat postinflammatory hyperpigmentation, whereas Q-switched lasers would be considered for nevi of Ota. Furthermore, a dermatologic surgeon may not offer the same procedures to a patient with Fitzpatrick skin type VI as she or he would to a patient with Fitzpatrick skin type II, given the greater risk of hyperpigmentation and scarring in darker skin types.

One of the keys to good rapport and great outcomes in aesthetic procedures is frank discussion of the expected outcomes and potential complications. Unreasonable expectations by the patient and unreasonable promises by the physician can lead to patient dissatisfaction, not to mention medicolegal suits against the physician. Patients should be educated using the average patient experience as an example. The best results ever experienced in the literature from the procedure should never be touted as a likely result. Patients must also understand that the procedure may have less benefit for them than for the average patient. Any expected transient side-effects and potential short- and longer-lasting adverse effects should be communicated clearly to the patient. This not only educates the patient about inherent risks of the procedure but also allows the patient to prepare for any "downtime" the procedure may entail. Furthermore, many noninvasive dermatologic procedures, such as botulinum toxin and dermal fillers, provide nonpermanent benefits. The typical duration of effects of these procedures must be discussed with the patient. Similarly, patients need to realize that some noninvasive procedures, such as laser photorejuvenation and hair removal, typically require multiple treatments to achieve optimal results. Given individual variability, it is helpful for the treating physician to state that "patients typically need at least 'X' number of laser treatments, but some patients may require more."

Professional office support staff and informative printed literature are often helpful adjuncts in providing education for the cosmetic patient. Well informed and well trained office and nursing staff can be valuable in providing basic information about the nature of the procedure and perioperative care. In addition, they can assist the physician by delineating the costs of the procedures and scheduling patients in a timely manner. Lastly, providing patients with printed pamphlets describing various procedures is helpful, particularly when multiple procedures are discussed during the consultation. This gives the patient an opportunity to review the information given during the consultation and to reconsider his or her options.

Photo-documentation

Patient photography has become one of the mainstays of cosmetic dermatology documentation. Not only is it a good source of legal documentation, but also it allows for better patient care. Following the patient's progress, or lack thereof, can be done in a more objective manner with photographs than by traditional written charting. Traditional written documentation and patient questioning can be more subjective and allow more room for physician and patient bias when evaluating response to therapy.

With appropriate, high-quality photography, response to treatment can be well assessed by both the physician and the patient. Further treatment courses can be modified based on evaluation of this objective measure of patient response. These photographs can greatly improve the level of patient satisfaction, because patients may not recall or appreciate their improvement without them. In addition, subtle imperfections present at initial consultation can be documented should they become more apparent or bothersome with correction of more significant cosmetic flaws. Photo-documentation of these preexisting conditions can also be valuable should the patient later attribute them to the procedure.

There are several important factors that can affect the quality and standardization of patient photographs. Some of these factors can be controlled for, but others are more difficult to standardize. The patient should always be photographed with the same background. A felt sheet that does not provide glare with flash photography serves as a good background. For better contrast, lighter-skinned patients should be photographed with a darker background, such as blue or black. Darker-skinned patients should be photographed with a lighter background, such as light blue or white. The same camera and same camera settings should be used for all visits. In general, flash photography provides the best and most standardized results, as ambient lighting can change from visit to visit. The area treated (e.g. the face) should fill the picture frame, and this should be standardized for all follow-up photos of the same patient.

It is helpful to standardize facial photos using the Frankfort horizontal position, in which the infraorbital rim is at the same level as the supratragal notch. Full-face frontal, right and left 45° oblique, and right and left lateral photos are typically obtained in a facial series.

Some aspects of patient photography are difficult to standardize. Patients' wrinkles and facial volume can vary significantly at different times of the day depending on level of fatigue, hydration status, and other factors. Use of different topical products, degree of tanning, and weight gain or loss between visits can significantly alter physical appearance. This may confound evaluation of the therapeutic effect of the treatments performed. These variables should be kept in mind when evaluating patient photographs.

There are multiple companies that now provide the tools for in-office photography for the practicing dermatologist. They provide the equipment as well as the software to take and store patient photographs efficiently and accurately. The photographs are stored in individual patient files, in a safe and Health Insurance Portability and Accountability Act (HIPAA) compliant manner.

Informed consent

Obtaining informed consent is an extremely important aspect of any medical procedure. It is an ethical responsibility and legal obligation prior to performing any procedure. After communication between the treating physician and patient, the patient must understand and agree to undergo a specific medical intervention. During the discussion, the treating physician must advise the patient, using the reasonable standard of care, regarding the diagnosis, nature, risks, and benefits of the proposed procedures, as well as similar details of alternative treatments. The patient must be given the opportunity to ask questions in order to gain a better understanding of the procedures.

The patient must demonstrate their understanding of the preoperative discussion before therapy is initiated. Evidence of this awareness is obtained with a signed consent form that outlines key aspects of the discussion. A written consent form is a legal document that includes the name and signature of the patient and medical provider, and the date on which the form was signed. It is ideal for the provider doing the procedure, rather than an assistant, to provide information. This allows less room for misunderstanding between the patient and the provider should any adverse event occur. The consent form should include the procedure, benefits, and possible risks of the procedure. The most common and expected adverse effects should be listed.

All treating physicians should understand that, although the consent form is a medicolegal document, it does not absolve the provider from all guilt should an adverse event occur. Consent forms are most protective for the provider in instances where unpredictable adverse events occur after appropriate treatment.

If the patient can prove, in a court of law, that the provider did not act according to the standard of medical care, then the consent form will not protect the provider. Many legal settlements involving cosmetic procedures are based on "breach of contract" issued against the treating physician who did not generate the promised results. Given the elective and imperfect nature of cosmetic procedures, selecting appropriate patients and interventions, setting realistic expectations, and discussing potential positive and negative outcomes are imperative for optimal surgical outcomes and patient satisfaction.

Further reading

American Medical Association. Professional resources: informed consent. Available at: http://www.ama-assn.org/ama/pub/category/4608.html (accessed 1 June 2007).

American Society for Aesthetic Plastic Surgery. Cosmetic surgery national data bank statistics, 2006. Available at: http://www.surgery.org/download/2006stats.pdf (accessed 1 May 2007).

Castle DJ, Honigman RJ, Phillips KA. Does cosmetic surgery improve psychosocial wellbeing? Med J Aust 2002;176:601–604.

Glogau RG. Aesthetic and anatomic analysis of the aging skin. Semin Cutan Med Surg 1996;15:134–138.

Grammer K, Thornhill R. Human (*Homo sapiens*) facial attractiveness and sexual selection: the role of symmetry and averageness. J Comp Psychol 1994;108(3):233–242.

Halberstadt J, Rhodes G. It's not just average faces that are attractive: computer-manipulated averageness makes birds, fish, and automobiles attractive. Psychon Bull Rev 2003;10(1):149–156.

Ho Tang, Brissett AE. Preoperative assessment of the aging patient. Facial Plast Surg 2006;22:85–90.

Honn M, Goz G. The ideal of facial beauty: a review. J Orofac Orthop 2007;68(1):6–16.

Klein JA, Kassarjdian N. Lidocaine toxicity with tumescent liposuction. A case report of probable drug interactions. Dermatol Surg 1997;23(12):1169–1174.

Powell D, Hobgood T. Detection and management of the unstable patient. Facial Plast Surg Clin North Am 2003;11:307–318.

Ratner D, Thomas CO, Bickers D. The uses of digital photography in dermatology. J Am Acad Dermatol 1999;41(5 Pt 1):749–756.

Scheinfeld N. Photographic images, digital imaging, dermatology, and the law. Arch Dermatol 2004;140(4):473–476.

Scheinfeld NS, Flanigan K, Moshiyakhov M, Weinberg JM. Trends in the use of cameras and computer technology among dermatologists in New York City 2001–2002. Dermatol Surg 2003;29(8):822–825.

Shackelford TK, Larsen RJ. Facial asymmetry as an indicator of psychological, emotional, and physiological distress. J Pers Soc Psychol 1997;72(2):456–466.

Starr JC. Integrating digital image management software for improved patient care and optimal practice management. Dermatol Surg 2006;32(6):834–840.

Synnott A. The beauty mystique. Facial Plast Surg 2006;22(3):163–174.

Zachariae H. Delayed wound healing and keloid formation following argon laser treatment or dermabrasion during isotretinoin treatment. Br J Dermatol 1988;118:703–706.

Cosmeceuticals

Lily Talakoub, Isaac M. Neuhaus,
and Siegrid S. Yu

Introduction

The Food, Drug, and Cosmetic Act defines drugs as products that cure, treat, mitigate or prevent disease, or affect the structure or function of the human body. The dermatology and cosmetic industries recognize "cosmeceuticals" as cosmetics that have drug-like benefits. The term cosmeceutical was first used by Albert Kligman to describe a cosmetic product that exerts a therapeutic benefit in the appearance of the skin, but not necessarily a biologic effect on skin function, which would then classify it as a drug. The Food and Drug Administration (FDA) does not recognize or regulate cosmeceuticals. The symbiotic relationship between a drug and a cosmetic has become increasingly evident with the rapid growth of the cosmeceutical industry over the past decade. There are now both prescription and over-the-counter cosmeceuticals available to consumers. This arbitrary distinction varies in different countries. For example, drugs such as tretinoin, available only by prescription in the USA, are sold as over-the-counter cosmeceuticals in Central America. Antiperspirant is also regulated as a drug in the USA, while being considered a cosmetic in Europe.

The market for cosmeceuticals in the USA has grown substantially over the past 10 years as the median age of the population increases and the market for noninvasive rejuvenation expands. Skin care companies often make miraculous claims based on little scientific evidence. In the modern era of direct to consumer advertising, claims can be misleading, causing the false belief that these products are subject to the same standards and vigorous testing for safety and efficacy as drugs.

Whether in an academic, medical, or surgical dermatology setting, many patients and colleagues inquire about these products. As professionals and leaders in the field of skin care, dermatologists must develop a solid knowledge base to inform and educate patients and peers regarding the use of skin care cosmeceuticals.

This chapter briefly summarizes skin barrier function and provides an overview of the most common cosmeceuticals available on the US market. As previously alluded to, little scientific evidence exists for many of the products mentioned. The best available evidence is reviewed, although many of the purported benefits highlighted in this chapter are anecdotal.

The skin barrier

Key Points

- The stratum corneum provides the permeability barrier of the skin.
- Cholesterol, free fatty acids, and glucosylceramides are the essential lipids providing the permeability barrier.
- Genetic and environmental factors alter lipid production and the skin barrier repair mechanism.

One of the integral roles of the skin is to maintain a barrier between the body and the external environment. Its varied roles include preventing the loss of body fluids and electrolytes, regulating body temperature, and protecting against ultraviolet radiation, oxidants, and microbes. Despite the great advances in basic science and pharmacology, limited products and drugs have been developed that can penetrate this sophisticated, highly organized, biologic membrane.

The stratum corneum serves as the permeability barrier of the skin. Disorders of its maintenance and repair remain among the leading causes of skin diseases. A measure of barrier integrity is the calculation of transepidermal water loss (TEWL). TEWL is an objective measure of water loss from the skin (in $g/m^2/h$), excluding losses due to sweating. Normal daily TEWL in adults ranges between 3.9 and 7.6 $g/m^2/h$. In disorders of cornification or barrier function, such as ichthyosis or atopic dermatitis, the levels may be above $15\,g/m^2/h$. Studies have shown that the repair mechanism of the stratum corneum responds to detergents, solvents, and trauma by increasing the machinery needed for lipid synthesis and secretion to minimize the TEWL. Aging and ultraviolet (UV) B radiation are among the many other stressors to the skin that decrease skin barrier function and increase TEWL.

The stratum corneum is made of keratinocytes embedded in a structurally and biochemically diverse matrix of parallel lamellar membranes containing cholesterol, free fatty acids, and glucosylceramides. The corneocytes form the cohesion of the cornified envelope, whereas the lipid matrix is the essential element of the stratum corneum's barrier function. The barrier repair mechanism relies on the synthesis and regulation of these three components, that work symbiotically to regenerate new lamellar bodies.

Hydration of the skin is dependent on the corneocyte natural moisturizing factor (NMF) and the lamellar bodies of the extracellular matrix. Once the stratum corneum's water levels fall below a critical point, measured as a 1% increase in TEWL, the enzymatic function required for desquamation is impaired. This results in increased corneocyte adhesion, resulting in the accumulation of scale and the appearance of dry, flaky skin.

Exfoliation of the skin is a tightly controlled mechanism required for hydration, flexibility, and tissue integrity. A complex series of enzymatic hydrolytic reactions disrupts the desmosomal attachments between corneocytes. This highly controlled mechanism is regulated predominantly by the pH and water content of the stratum corneum, as well as the corneocyte-derived NMF, derived from the hydrolysis of the protein fillagrin. The homeostasis of the stratum corneum is dependent on many signaling mechanisms, including water content, pH, calcium levels, and cytokine milieu, all of which promote a cascade of events leading to exfoliation, barrier repair, and recovery.

Many genetic and environmental factors alter lipid production and the skin barrier. UV radiation, aging, atopic dermatitis, oral glucocorticoids, disease, diet, stress, and humid or dry environments play a role in the perturbation and delayed repair of the epidermal barrier. Studies also demonstrate racial differences in skin barrier function. As repair normally functions at an acidic pH, neutralization of this pH delays the normal repair mechanism and increases the abnormalities in corneocyte adhesion. Successful treatment of these perturbations relies upon the understanding of the barrier mechanism and the underlying structural and physiologic mechanisms behind normal, dry, oily, and so-called "sensitive" skin (Fig. 2-1).

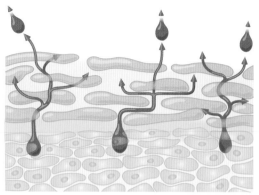

Figure 2-1 The skin barrier: bricks and mortar illustration

Skin type

Key Points

- Skin type is defined by a balance of re-epithelialization and desquamation, sebum secretion, and hydration.
- Skin type can be measured objectively, but is often a subjective assessment of tangible or visible areas of disequilibrium.

Normal skin is defined as skin with a balance of re-epithelialization and desquamation, sebum secretion, and hydration. There are therefore no tangible or visible areas of disequilibrium. A minority of individuals present with normal skin type, and normal skin characteristics can easily change with age, ambient temperature, humidity, and mechanical or chemical stresses. Oily, greasy, or shiny skin can be due to an increase in sebum production during adrenarche, the presence of acne due to a shift in androgen production, abnormal keratinization and *Propionibacterium acnes* proliferation, or seborrhea. Self-perceived dry skin is usually due to a defect in the barrier function of the stratum corneum with an increase in TEWL and a subsequent feeling of chapped, tight, scaly skin. Dry skin is usually a secondary manifestation of excessive cleansing, stripping the stratum corneum from natural lipids, UV radiation, exposure to extreme climates, or treatment with agents such as retinoids. Sensitive skin has a low threshold for irritancy. Patients with sensitive skin develop stinging, burning, or widespread dermatitis from topical applications of products, particularly those with fragrance, acid or alkaline pH, or preservatives.

Skin type can be assessed by meticulous methods of measuring TEWL, sebum production, and mathematical calculations of skin pigment color and elasticity. However, even objective measurements may be an inaccurate representation of a patient's self-perceived skin type.

Moisturization

Key Points

- Moisturizers contain lipids and ingredients with emollient, humectant, and occlusive properties.
- Selecting an optimal moisturizer depends on the skin type, vehicle, and the needs of the patient.

Moisturizers function to restore the hydration of the epidermal barrier. Water within a moisturizer produces only a transient increase in the hydration of the stratum corneum. Physiologic lipids, when applied together in equimolar concentrations, enhance the stratum corneum's own lipid synthesis mechanism. Nonphysiologic lipids do not penetrate the stratum corneum, but rather provide barrier protection by intercalating between corneocytes, creating a diffuse hydrophobic impermeable surface. Neither of these lipid categories, when applied externally, retards the normal production of lipids within the stratum corneum. Moisturizers available today have different combinations of these physiologic and nonphysiologic lipids, as well as ingredients with emollient, humectant, and occlusive properties (Tables 2-1 & 2-2).

Occlusives are agents designed to reduce TEWL by forming a hydrophobic film on the skin between the corneocytes. Occlusive ingredients are greasy, and function best when applied to slightly dampened skin. Petrolatum can reduce TEWL by 98% and is the most effective occlusive agent. Mineral oil and lanolin are also used widely in over-the-counter skin care products, but are less efficacious in preventing TEWL compared with petrolatum. Mineral oil is the main ingredient excluded in oil-free products. Lanolin has been implicated in many cases of allergic contact dermatitis. Silicone derivatives are smoother in texture and less greasy, but also have limited ability in preventing TEWL.

Humectants attract and trap water from the dermis and the humid environment for the stratum corneum. They can, however, paradoxically cause this water to be lost into the environment and thus need to be used in conjunction with an occlusive agent to prevent further TEWL. The most effective humectant, glycerol, binds and holds water in the stratum corneum, glycerol also aids in the proteolysis of the corneocyte desmosomes, thereby aiding in desquamation. NMF components such as sodium pyrrolidone carboxylic acid, lactate, and urea have also been shown to decrease TEWL and increase skin capacitance

(Box 2-1). In particular, moisturizers with urea have been shown to decrease TEWL in atopic and ichthyotic patients.

Emollients are generally lipids and oils, which play a role in filling the crevices between desquamating corneocytes, thereby causing the appearance of a smooth skin texture, enhanced flexibility, and skin softness. Not only do these products provide instant lubrication and moisturization, they have also been shown to improve barrier repair. These agents correlate with consumer satisfaction as they provide the instantaneous feel of moisturization.

Most moisturizer formulations consist of lotions or creams with a combination of an occlusive, humectant, and emollient. A lotion is an oil-in-water emulsion, whereas a cream is a water-in-oil emulsion. Cosmetically elegant lotions are a thinner consistency than creams, and are often used as day moisturizers. These products also contain mineral oil, propylene glycol, and water. Creams are thicker and greasier than lotions, and are made of petrolatum or lanolin derivatives, mineral oil, and water. There are also complicated emulsions consisting of oil-in-water-in-oil emulsions, as well as gels, foams, and sprays. Emulsion lipids consist of long-chain saturated fatty acids including stearic, linoleic, oleic, and lauric acid, found. Other oils used as emollients include fish oil, petrolatum, shea butter, and sunflower seed oil.

Selecting an optimal moisturizer thus depends on the skin type, vehicle, and the needs of the patient. For example, dry skin may require a

BOX 2-1

Components of the natural moisturizing factor within corneocytes

Urea/uric acid

Sugars

Sodium

Glucoasamine

Lactate

Amino acids

Formate

Pyrrolidone carboxylic acid (PCA)

Ammonia

Citrate

Creatinine

Chloride

Calcium

Magnesium

Phosphate

higher oil-to-water concentration and heavier occlusive agents. On the other hand, oily skin would benefit from lower oil to water ratios and from nongreasy emollients such as silicone, used in combination with oil-absorbent compounds such as talc.

Table 2-1 Physiologic and nonphysiologic lipids

Physiologic lipids	Nonphysiologic lipids
Ceramides	Petrolatum
Cholesterol	Bees wax
Free fatty acids	Lanolin
	Squalene

Table 2-2 Properties of moisturizers

Moisturizer property	Ingredient
Occlusive	Petrolatum
	Mineral oil
	Paraffin
	Squalene
	Silicone derivatives (dimethicone and cyclomethicone)
	Lanolin
	Caprylic/capric triglyceride
	Caranuba and candelilla wax
	Lecithin
	Cholesterol
	Propylene glycol
	Stearic acid
	Cetyl and stearyl alcohol
Humectant	Glycerin (glycerol)
	Sodium pyrrolidone carboxylic acid
	Sodium lactate
	Propylene glycol
	Sorbitol
	Ammonium lactate
	Potassium lactate
	Sorbitol
	Urea
	Panthenol
	Honey
	Gelatin
	Hyaluronic acid

Table 2-2 Properties of moisturizers—cont'd

Moisturizer property	Ingredient
Emollient	Dimethicone and cyclomethicone
	Propylene glycol
	Glycol stearate
	Glyceryl stearate
	Lanolin
	Soy sterol
	Sunflower seed oil glycerides
	Octyl dodecanol
	Hexyl dodecanol
	Oleyl alcohol
	Oleyl oleate
	Octyl stearate
	PEG-7 glyceryl cocoate
	Coco-caprylate/caprate
	Myristyl myristate
	Cetearyl isononanoate
	Isopropyl myristate

PEG, polyethylene glycol.

Cleansers

Key Points

- Soaps and cleaners contain surfactants that lift dirt and aid in the solubility and absorption of oils.
- Mild synthetic detergents (syndets) combine a mild surfactant with a moisturizer.
- Cleansers with emollient properties provide superior stratum corneum moisturization.

Cleansers are products designed to remove debris, make-up, secretions, sweat, sebum, and bacteria while aiding in the exfoliation of the stratum corneum. Cleansers are formulated with surfactants that lift dirt and aid in the solubility and absorption of oils. Surfactants can be harsh to the proteins and lipids in the stratum corneum, potentially causing barrier damage and dryness. New milder cleansers, however, are made to minimize this damage while providing additional moisturization to the skin.

Soaps were the earliest form of skin cleansers, and are still widely in use. New developments in liquid cleansers and body washes include mild synthetic detergents (syndets) which combine a mild surfactant with a moisturizing lotion containing a humectant, emollient, and occlusive. These moisturizing washes contain more emollient than surfactant in their list of ingredients, with water being the first ingredient listed and oils or petrolatum the second. Thus, using a cleanser with an emollient provides superior stratum corneum

Table 2-3 Components of soaps and syndets	
Syndet	Soap
Sodium cocoyl isethionate	Sodium tallowate
Stearic acid	Sodium cocoate
Sodium stearate	Palm kernelate
Cocamido propyl betaine	Sodium palmitate
Polyethylene glycol (PEG)	Water
Sodium isethionate	PEG-6 methyl ether
Coconut fatty acid	Palm acid or tallow acid
Natural oils	Fragrance
Salts	Glycerine
Sequestrant	Sorbitol
Titanium dioxide	Sodium chloride
	Pentasodium pentetate
	Tetrasodium etidronate
	Butyl hydroxyl toluene (BHT)
	Titanium dioxide

moisturization compared with using a soap or mild cleanser without an emollient.

Soaps and syndets generally contain different ingredients and differing pH. Syndets are neutral or acidic. In contrast, soaps are alkaline and proven to be more irritating to lipids in the stratum corneum (Table 2-3). Studies of patients with atopic dermatitis, acne, rosacea, retinoid sensitivity, and post-chemical peel reveal similar cleansing capabilities for soaps and syndets. However, the use of syndets and mild cleansers provides improved skin softness and reduced irritation compared with soaps.

Other skin care products: masks and astringents

Key Points

- Masks provide mechanical exfoliation.
- Toners and astringents are products that are used primarily in anti-acne regimens or for antiseptic and antimicrobial functions.
- Toners that are alcohol based can be irritating to the skin.

The skin care market has expanded greatly over the past decade owing to the inclusion of other skin exfoliating products. These products often contain numerous other cosmeceutical ingredients including salicylic acid, vitamins, minerals, and botanicals.

Masks, originally derived from mud baths, are made from polyvinyl alcohol (allowing them to be peeled off), or are clay-based (allowing them to dry on the skin and be rinsed off). Masks can be used for chemical or mechanical exfoliation, or as a vehicle to deliver a therapeutic agent. Most masks are applied weekly to improve skin hydration, exfoliate, and unclog pores. Physical abrasive agents are also added to enhance mechanical exfoliation. There is a diversity of masks on the market. Anti-acne masks may include ingredients such as salicylic acid or sulfur, whereas soothing masks contain honey or green tea. Other masks are manufactured with algae, cucumber, essential oils, and soy.

Toners are products used after skin cleansing to clean soap or cleanser residue and remove remaining sebum and make-up incompletely removed with cleansers. Inconsistent nomenclature leads to confusion, as toners are also referred to as astringents, skin fresheners, toning lotions, clarifying lotions, or pore lotions. Toners are either alcohol or nonalcohol based. Their use in dermatology is predominantly integrated in anti-acne regimens, or for antiseptic and antimicrobial functions. Different formulations developed for anti-acne benefits contain salicylic acid or high tannin contents. Toners developed for dry skin contain honey, allantoin, and aloe vera. Witch hazel, tea tree oil, eucalyptus, and α-hydroxy acids are also in many new over-the-counter astringents and toners. Side-effects include contact dermatitis and irritation, depending on concentration of alcohol or solvents that disrupt the epidermal barrier function. Regardless of nomenclature, these products are used widely and, because of the aesthetically pleasing feeling they give to the skin, are generally well accepted by patients.

Photoaging

Key Points

- Photodamage is the visual and tangible effects of UV radiation.
- UV radiation damages collagen, increases elastin breakdown, and alters extracellular membrane proteins in the skin.
- Photodamage also produces free radicals, which break down cell membranes, proteins, and DNA.

The concept of photodamage encompasses visual and tangible damage to the skin as a result of UV radiation. Sun-exposed skin can develop fine rhytides, roughness, dyschromia, and skin cancer. UV exposure causes epidermal thickening and disruption of the normal architecture of connective tissue within the dermis. It damages the crosslinked structure of collagen and elastin fibers, and decreases the amount of glycosaminoglycans (GAG), particularly hyaluronic acid, within the dermis. Chronic UV damage causes the accumulation of abnormal elastin and fibrillin, referred to as solar elastosis. UV radiation also disrupts the extracellular membrane proteins, namely the

GAGs that bind to water and help hydrate and support the skin. In photodamaged skin, GAGs are preferentially deposited in the elastotic areas rather than in their normal location between collagen and elastin fibers, thus causing the characteristic leathery appearance. Photodamage produces free radicals, which break down cell membranes, proteins, and DNA. Research has shown that these changes reflect upregulation of activating protein (AP)-1 transcription factor, which activates collagen breakdown and blocks collagen gene expression, further impairing collagen synthesis. Free radicals also cause the upregulation of nuclear factor (NF)-κB transcription factor, which stimulates the release of pro-inflammatory cytokines such as tumor necrosis factor (TNF)- α, interleukin (IL)-1, IL-6, and IL-8. Within the dermis, this loss of collagen results in the appearance of fine lines and saggy, thinner skin. The complex changes of aged skin reflect decreased cell adhesion and differentiation, loss of collagen and GAG, and increased elastic tissue breakdown.

Retinoids

Key Points

- Retinoids are vitamin A derivatives that bind to nuclear retinoic acid receptors and modify gene expression.
- Retinoid derivatives are found in many prescription and over-the-counter products.
- Retinoids have been shown to be effective in the treatment of acne and the improvement of photoaging.
- Patient education regarding their proper use can enhance compliance and decrease skin irritation.

Over 20 years of research has confirmed the importance of retinoids for the integrity of mucosal and epithelial surfaces. Retinoids (Table 2-4) are an example of a group of products that are both a drug and a cosmeceutical. The delineation between drug and cosmeceutical depends on the concentration of the product, the formulation, and the vehicle in which the retinoid is delivered.

Retinol (vitamin A), its derivatives, and oxidized metabolites that possess vitamin A activity are formulated as both naturally occurring and synthetic chemicals in cosmeceuticals. Vitamin A is a naturally occurring derivative of β-carotene. However, synthetics are now formulated to mimic the pharmacologic properties of vitamin A in varying degrees and with lower irritancy profiles.

Oxidized retinol, or retinoic acid, is the active ingredient in most cosmeceuticals (all-*trans*, 9-*cis*, and 13-*cis* retinoic acids). Retinol, or its oxidized form, binds three isoforms of nuclear family receptors known as retinoic acid receptors (RARs) and retinoid X receptors (RXRs). RARs bind all-*trans* retinoic acid, and RXRs bind 9-*cis* or 13-*cis* retinoic acid. Upon binding, a heterodimer is formed which translocates into the nucleus to bind retinoic acid response elements on DNA, thereby modifying gene expression.

In the skin, through a series of enzymatic reactions, retinol is metabolized to retinaldehyde, all-*trans* retinoic acid, and finally to 9-*cis* and 13-*cis* retinoic acids. By-products of this multistep process produce storage forms known as retinyl esters (retinyl palmitate and retinyl propionate). Both the metabolites and the storage forms have some biologic activity, are less irritating, and have been used in cosmeceuticals for their ability to convert to retinoic acid when applied exogenously (Fig. 2-2).

Several well controlled trials have demonstrated the benefits of retinoids in reducing fine lines, roughness, and dyspigmentation. Retinol has been used widely in cosmeceuticals for its ease of penetration, ability to convert to tretinoin, and lower irritancy profile. Studies have also shown retinol's efficacy in increasing dermal collagen, GAG, and anchoring fibrils, protecting from oxidative damage, inhibiting lipid peroxidation, increasing keratinocyte differentiation and cell turnover, and decreasing the number of sebocytes. However, use of retinol in over-the-counter preparations has not been shown to be as effective in anti-acne preparations and in reducing the signs of photoaging as prescription tretinoin. Retinaldehyde,

Table 2-4 Types of retinoid S	
Naturally occurring	Metabolic and synthetic derivatives
Retinol (vitamin A alcohol)	Tretinoin (all-*trans*-retinoic acid)
Retinal (vitamin A aldehyde)	Isotretinoin (13-*cis*-retinoic acid)
Retinoic acid (vitamin A acid)	Etretinate
	Etretin
	Arotinoid
	Adapalene

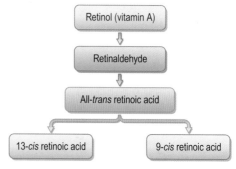

Figure 2-2 Retinol metabolism

which converts to tretinoin, has also been shown to improve signs of aging.

Many third-generation retinoids have been developed. Adapalene and tazarotene are both regulated as drugs, and have similar action to tretinoin. Adapalene is approved only for topical acne and has a decreased irritancy profile compared with tretinoin. No studies have shown any benefit for these agents with regard to efficacy in treating signs of photoaging. Tazarotene, approved for plaque-type psoriasis and acne, is effective in the treatment of acne, but can be irritating to the skin and has not been proven effective for photoaging.

The main side-effects of retinoids are their potential for teratogenicity and their irritancy. This irritation can be minimized by decreasing dosing frequency as well as slow upward titration of the dosage upon initiation of use. A thorough conversation with patients regarding application techniques can enhance patient compliance and decrease frustration. Patients should be educated carefully regarding optimal application of retinoids, including the application of a small "pea-sized" amount to the entire face at night 20 min after washing the treatment area. Patients should also be warned about teratogenicity and photosensitivity reactions with the use of these medications.

Antioxidants

Key Points

- UV radiation induces the formation of reactive oxygen species in the skin.
- Reactive oxygen species are implicated in skin cancer and cutaneous photoaging.
- Vitamins, minerals, and natural products with antioxidant properties have been widely incorporated into skin care products.
- Further research is needed to identify the ability of these agents to scavenge free radicals when applied topically.

The skin is subject to daily exogenous reactive oxygen species (ROS) such as pollution, UV radiation, and drugs. UV radiation induces the formation of ROS in the skin and impairs the skin's ability to neutralize these ROS. The skin has the ability to cope with ROS by endogenous mechanisms that scavenge free radicals, bind metal ions, and remove oxidatively damaged compounds.

Extensive studies have been performed over the past decade on ROS and aging. ROS are superoxide anions, peroxide, and singlet oxygen, all of which are generated by exposure of skin to UV radiation. In vitro studies illustrate ROS-induced upregulation of transcription factor AP-1, increases the activity of matrix metalloproteinases (MMPs), causing collagen breakdown and NF-κB-induced inflammatory mediators, all of which contribute to the aging process.

This section reviews the many vitamins, minerals, and natural products with antioxidant properties (Table 2-5 & Box 2-2). Many of the benefits mentioned are anecdotal and cannot be measured quantitatively when these agents are applied topically. Well designed trials are lacking, and correlations to topical applications are often made from studies of these agents following oral administration.

Vitamin B3: niacinamide

Vitamin B3, also known as niacinamide, is the precursor to the ubiquitous molecule nicotinamide adenine dinucleotide (NAD) and NADP. The reduced forms, NADH and NADPH, are potent intracellular antioxidants. NAD and NADP are the primary mediators in cell redox reactions, and prevent the protein glycation mechanism that occurs when sugars crosslink with proteins. Vitamin B3 is amongst the water-soluble vitamins that easily penetrate the stratum corneum when applied topically.

Studies that highlight the numerous roles of niacinamide on the skin include prevention of photoimmunosuppression, photocarcinogenesis, reduction of acne severity, reduction in TEWL, and decreased appearance of photoaging. Vitamin B3 has been shown to inhibit melanosome transfer from melanocytes to the keratinocytes. In vitro studies also elucidate its role in collagen synthesis, synthesis of ceramides for barrier protection, increasing involucrin and filaggrin, decreasing sebum production, and preventing TEWL.

Vitamin B5: panthenol

Vitamin B5, also known as pantothenic acid, is a component of the coenzyme A complex that plays an integral role in fatty acid synthesis and gluconeogenesis. Vitamin B5 is water soluble and easily absorbed topically through the stratum corneum. It is currently used topically in the treatment of wounds, bruises, scars, pressure and dermal ulcers, thermal burns, postoperative incisions, and radiation dermatitis.

Panthenol, the alcohol of panthanoic acid, is currently found in many skin care products and cosmetics. Its functions include the promotion of fibroblast proliferation for wound healing, increased lipid synthesis, and improvement of signs of photoaging and hyperpigmentation. It is often used in hair products as it improves elasticity and augments softening of the hair.

Vitamin C

Vitamin C is a water-soluble, essential nutrient necessary for the normal structure and function of the skin. The antioxidant properties of vitamin C are due to its ability to donate electrons to neutralize free radicals. Vitamin C also helps to regenerate another antioxidant, vitamin E. Vitamin C is necessary in the hydroxylation of proline and lysine during collagen crosslinking, and the transcriptional regulation of collagen synthesis. Vitamin C also inhibits the elastin biosynthesis seen in aged elastotic skin.

The role of vitamin C in photoaging is linked to its ability to stimulate collagen repair as well as to prevent UVB-induced erythema and sunburn cell formation, both markers of photodamage. Several well controlled studies have shown its benefits in decreasing the appearance of fine lines, Vitamin C increases type I collagen mRNA, aids in elastic tissue repair, and clinically improve skin texture and pigmentation.

Patients who applied 5% L-ascorbic acid to one arm and vehicle to another arm showed a biopsy-proven increase in mRNA levels of collagen I and III, and increased levels of MMP-1.

There are three forms of vitamin C: L-ascorbic acid (least stable, oxidized by air), ascorbyl-6-palmitate, and magnesium ascorbyl phosphate (most stable). Although oral supplementation is available, little absorbed vitamin C is delivered effectively to the skin. Topical preparations are also difficult to formulate as vitamin C is oxidized in air and degraded by light and heat. Topical preparations of L-ascorbic acid or its ester derivatives are absorbed percutaneously, depending on the concentration of the ascorbic acid and its pH. The pH of the topical preparation must be less than 3.5 to allow it to penetrate the thick stratum corneum.

Other vitamin C derivatives have similar properties to L-ascorbic acid. Magnesium ascorbyl phosphate also functions as an antioxidant, stimulates type I collagen production, and protects against UVB-induced lipid peroxidation. Ascorbyl-6-palmitate, the fat-soluble analog of L-ascorbic acid, can penetrate the stratum corneum better than L-ascorbic acid and has a lower irritancy profile owing to its neutral pH.

Vitamin E

Vitamin E, known as α-tocopherol, is also an essential nutrient that cannot be synthesized endogenously. It is normally found in vegetables, vegetable oils, cereals, and nuts. Vitamin E is a lipophilic antioxidant, and the most abundant antioxidant in the skin. Although there are few well controlled studies effectively delineating the functions of vitamin E in normal tissues, some of its purported benefits include its ability to prevent lipid membrane peroxidation.

Synergistic functions of Vitamin C & E include the ability of vitamin C to regenerate vitamin E and to enhance the antioxidant capacity of vitamin E. These two vitamins work symbiotically to provide photoprotection against UV radiation. Small studies have shown decreased erythema, edema, DNA adduct formation, lipid peroxidation, and sunburn cell formation when vitamin E is applied before UV exposure. Decreased skin rhytidosis and skin tumor incidence has also been reported following topical vitamin E administration.

Oral vitamin E supplementation can increase the delivery of vitamin E to the skin via sebaceous gland secretion. However, the vitamin E supplied would be available only to the upper epidermis at the level of the pilosebaceous units. Topical preparations range in concentration from 0.1% to 20%, although there is no dose–response relationship and thus no proof regarding the amount of vitamin E that is required to achieve clinical efficacy. Side-effects of topical preparations include irritant allergic contact dermatitis, urticaria, and erythema multiforme-like eruptions.

Ubiquinone

Ubiquinone, also known as coenzyme Q, is a ubiquitous lipid-soluble antioxidant that is present in the mitochondria of all living cells and is utilized in the synthesis of ATP. It has been shown to reduce peroxidation of low-density lipoproteins, regenerate endogenous vitamin E, and protect cells against UV-induced oxidative stress.

Topical preparations decrease UV-induced DNA damage, increase levels of GAG, and protect against UV-induced collagen degradation. Clinically, ubiquinol cream has been shown to decease wrinkle depth, compared with vehicle cream in split-face trials.

α-Lipoic acid

α-Lipoic acid (ALA) is an endogenous antioxidant that is a potent free radical scavenger. Similar to ubiquinone, it is made in the mitochondria of human cells. Little ALA is active in circulation as most of the soluble lipoic acid is bound to lysine. Free ALA is either transported to tissues or converted to dihydrolipoic acid (DHLA).

Lipoic acid acts as a cofactor in the citric acid cycle and in nucleic acid and protein synthesis. It is a small molecule, both lipid and water soluble, and thus readily penetrates the stratum corneum. Both ALA and DHLA scavenge ROS and regenerate endogenous antioxidants such as vitamin E, vitamin C, glutathione, and ubiquinol; these are important functions in the protection of UV-induced damage. ALA's antioxidant and anti-inflammatory properties are due to the selective inhibition of NF-κB activation and inhibition of pro-inflammatory mediators such as TNF-α and interleukins.

There are no well controlled trials delineating the benefits of ALA for cutaneous photodamage. Anecdotal evidence suggests its role in the reduction of fine wrinkles and improved skin texture.

Dimethylaminoethanol (DMAE)

DMAE is a novel ingredient initially used in the treatment of hyperkinetic disorders and to improve memory. It is now being used in cosmeceutical products, gaining popularity from its activity as a precursor to acetylcholine. Initially utilized as a firming and anti-aging product, new functions, including anti-inflammatory and antioxidant activities, have now been elucidated. In vitro, DMAE inhibits IL-2 and IL-6 secretion in addition to its actions as a free radical scavenger. Although the exact mechanism of action of DMAE is unclear, its acetylcholine-like functions increase contractility and cell adhesion in the epidermis and dermis, resulting in the appearance of firmer skin.

Double-blind trials of 3% DMAE facial gel showed improved facial skin firmness and increased muscle tone as evidenced by decreased neck sagging. Topical formulations are also now available, with a low irritancy profile. Few well controlled studies exist documenting its long-term efficacy and toxicity.

Genistein

Derived from the soybean, this antioxidant when taken orally has been shown to protect against bladder, breast, colon, liver, lung, prostate, and

Table 2-5 Other antioxidants

Antioxidant	Description
Melatonin	Melatonin is an endogenous hormone secreted by the pineal gland, with an ability to scavenge free radicals. Anecdotal studies have shown an ability of melatonin to suppress UV-induced erythema. No well controlled studies exist regarding its efficacy in cosmeceutical preparations
Catalase	Catalase is an endogenous antioxidant present in all human cells. Biochemically, its function resides in its ability to catalyze the decomposition of hydrogen peroxide to water and oxygen
Glutathione	Glutathione is a ubiquitous water-soluble peptide present in all human cells, made of glutamic acid, cysteine, and glycine. It also functions as an antioxidant by scavenging free radicals induced by UV radiation
Glucopyranosides	Glucopyranosides are potent antioxidants also known as resveratrol and polydatins. They are often found in fruits and vegetables, with the highest proportion in grape skins. They function to prevent lipid peroxidation of cell membranes
Cysteine	Commonly known as N-acetylcysteine (NAC), a precursor to glutathione, cysteine is a potent endogenous antioxidant. NAC has been shown to protect against UV-induced immunosuppression and can modulate the expression of oncogenes and tumor suppressor genes
Furfuryladenine	Furfuryladenine (Kinerase®) is a growth factor found in plants that slows the natural aging process of plants. Cut leaves exposed to furfuryladenine remain green, while unexposed leaves turn brown. It is used in anti-aging skin products, as in vitro studies have shown some anti-aging benefits. Few well controlled trials have been performed regarding its efficacy in vivo
Carnosine	Carnosine (β-alanyl- L-histidine) complexes with metal ions. It is believed to rejuvenate senescent cultures of human fibroblasts
Uric acid	Uric acid, a product of purine metabolism, is thought to function by scavenging iron and copper

skin cancers in animal studies. Topical genistein scavenges free radicals, protects against lipid peroxidation, and decreases UV-induced erythema and photodamage. Of particular interest is the ability of genistein to inhibit tyrosine protein kinases and the UV-induced expression of proto-oncogenes necessary for tumor growth and progression.

Spin traps

Spin traps are nitrone derivatives that include DMPO (5,5-dimethyl-1-pyrroline-N-oxide), DEPMPO (5-diethoxyphosphoryl-5-methyl-1-pyrroline-N-oxide), TEMPONE-H (1-hydroxy-2,2,6,6-tetramethyl-4-oxo-piperidine), and POBN (α-(4-pyridyl-1-oxide)-N-tert-butyl nitrone). The formation of free radicals is secondary to electrons that spin out of the ground state to a less stable, free radical state. Spin traps are free radical scavengers that trap these spinning electrons and bring them back to a state of stability. These agents, when added to creams and sunscreens, scavenge free radicals and prevent oxidative damage.

Hydroxy acids

Key Points

- Chemoexfoliation is the mechanism by which synthetic products are used to slough cohesive corneocytes.
- Three main chemoexfoliants used in dermatology include: α-hydroxy acids, β-hydroxy acids, and poly-hydroxy acids.
- These agents have been shown to improve skin texture, skin barrier function, and the appearance of photoaging.

Aging and many skin disorders are due to defects in the ability of the stratum corneum to desquamate. There are thermal, mechanical, and chemical exfoliating techniques. This section focuses on chemoexfoliation, a mechanism by which natural or synthetic products are used to slough cohesive corneocytes. These chemicals include α-hydroxy acids (AHAs), β-hydroxy acids (BHAs), and poly-hydroxy acids (PHAs) (Table 2-6).

Table 2-6 Types of hydroxy acid		
α-Hydroxy acids	β-Hydroxy acids	Poly-hydroxy acids
Glycolic acid	Salicylic acid	Gluconic acid
Lactic acid	β-Lipohydroxy acid (β-LHA)	Lactobionic acid
Tartaric acid	Tropic acid	Galactose
Citric acid		

AHAs are carboxylic acids derived from plants and synthetically made for use in chemical exfoliating products. Many of these naturally occurring acids are neutralized for over-the-counter use. At low concentrations, these products reduce corneocyte adhesion, thereby decreasing scale. When applied in higher concentrations and at low pH values, these same AHAs cause epidermolysis via cleavage of the desmosomal attachment sites of the basal layer. This effect can then produce varying degrees of exfoliation of the skin. The different AHAs include glycolic acid (derived from sugar cane), lactic acid (derived from sour milk), citric acid (derived from citrus fruits), mandelic acid, malic acid, and tartaric acid (derived from grapes).

AHAs are useful in the management of various cosmetic and dermatologic conditions, including dry skin, seborrheic dermatitis, callosities, acne scarring, actinic and seborrheic keratoses, warts, and photodamaged skin. The cosmetic use of AHA has gained great attention over the past decade as studies have shown improvement of the skin texture as a thinner epidermis has better light reflectance qualities.

BHAs, the most well known of which is salicylic acid, also increase epidermal shedding. Other BHAs include β-lipohydroxy acid (B-LHA) and tropic acid. The primary role of these agents is to enhance corneocyte shedding without any significant benefit in the deeper dermis. Salicylic acid is lipophilic and can penetrate the sebum-enriched follicular infundibulum of the pilosebaceous unit. It is used widely in over-the-counter acne products as it has been shown in multiple studies to have the ability to dislodge comedones and prevent the formation of new comedones.

PHAs are a new generation of hydroxy acids developed to provide similar beneficial effects with less irritancy than AHAs. The polyhydroxy acids include lactobionic acid, galactose, and gluconic acid. In comparison with AHAs, which are single-strand molecules, PHAs acids are larger, multiple-strand molecules with slower skin penetration, slower absorption, and reduced irritancy. PHAs can be used on patients with sensitive skin, including those with rosacea and atopic dermatitis. PHAs also have humectant properties and can enhance the barrier function of the stratum corneum. Similar to AHAs, PHAs possess antioxidant properties and are used to improve the appearance of photoaged skin.

Mechanism of corneocyte shedding

The precise mechanism of corneocyte shedding is still under investigation. Some authors claim that AHAs and BHAs have the ability to bind calcium in tissues, and reduce calcium at cell–cell adhesions. Alternative hypotheses for the mechanism of chemical exfoliation include the induction of keratinocyte apoptosis.

Mechanism of skin moisturization

AHA has been shown in small studies to increase the synthesis of dermal GAG, improve the quality of elastic fibers, and increase the density of collagen. These changes are thought to be due to an increased collagen mRNA and hyaluronic acid content of the epidermis and dermis. Studies have shown that 2% glycolic acid results in an increase in hyaluronic acid content in the epidermis and dermis, and an increase in collagen mRNA gene expression at AHA-treated sites compared with vehicle treatment alone.

Mechanism in barrier repair

Despite their exfoliative properties, repeated AHA and BHA use over 4 weeks has been shown to have no effect on TEWL. Studies evaluating mice treated with daily glycolic or lactic acid showed that the treated mice had a thinner stratum corneum with no change in TEWL and a paradoxical increase in lamellar bodies compared with untreated controls. Thus, despite their ability to induce corneocyte shedding and desquamation, AHA and BHA in fact help to improve the barrier function of the skin.

Mechanism of antitumorigenesis

Glycolic and tartaric acid have distinct antitumorigenic properties. Glycolic acid has been shown to block UV-induced apoptosis in mice treated twice daily after UV exposure. Treated mice had lower activation of AP-1 and NF-κB, and an approximately 20% reduction in skin tumor incidence, compared with untreated controls. Similarly, mice irradiated with UVB and given 30% salicylic acid for 18 weeks had a decreased number of skin tumors compared with untreated animals.

Mechanism of skin lightening

Both glycolic and lactic acids can inhibit tyrosinase activity, thus suppressing melanin formation. Secondary effects are increased penetration of lightening agents by increasing epidermal turnover and improvement in the appearance of hyperpigmentation by increasing keratinocyte shedding. AHA 10–40% nightly can be compounded with 4% hydroquinone to treat photoaged skin and dyspigmentation.

Other benefits for photoaged skin

Glycolic acid improves skin texture, fine wrinkling, and hyperpigmentation. Well controlled trials of 8% glycolic and 8% L-lactic acid creams showed a decrease in mottled hyperpigmentation, roughness, and overall sallowness of photoaged skin. AHA at a 25% concentration increased dermal acid mucopolysaccharides, elastic fibers, and collagen density. These agents further enhance the appearance of acne and photoaging when used in combination with tretinoin, with no added irritancy compared with tretinoin alone.

Although the keratolytic properties of AHA are stronger than those of BHA, careful use of both of these harsh chemicals is warranted as their acidic properties can induce significant photosensitivity, epidermal damage, and scarring. Although these agents decrease tumorigenicity induced by UV radiation, the high epidermal turnover rate increases the intensity of the exposure of the epidermis and dermis to UV. Salicylates that are absorbed percutaneously also pose the potential risk of salicylate toxicity if applied over a large body surface area or to a compromised epidermal barrier. These risks are typically evident with the use of high concentrations of salicylic acid ointment or salicylic acid, not at the concentrations or body surface areas used in over-the-counter acne treatments. These products are category B (lactic and glycolic acid) and C (salicylic acid), and thus should be used with great caution in pregnancy, lactation, and in young children.

The multifaceted effects of hydroxy acids all contribute to the ability of these agents to improve signs of aging, including the appearance of fine lines, hyperpigmentation, and skin texture.

Botanicals

Key Points

- There has been increasing demand for botanical agents in skin care products.
- Botanicals are chemicals extracted from the leaves, barks, roots, and flowers of plants.
- There are thousands of botanical agents with purported therapeutic benefits; however, their use in skin care products varies considerably based on harvest and extraction techniques.
- Further research is needed to define the optimal concentration, beneficial properties, and side-effects when botanicals are used in topical preparations.

Over the past 5 years there has been increasing demand for botanical products and their development. Consumers are more aware of ingredients in the products they use and natural ingredients are now a part of most skin care products in the US market. Some botanicals have proven physiologic benefits, whereas many others are synthetic variants of plant extracts that may or may not have the same benefits of naturally occurring ingredients.

Botanicals are extracted from the leaves, barks, roots, and flowers of plants. They undergo grinding, distilling, pressing, and drying to make a liquid, powder paste, syrup, or crystal, and are then further processed chemically – often heated to derive the essential oils incorporated into products. Through the aforementioned vigorous processing and heating, many natural extracts lose their beneficial properties. Additionally, the amount extracted from each plant may not be sufficient to deliver the purported benefits.

There are thousands of naturally occurring extracts of plants with physiologic benefits, with each natural extract containing a large number of active components. Many of the extracts work synergistically to provide a therapeutic benefit. As opposed to synthetic products that are made under standardized conditions, botanicals differ in efficacy and toxicity depending on time of harvest, weather, preparation of the herb, and final extraction. The efficacy of botanical products is based primarily on anecdotal evidence rather than scientific investigation, and they are considered dietary supplements or food additives, excluding them from FDA regulations. This chapter focuses on the most widely used botanicals in skin care products.

Most botanicals may be classified into categories comprising their suggested benefit. The botanical antioxidants are further subclassified into flavenoids, carotenoids, and polyphenols (Table 2-7).

Soy

Soy is a naturally occurring isoflavone comprised of genistein and daidzein. It is also classified as phytoestrogen, owing to its structural similarity to

Table 2-7 Botanical antioxidants	
Flavones	Rutin (apples, blueberries)
	Quercetin (apples, blueberries)
	Hesperidin (lemons, oranges)
	Diosmin (lemons, oranges)
	Soy
	Silymarin (milk thistle)
Xanthones	Mangiferin (mango plant)
	Mangostin (bilberry plant)
Carotenoids	Astaxanthin (tomatoes)
	Lutein (tomatoes)
	Lycopene (tomatoes)
Polyphenols	Rosmarinic acid (rosemary)
	Hypericin (St John's wort)
	Ellagic acid (pomegranate fruit)
	Chlorogenic acid (blueberry leaf)
	Oleuropein (olive leaf)
	Curcumin (tumeric root)
	Pycnogenol (marine pine bark)
	Terpenoids (ginko biloba)
	Procyanidin (grape seed)
	Epigallocatechin (green tea)

estrogen. Soy has received significant attention as a result of studies suggesting preventive benefits in cardiovascular disease and breast cancer in the Asian population. Like estrogen, soy also has the ability to increase skin thickness and promote collagen gene expression. The genistein component of soy products provides the antioxidant effects by acting as a scavenger of free radicals and an inhibitor lipid peroxidation.

Curcumin

Curcumin is derived from tumeric root and has been used for years as a food additive and spice. Curcumin is a polyphenol antioxidant with many other anti-inflammatory functions. Several human studies have shown curcumin's anti-inflammatory activity as an inhibitor of leukotriene, lipo-oxygenase, and cyclo-oxygenase, as well as an inhibitor of platelet aggregation and stabilizer of neutrophilic lysosomal membranes. It has also been shown to inhibit collagenase, elastase, and hyaluronidase. The hydrogenated form, tetrahydrocurcumin, is also a potent antioxidant and the form most often added to products.

Silymarin

Silymarin is extracted from the fruit, seeds, and leaves of the milk thistle plant, *Silybum marianum*. It is a mixture of three types of flavenoids: silybinin, silydianin, and silychristine. All function as potent antioxidants by scavenging free radicals, preventing lipid peroxidation, and decreasing the production of pyrimidine dimers. Hairless mice treated with silymarin prior to UVB exposure showed a significant decrease in the number of skin carcinomas, an effect thought to be due to the ability of silymarin to prevent the formation of pyrimidine dimers and angiogenesis.

Pycnogenol

Derived from the French marine pine bark, *Pinus pinaster*, pycnogenol is a water-soluble polyphenol that functions as a free radical scavenger and antioxidant. Pycnogenol also augments the antioxidant effects of vitamins C and E. It is used orally for the prevention of cardiovascular disease, and is used topically for the prevention of cutaneous oxidative damage. There have been no reported adverse effects from topical or oral use of pycnogenol.

Kinetin

Kinetin is a cytokinin, or adenine derivative, found in various plants and human cells. This product, referred to in skin care products as N^6-furfuryladenine, has been shown to improve the appearance of photoaging by decreasing fine wrinkles, improving pigmentation, and increasing skin smoothness. It is a strong antioxidant used to slow the yellowing of leaves and the over-ripening of fruits. Although the exact mechanism of action is unknown, kinetin provides benefits in DNA repair, prevents oxidative protein damage, and decreases TEWL when applied topically.

Ginkgo biloba

Ginko biloba is an extract of the plant group known as terpenoids. It is a polyphenol antioxidant known to increase superoxide dismutase activity in the epidermis after topical application. Studies in fibroblast models suggest its role as a free radical scavenger and its ability to prevent lipid peroxidation, Ginkgo biloba has also been shown in vitro to stimulate human fibroblast proliferation and to increase collagen and fibronectin formation. There have been no large in vivo studies evaluating its anti-aging effects.

Teas

Tea leaves are a rich source of polyphenols. They are strong natural antioxidants, able to scavenge singlet oxygen, superoxide radicals, hydroxyl radicals, and hydrogen peroxide. Teas have been shown in numerous in vitro studies to inhibit UV-induced skin cancer formation. They have the ability to regenerate vitamin E, reduce the number of UV-induced pyrimidine dimers, inhibit angiogenesis factors such as vascular endothelial growth factor (VEGF), and prevent against UV-induced erythema and sunburn cell formation.

Tea tree oil

Tea tree oil is an essential oil consisting of terpene. It has antimicrobial properties for Gram-positive and Gram-negative infections, herpes simplex virus, candida, and *Trichophyton*. Topical applications of tea tree oil are used for the treatment of acne and onychomycosis. Tea tree oil has the ability to reduce histamine-induced type I hypersensitivity reactions. As it is a sun sensitizer and can be cytotoxic to epidermal cells exposed to UV radiation. Tea tree oil should not be used for burns or on sunburned skin. It is also a common cause of allergic contact dermatitis.

Grape seed

Grape seed oil is derived from the maritime pine bark, *Pinus pinaster*. Grape seed extract is a polyphenol composed of procyandins (proanthocyandin, leukocyandin, and tannins). Procyandins have potent antioxidant, anti-inflammatory, and anticarcinogenic properties. Although no clinical trials have been performed, anecdotal reports suggest beneficial effects of grape seed for hair growth, wound healing, UV protection, and the stabilization of elastin and collagen by inhibition of MMPs. Topical formulations of grape seed extract have been used for years because of its ability to inhibit histamine synthesis, promote wound healing, improve photoaging, reduce postoperative edema, reduce venous insufficiency, and reduce UV-induced sunburn cell formation and immunosuppression.

Soothing agents

Soothing agents include prickly pear, aloe vera, allantoin, witch hazel, and papaya. These agents contain 80% water, 10% sucrose, tartaric acid, citric acid, and other mucopolysaccharides. The evaporation of water from topical application of these agents causes cooling of the skin, and the mucopolysaccharides provide a protective coating over wounded skin.

Aloe vera

Aloe vera is one of the most widely used botanical agents. It is made from a colorless gel extracted from the aloe vera plant. It is composed of 99.5% water and a complex mix of mucopolysaccharides, amino acids, hydroxyquinone glycosides, and minerals. Aloe vera has been shown to accelerate wound healing and to protect and soothe the skin. It is antibacterial to *Staphylococcus* species, *Helicobacter pylori*, and dermatophyte fungi. Aloe vera increases blood flow, reduces inflammation, and enhances wound healing. In topical preparations, it has been shown to increase collagen synthesis in wounds. Aloe vera is found in a wide range of over-the-counter products including soaps, shampoos, and moisturizers. Side-effects include allergic contact dermatitis and potential carcinogenic properties, use in pregnancy and lactation is contraindicated.

Allantoin

Allantoin is extracted from the comfrey root and is often synthetically derived. It is added to many products to treat burns, dermatitis, wounds, acne, and impetigo. Allantoin is also added to sensitive skin moisturizers and hand sanitizers, and in topical formulations for the treatment of scars and keloids. It is carcinogenic and thus contraindicated in pregnancy and lactation, and can be fatal when orally consumed.

The growing consumer demand for all-natural ingredients in foods and over-the-counter products has increased interest in botanicals for skin care (Table 2-8). There is little evidence from human trials to support their efficacy, and the rigorous processing prior to their inclusion in cosmeceuticals often depletes the beneficial properties of the extract. Despite this, the use of botanicals is widespread and will continue to expand as the demand for natural products increases.

Table 2-8 Other botanicals

Witch hazel	Derived from the leaves of the witch hazel plant, the witch hazel extract contains a high proportion of tannins, which function as topical vasoconstrictors. Witch hazel is used as an astringent for oily skin and is useful for the treatment of venous varicosities and spider veins
Glycyrrhizin	Glycyrrhizin is found in licorice root and inhibits the pro-inflammatory activities of prostaglandins and leukotrienes
Ginseng	Ginseng is one of the steroidal saponins known as ginsengosides. Ginseng enhances immunity, increases protein synthesis, and has antioxidant, antiviral, and antitumor properties
Capsaicin	Extracted from cayenne peppers, capsaicin inhibits substance P. It is often used for the treatment of pruritus and pain
Podophyllotoxin	Podophyllotoxin is extracted from the may apple. It has viricidal properties and is used for the treatment of condyloma and verruca vulgaris
Echinacea	Echinacea extract is derived from the echinacea plant. It has been shown anecdotally to stimulate immunity and protect collagen. It has antioxidant and antimicrobial properties. Its widespread uses include the treatment of stomatitis, wounds, burns, prevention of infection, and treatment of ulcers and photoaging
Garlic	Garlic is an alliin and allicin polysaccharide. It contains saponins and vitamins A, B2, and C. Garlic has antimicrobial and antioxidant properties, as well as anti-yeast and anti-dermatophyte activity
Saw palmetto	Saw palmetto is also a flavenoid antioxidant. It has antiandrogenic, antiestrogenic, and anti-inflammatory activities
St John's wort	St John's wort is a wound healing agent with anti-staphylococcus and anti-inflammatory activity
Pomegranate	Pomegranate consists of 25% tannin polyphenols such as ellagic acid, in addition to ascorbic acid, niacin, and piperidine alkaloids. It inhibits Gram-negative bacteria, fungi, parasites, and viruses, and has photoprotective properties
Chamomile	Chamomile, a member of the composite family, is an anti-inflammatory, antiallergic, antimicrobial, and antioxidant analgesic botanical. It inhibits the release of histamine, lipo-oxygenase, and cyclo-oxygenase. Its ability to stimulate granulation tissue formation has led to its use in wound healing
Lavender	Lavender is also a plant extract that has anti-inflammatory, antimicrobial, and antiallergic properties. It has been shown to inhibit mast cells. Lavender's wide range of uses includes topical preparations therapeutic for bites, burns, wounds, acne, psoriasis, herpes simplex virus, and fungal infections

Skin lightening

Key Points

- Skin lightening agents include phenolic and nonphenolic compounds.
- The mechanism of skin lightening by topical agents includes decreased tyrosinase synthesis, increased tyrosinase degradation, melanocyte toxicity, increased keratinocyte desquamation, or decreased melanosome transfer to keratinocytes.
- There are no reliable, safe, and universally effective skin depigmenting agents.
- Increased debate over the safety of hydroquinone has stimulated research into alternative, safer, agents for skin lightening.

Table 2-9 Mechanism of action of depigmenting agents

Action	Agents
Inhibition of tyrosinase synthesis	Retinol, kojic acid, hydroquinone, arbutin, glabridin, ellagic acid, paper mulberry, azaleic acid, monobenzyl ether of hydroquinone
Decreased tyrosinase synthesis	Ascorbic acid, aloesin
Decreased tyrosinase transfer	Glucosamine, tunicamycin
Tyrosinase degradation	Linoleic acid
Toxicity to melanocytes	Hydroquinone, monobenzyl ether of hydroquinone
Increased desquamation of keratinocytes	Retinoids, α- and β-hydroxy acids, linoleic acid
Decreased melanosome transfer to keratinocytes	Niacinamide, retinol, soy

Hyperpigmentation results from an increased number of melanocytes or increased production of melanin. Despite the many acquired or hereditary disorders of pigmentation, few products have been developed that can effectively and evenly depigment the skin. Some of the most prevalent patient concerns in dermatology involve pigmentation from UV radiation, drugs, melasma, post-inflammatory pigmentation, acne scarring, poikiloderma of Civatte, ephilides, and solar lentigos. Management focuses on photoprotection and topical skin lightening agents available in skin care products (Tables 2-8, 2-9 & 2-10).

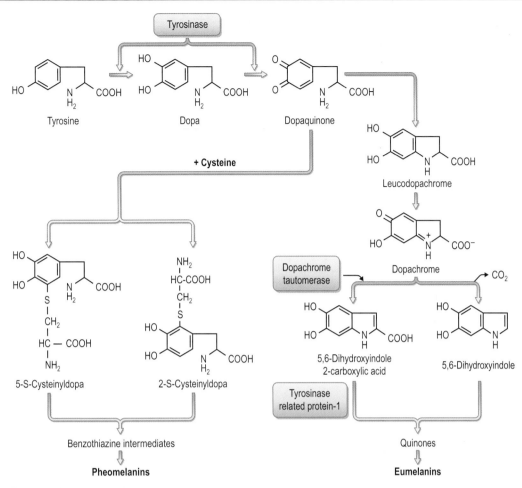

Figure 2-3 Tyrosinase pathway

Phenolic agents

Hydroquinone

Hydroquinone is a skin lightening agent available as either a pharmaceutical or a cosmeceutical. Its mechanism of action depends on its ability to inhibit tyrosinase synthesis, thereby inhibiting the production of melanin (Fig. 2-3). Other functions of hydroquinone include its ability to inhibit DNA and RNA synthesis, and to degrade melanosomes. Products sold at 2% concentration are available in more than 100 over-the-counter products, whereas those with a 3–10% concentration are prescription products and regulated as drugs. New products on the market today use hydroquinone in combination with topical retinoids and topical steroids for treatment of melasma and photopigmentation.

Hydroquinone has received scrutiny recently owing to its risk of ochronosis, a severe but rare side-effect. Endogenous ochronosis is a manifestation of a rare metabolic disorder known as alkaptonuria, which results from a deficiency of homogentisic acid oxidase. Exogenous ochronosis is a rare cutaneous side-effect of the long-term use of topical depigmenting agents such as hydroquinone. Ochronosis is characterized by an asymptomatic blue–black pigmentation of skin and cartilage. Although the exact cause of ochronosis from topical hydroquinone is not known, studies suggest that hydroquinone may inhibit homogentisic acid oxidase in the dermis, with the accumulation of homogentisic acid in the dermis causing ochronotic pigment deposition. Other agents reported in the literature to cause exogenous ochronosis are antimalarials, resorcinol, phenol, mercury, and picric acid.

A recent literature review revealed only 22 reported cases of ochronosis with hydroquinone use in more than 10 000 patient exposures over 50 years. This is an extremely low risk, and hydroquinone can be used safely in patients. Most cases of ochronosis reported are with long-term use of hydroquinone in doses greater than those in topical over-the-counter preparations. Although cases of ochronosis with the use of 2% hydroquinone have been reported, dermal absorption of hydroquinone up to 4% has been shown to be equivalent to that

Table 2-10 Skin lightening agents

Type	Agents
Phenolic	Hydroquinone
	Monobenzyl ether of hydroquinone
	4-methoxyphenol
	4-isopropylcatechol
	4-hydroxyanisol
	N-acetyl-4-S-cysteaminylphenol
Nonphenolic	Corticosteroids
	Retinol
	Azelaic acid
	N-acetylcysteine (NAC)
	L-ascorbyl-2-phosphate
	Kojic acid
	Niacinamide
	Ascorbic acid
	Arbutin
	Paper mulberry
	Soy
Combination	Kligman's formula: 5% hydroquinone, 0.1% tretinoin, 0.1% dexamethasone in hydrophilic ointment
	Pathak's formula: 2% hydroquinone, 0.05–0.1% tretinoin
	Westerhof's formula: 4.7% NAC, 2% hydroquione, 0.1% triamcinolone acetonide

absorbed from ingestion of common foods containing hydroquinone. The risk of ochronosis is reportedly greater in African American women, when the product is used on large surface areas at concentrations greater than 4% for extended periods of time.

Hydroquinone at 2% concentration is widely used in topical cosmeceutical preparations. The current recommendations for its use are on hyperpigmented lesions for approximately 4–6 weeks. The benefits of hydroquinone are reportedly evident in the first 4–6 weeks of use, and plateau at 4 months. Use beyond 4 months is generally not recommended.

Combination products containing hydroquinone include the Kligman formula, which contains 5% hydroquinone with 0.1% retinoic acid and 0.1% dexamethasone in a hydrophilic ointment base. Newer products such as Tri-Luma® cream (Galderma laboratories, Fortworth, TX) contain 0.01% fluocinolone, 4% hydroquinone, and 0.05% tretinoin.

The FDA has proposed warnings regarding the carcinogenic potential of hydroquinone. Hydroquinone, a metabolite of benzene, is an inhibitor of DNA and RNA synthesis. High doses of hydroquinone used for extended periods of time have been shown in laboratory animals to cause hepatic adenoma, renal adenoma, and leukemia. Allegations of hepatic and renal adenomas stem from murine studies and have not been reported in humans treated with oral or topical hydroquinone. Additionally, hydroquinone has been implicated in animal studies to cause mononuclear cell leukemia. The leukemogenic potential is only in the presence of phenol, and has been described in murine studies only after high-dose oral intake for over 2 years. No mononuclear cell leukemia has been reported with topical use of hydroquinone.

In conclusion, the FDA's proposed ban on the use of hydroquinone in over-the-counter preparations is based on carcinogen studies not validated in human trials. Ochronosis is, however, a documented side-effect of hydroquinone use and all patients should be advised against the long-term use of hydroquinone-containing products.

Arbutin

Arbutin, hydroquinone-β-D-glucopyranoside, is a crystallized extract of the bearberry plant. Its mechanism, similar to that of hydroquinone, involves the inhibition of tyrosinase activity. However, unlike hydroquinone, it does not inhibit the synthesis of tyrosinase; rather it inhibits tyrosinase activity by acting as a molecular mimic to the amino acid tyrosine.

N-acetyl-4-S-cysteaminylphenol

N-acetyl-4-S-cysteaminylphenol is a phenolic thioether skin lightening agent used in the treatment of solar lentigos. It is cytotoxic to melanocytes that are actively producing eumelanin. A few studies have also suggested an antitumor effect against the proliferation of melanoma cells in vitro. N-acetyl-4-S-cysteaminylphenol is more stable and less irritating than hydroquinone. Combination products containing N-acetyl-4-S-cysteaminylphenol and tretinoin are also available.

Nonphenolic agents

Retinoids

Retinoids have also been shown to decrease the pigmentation of melasma and post-inflammatory pigmentary alterations. Studies have shown that retinoids disperse the melanin pigment in keratinocytes with a loss of supranuclear caps in the basal layer. Retinoids also function to impede melanosome transfer to keratinocytes and increase epidermal turnover.

Kojic acid

Kojic acid is derived from *Aspergillus* and *Penicillium* fungi. It also functions as a tyrosinase inhibitor by chelating copper ions needed for tyrosinase function. This agent has been used in the food industry to prevent browning of foods and to redden unripe tomatoes. It is available in concentrations of 1–4%. Unlike hydroquinone, it has a high incidence of irritant contact dermatitis and is often used in combination products with corticosteroids to reduce its irritant profile. Kojic acid is also reportedly a potent scavenger of ROS and is consumed orally for its proposed anti-aging and anticancer benefits.

Licorice extract

Licorice extract is also known as glabridin. The licorice root is a tyrosinase inhibitor derived from the root of the tree, *Glycyrrhiza glabra linneva*. A combination product containing 0.4% glabridin, 0.05% betamethasone, and 0.05% retinoic acid has been shown to be effective in the treatment of melasma; however, it is not available in the USA. No specific adverse effects have been reported.

Paper mulberry

Paper mulberry is also a tyrosinase inhibitor extracted from the root bark of *Broussonetia papyrifera*. No long-term studies have provided any data on its efficacy. No significant adverse effects have been reported.

Soy

As mentioned above, soybeans have many clinically significant properties. The skin lightening function of soy is due to the inhibition of the phagocytosis of melanosomes by keratinocytes.

Vitamin C

Vitamin C interferes with pigment production at various stages of the melanin synthesis pathway. It interacts with copper ions at the tyrosinase active site, blocking the formation of melanin.

Melatonin

Melatonin is an endogenously produced hormone synthesized by the pineal gland in response to sunlight and diurnal rhythms. Its skin lightening functions are secondary to the inhibition of tyrosinase in melanocytes.

Glycolic acid

Glycolic acid is derived from sugarcane and is used most commonly as an exfoliating agent. Glycolic acid in high concentrations can function to lighten skin by stimulating corneocyte desquamation. By stimulating the shedding of the top layers of the skin, it also enhances the penetration of other topical skin lighteners.

Aloe

Aloe vera is a noncompetitive inhibitor of tyrosinase and a competitive inhibitor of dihydroxyphenylalanine (DOPA) oxidation. Aloe vera has been shown to inhibit UV-induced melanogenesis.

Niacinamide

Niacinamide, vitamin B3, inhibits the transfer of melanosomes to keratinocytes.

Azaleic acid

Azaleic acid is a naturally occurring dicarboxylic acid isolated from *Pityrosporum ovale*. It is a weak competitive inhibitor of tyrosinase activity. Azaleic acid also inhibits thioredoxin reductase, an enzyme needed for DNA synthesis, and thus has additional antiproliferative and cytotoxic effects on melanocytes. Azaleic acid used topically in a 20% cream has a variety of therapeutic uses including treatment for acne, rosacea, lentigines, and hyperpigmentation.

Despite many years of research and significant scientific interest in skin lightening agents, there are no reliable, safe, and universally effective skin depigmenting agents. Synthetic products and botanical agents show some promise, but studies evaluating their safety and efficacy are lacking. The debate over the safety of hydroquinone will continue to stimulate researchers and industry to find a safer alternative in years to come.

Metals

Key Points

- Metals play a critical role in the integrity of skin, hair, and nails.
- Their use in sunscreens and antimicrobial agents has been well elucidated, but further research is needed to define their benefits in topical antiaging preparations.

Many skin disorders are due to metal deficiencies. These include zinc deficiency (acrodermatitis enteropathica) and copper deficiency (Menkes' disease). These deficiency dermatides illustrate the integral role of metals in the maintaining integrity of skin, hair, and nails.

Zinc

Zinc is a ubiquitous metal critical to the stability and activity of enzymes required for DNA replication, gene transcription, and protein synthesis. It is essential for proper wound healing, signaling, and structure of the extracellular membrane. Zinc is used in topical preparations for barrier protection, wound healing, and treatment of inflammatory disorders. Its use as a broad-spectrum sunscreen has been documented in studies that illustrate decreased oxidative stress on UV-irradiated skin fibroblasts treated with topical zinc preparations. Antifungicidal properties of zinc pyrithione have also stimulated its use in antidandruff shampoos.

Copper

Copper is an essential cofactor necessary for the proper functioning of many enzymes. Copper plays an instrumental role in the function of tyrosinase necessary for melanin synthesis and the function of lysyl oxidase required for collagen synthesis. Additionally, copper is a cofactor for superoxide dismutase, which scavenges free radicals that cause oxidative damage to the skin. Topically applied copper has been shown in small studies to improve skin roughness, increase collagen synthesis, and improve the appearance of fine lines and photodamage.

Selenium

Selenium is an essential element in plants. It is required for the function of glutathione peroxidase and thioredoxin reductase, both of which protect cells against oxidative damage. Selenium has strong antioxidant abilities, protecting cells against DNA oxidation, lipid peroxidation, and UV-induced DNA damage. Selenium's antimicrobial properties are beneficial in antidandruff treatments.

Anticellulites

Key Points

- There is no clear consensus as to the etiology of cellulite.
- Topical preparations have been designed to alter fat breakdown mechanisms; however, none has been proven in well controlled studies to provide reproducible benefit.

There is no consensus as to the etiology of cellulite or its female predilection, and no criteria that can effectively measure its improvement.

Topical treatments are designed to change the metabolism of adipocytes by slowing down lipogenesis or increasing lipolysis. Fat breakdown or lipolysis is inhibited by α_2-adrenergic receptors and stimulated by β-adrenergic receptors. Agents that stimulate β-adrenergic receptors thereby increase fat breakdown. These agents include theobromine, theophylline, aminophylline, caffeine, isopropylarterenol hydrochloride, and epinephrine. Agents that inhibit α_2-adrenergic receptors and thereby prevent the inhibition of lipolysis include yohimbine, piperoxan, phentolamine, and dihydroergotamine.

During the past decade, many new cosmeceuticals have been developed for over-the-counter products that claim to improve the appearance of cellulite (Box 2-3). Few such products have been studied in well controlled trials.

BOX 2-3

Anticellulite cosmeceuticals

Isopropylarterenol hydrochloride

Epinephrine

Yohimbine

Piperoxan

Theophylline

Barley

Butcher's broom

Centella

Witch hazel

Algae

Aminophylline

Caffeine

Phentolamine

Dihydroergotamine

Theobromine

Gingko

Green tea

Ivy

Thistle

Enzymes

Key Points

- Topically applied enzymes are now being developed, with anecdotal benefits for photo-damaged skin.
- Further research is needed to evaluate the absorption of these large molecules when used in topical preparations.

Topical lotions with DNA repair enzymes applied to UV-exposed skin have been shown to decrease the development of actinic keratoses and basal cell carcinomas. Additionally, topical application of photolyase-containing liposomes decreases UV-induced cyclobutane dimer formation and UV-induced immunosuppression, erythema, and sunburn cell formation. The most common topically applied enzymes include papain and DNA repair enzymes.

Papain

Papain, derived from the papaya fruit, is an enzyme that digests intracellular protein bonds. When used topically, papain can improve epidermal exfoliation and may be used in the treatment of hypertrophic scars.

DNA repair enzymes

Bacteria-derived DNA repair enzymes have been reported to decrease skin cancer by inhibiting the formation of UV-induced cyclobutane pyrimidine dimers. The clinical applications of DNA repair enzymes are still limited, as many cannot be absorbed topically.

Growth factors

Key Points

- Growth factors are cytokines and proteins that regulate intercellular signaling, cell growth, cell development, and tissue repair.
- Growth factors developed for skin care products include epidermal growth factor, transforming growth factor, and platelet-derived growth factor.
- The ability of these large proteins to penetrate the stratum corneum is limited, and thus further research is needed to define their role in topical skin care preparations.

Growth factors are naturally occurring cytokines and proteins that regulate intercellular signaling, cell growth, cell development, and tissue repair. They are derived from epidermal cells, culture fibroblasts, placental cells, and plants. Their interactions stimulate tissue repair and immune responses, and increase the synthesis of collagen, elastin and GAGs.

Growth factors included in skin care products include epidermal growth factor (EGF), transforming growth factor (TGF), and platelet-derived growth factor (PDGF). EGF, found in plasma, sweat, urine, saliva, and semen, stimulates epidermal re-epithelialization and differentiation, and has been used for the treatment of burns and surgical wounds. TGF augments the production of extracellular matrix proteins for epithelial repair, promotes angiogenesis, and accelerates wound healing.

Studies evaluating topical growth factor mixtures applied to photodamaged skin have shown improvement in new collagen formation, epidermal thickening, skin hydration, roughness, dyspigmentation, and wrinkles. The wound healing benefits of growth factors have also been evaluated following ablative and nonablative laser resurfacing, with treated skin exhibiting less erythema and improved wound healing.

A controversial debate has arisen in the literature about growth factors such as VEGF. This concern stems from studies showing growth progression of in vitro melanoma cells with the addition of VEGF. In contrast, other studies have shown in vitro growth inhibition of squamous cell carcinoma with the addition of VEGF and TGF-β. Other potentially detrimental effects of growth factors include the ability of TGF-β to induce scar formation by activating fibroblasts and thus promoting the formation of keloidal scarring.

Debate has also arisen over whether or not large proteins such as growth factors can penetrate the stratum corneum. Studies are now under way to evaluate novel delivery systems that disrupt the stratum corneum, thereby allowing higher-molecular-weight molecules such as growth factors to penetrate the dermis. These investigated techniques include liposomal transdermal delivery, microporation, phonophoresis, and iontophoresis.

Hormones

Key Points

- Endogenous hormones play a key role in the integrity of human skin, hair, and nails.
- The exogenous application of estrogen and testosterone is under investigation; however, their use in topical preparations are currently limited.

The cutaneous manifestations of endocrinopathies, such as skin changes seen in menopause, hypothyroidism, hyperinsulinemia, and Addison's disease, have been well defined in the dermatology and endocrinology literature.

Many studies have shown the benefits of topical estrogen preparations, including improved skin texture, wrinkling, elasticity, and neovascularization. Small studies have also demonstrated biopsy-proven increase in type III collagen levels in estrogen-treated skin. However, long-term studies on the efficacy and toxicity of topical estrogens are lacking. Topical estrogen and estrogen–progestogen preparations are also currently used in Europe and are effective for the management of hormonal acne.

Testosterone creams have also gained increased acceptance, as recent studies have postulated that oral supplementation may improve memory and sexual function; however, limited studies have been carried out on the effects of topically applied testosterone. Side-effects of topically applied androgenic steroids, including acne and hirsutism, have limited their use in over-the-counter cosmeceuticals.

Peptides

Key Points

- Peptides are sequences of amino acids that mimic the amino acids in collagen and elastin.
- Three classes of peptide used in topical antiaging regimens include: signal peptides, carrier peptides, and neurotransmitter inhibiting peptides.
- The ability of these large molecular weight compounds to penetrate the stratum corneum is limited and thus few studies have shown any sustainable benefit.

Photoaged skin exhibits decreased synthesis of procollagen I mRNA in fibroblasts, thicker elastotic fibers, and increased MMP levels. Peptides are sequences of amino acids that mimic the amino acids in collagen and elastin, and are believed to increase collagen and elastin synthesis. One caveat of peptide use in skin products is the inability of these large-molecular-weight compounds to penetrate the stratum corneum.

Three types of peptide are used in cosmeceuticals: signal peptides, carrier peptides, and neurotransmitter inhibiting peptides.

Signal peptides

Signal peptides are short-chain amino acids that augment communication between cells. One example of a signal peptide in cosmeceutical products is valine-glycine-valine-alanine-proline-glycine (VGVAPG). This amino acid sequence has been shown to stimulate human skin fibroblast production, downregulate elastin expression, and promote the chemotaxis of fibroblasts in vitro. An alternative peptide, tyrosine-tyrosine-arginine-alanine-aspartame-aspartame-alanine, inhibits procollagen C proteinase, an enzyme that cleaves C-propeptide from procollagen-I and thereby decreases collagen breakdown. Alternatively, lysine-threonine-threonine-lysine-serine (Pal-KTTKS – Strivectin® and Regenerist®) is also a signal peptide found in type I procollagen. This pentapeptide has been shown to stimulate in vitro synthesis of collagen type I, IV, and fibronectin.

Carrier peptides

Carrier peptides are peptides with an ability to deliver metals to the skin. The tripeptide glycyl-L-histidyl-L-lysine facilitates copper uptake by the cell. Copper is a cofactor for lysyl oxidase, the enzyme needed for collagen synthesis. This tripeptide also increases levels of MMP-2 and increases the level of tissue inhibitor of metalloproteinases (TIMP-1 and TIMP-2).

Neurotransmitter inhibiting peptides

Neurotransmitter inhibiting peptides, such as the hexapeptide known as Argireline® (acetyl-glutamyl-glutamyl-methoxyl-glutaminyl-arginyl-arginylamide)(Lipotec OUP, Barcelona, Spain), functions in a manner similar to botulinum toxin. Argireline mimics the N-terminal domain of synaptosome-associated protein-25 kDa (SNAP-25), which blocks the formation of the soluble N-ethylmaleimide-sensitive factor attachment protein receptor (SNARE) protein complex that is needed for docking vesicles of acetylcholine release. This synthetically derived peptide is marketed to provide the same muscle relaxing and wrinkle reducing effects as botulinum toxin. However, when applied topically, these agents do not effectively penetrate the skin to reach the deeper muscles in the concentrations needed to provide benefits similar to those of botulinumtoxin injections. Limited safety and efficacy studies have been performed to prove any sustainable benefits.

The use of peptides in cosmeceuticals is still a novel concept with limited studies. The large size of these molecules limits their penetration through the stratum corneum. Although safety and efficacy data are lacking, many of these products are popularly used in over-the-counter anti-aging regimens.

Proteins

Key Points

- Proteins are agents developed to improve skin and hair hydration.

When applied topically, protein has the unique ability to bind and hold water in the skin. Similar to a humectant, the ability to hold water improves the appearance of aged skin by providing hydration and assisting in barrier repair. Proteins have also been added to many hair conditioners to restore hair shaft fractures induced by aging and repeated trauma. Proteins are also manufactured in hair-styling products as they neutralize the charge from static electricity often present on the hair shaft.

Anti-acne agents

Many of the products previously mentioned in this chapter, including retinoids, salicylic acid, and azelaic acid, are useful in the management of acne. As previously alluded to, salicylic acid is comedolytic, anti-inflammatory, and promotes epidermal desquamation and turnover. Retinol-based products eliminate microcomedones, enhance epithelial turnover, and decrease sebum production. Azalaic acid is a naturally occurring botanical with mild antimicrobial and mild keratolytic activity. Other naturally occurring cosmeceuticals include niacinamide, which increases desquamation and decreases sebum production.

Over-the-counter benzoyl peroxide preparations are commonly used for their antimicrobial and anti-inflammatory benefits. Topical preparations containing 1–10% sulfur are mild keratolytics and bacteriostatic agents against *P. acnes*. Sodium sulfacetamide is also a bacteriostatic agent with activity against both Gram-positive and Gram-negative bacteria. Although many of these products have relatively mild side-effects, including irritation and dryness, sulfur-based products have been shown to induce life-threatening hypersensitivity reactions and should be avoided in patients with a sulfa allergy.

Anti-redness agents

Facial redness is multifactorial. Genetics, superficial telangiectasias, and cutaneous disorders including seborrhea and rosacea, all contribute to the appearance of flushed, red skin. Surface vasodilation and inflammation can be reduced by skin care products containing vasoconstricting and anti-inflammatory agents. Product ingredients used for erythema include soothing agents such as prickly pear and aloe vera, humectants such as panthenol, and anti-inflammatory agents such as green tea. Moisturizers and cosmetics have also been developed with green-tinted colorings to help camouflage erythema. Patients with facial redness should avoid products containing harsh acids, such as salicylic acid. Products with fragrance enhance irritancy and can potentially worsen facial erythema. Furthermore, sunscreens should be applied daily to prevent UV-induced erythema.

Irritancy

Key Points

- Irritant and allergic dermatitis is common with over-the-counter skin care products.
- Fragrances, preservatives, and vehicles are common culprits of irritancy or hypersensitivity.
- Patient education regarding product ingredients and their proper use can enhance compliance and decrease skin irritation.

Contact dermatitis, either irritant or allergic, is seen commonly with cosmeceuticals. The lack of reports of proven contact sensitivity is due to the lack of standardization of these products, and a lack of allergens available for testing.

Although many natural or synthetic products are potent skin sensitizers or irritants, the vehicles in which these products are made also contain preservatives, fragrances, and colorings that can cause irritant or allergic contact dermatitis.

To improve consumer satisfaction, many skin care products contain added fragrance. However, most product labels do not delineate these additives on their packaging. Additionally, chemicals such as benzyl alcohol and benzyl aldehyde, often used as a fragrance, can be added to products for their functions separate from their fragrance. These products are routinely used in "fragrance-free" cosmetics. Similarly, botanicals containing a natural fragrance are not labeled as containing a fragrance on product labels. Similarly, products labeled as "unscented" do not imply that no fragrance is used; this implies that no odor can be percieved. Unscented products contain masking fragrances designed to disguise the chemical odor of the agent.

Preservatives are also widely used to prevent bacterial growth and oxidation of cosmeceutical products. These agents, including formaldehyde, formaldehyde releasers, parabens, kathon CG, and Euxyl K 100, are also culprits of allergic contact dermatitis. Vehicles containing these preservatives are so widespread that it is often challenging for the patient who has developed an irritant or allergic reaction to these agents to identify depict the culprit ingredient effectively.

Patch testing is recommended for any patient with a suspected alergic contact dermatitis. Furthermore, educating consumers and patients about product ingredients is imperative, particularly when an unknown or treatment recalcitrant contact hypersensitivity develops.

The future of cosmeceuticals

The increasing demand for cosmeceuticals and the rapid growth of this industry have instigated the scientific evaluation of many synthetic and natural agents for skin care.

As the market for cosmeceuticals and the armamentarium for dermatologists and patients grows, there is an increased need for improved methods to evaluate the safety and efficacy of these products in well controlled trials. Calculations of skin TEWL, capacitance, and sebum production have furthered our knowledge and understanding of topical products. New developments to measure the aging process, including silicone impressions that analyze wrinkle depth, and optical profilometry, which measures changes in skin topography, are among the many new computer imaging techniques being used objectively to characterize photo aged skin. Skin color changes can also be measured objectively using tools such as tristimulus colorimeters, which use mathematical evaluations of color hue, and spectrophotometers, which use wavelengths reflected from the skin surface to quantify skin color. New technologies have also been developed to quantify skin firmness, blood flow, and skin hydration. These instruments are now in widespread use to quantify and measure objective parameters, and will be useful in our quest to provide evidence-based recommendations for our patients.

Conclusion

In 2006, the cosmeceutical market rose to nearly $8.2 billion in profits in the USA alone. The development, use, and marketing of these products will continue to rise as the aging population strives to find noninvasive alternatives to anti-aging regimens. Well designed, randomized, placebo-controlled trials and basic science research is lacking. Industry is leading the research behind much of the science we now know to influence the development of cosmeceuticals. As the market grows, so should our understanding of the products, as it is *our* patients who use these products. As leaders of the field of dermatology, we need to understand the science of cosmeceuticals in order to provide our patients with optimal education and skin care guidance.

Further reading

Agarwal R, Katiyar SK, Khan SG, Mukhtar H. Protection against ultraviolet B radiation-induced effects in the skin of SKH-1 hairless mice by a polyphenolic fraction isolated from green tea. Photochem Photobiol 1993;58(5):695–700.

Akhavan A, Bershad S. Topical acne drugs: review of clinical properties, systemic exposure and safety. Am J Clin Dermatol 2003;4:473–492.

Akiyama T, Ishida J, Nakagawa S, et al. Genistein, a specific inhibitor of tyrosine-specific protein kinases. J Biol Chem 1987;262(12):5592–5595.

Alam M, Dover JS. On beauty: evolution, psychosocial considerations, and surgical enhancement. Arch Dermatol 2001;137(6):795–807.

Angel P, Szabowski A, Schorpp-Kistner M. Function and regulation of AP-1 subunits in skin physiology and pathology. Oncogene 2001;20(19):2413–2423.

Arora RB, Kapoor V, Basu N, Jain AP. Anti-inflammatory studies on *Curcuma longa* (turmeric). Indian J Med Res 1971;59(8):1289–1295.

Ashcroft GS, Greenwell-Wild T, Horan MA, et al. Topical estrogen accelerates cutaneous wound healing in aged humans associated with an altered inflammatory response. Am J Pathol 1999;155(4):1137–1146.

Badreshia-Bansal S, Draelos ZD. Insight into skin lightening cosmeceuticals for women of color. J Drugs Dermatol 2007;6:32–39.

Bangha E, Elsner P, Kistler GS. Suppression of UV-induced erythema by topical treatment with melatonin (N-acetyl-5-methoxytryptamine). Influence of the application time point. Dermatology 1997;195(3):248–252.

Baran R, Maibach HI. Textbook of Cosmetic Dermatology, 3rd edn. London: Taylor & Francis, 2005.

Barel AO, Paye M, Maibach HI. Handbook of Cosmetic Science and Technology. New York: Marcel Dekker, 2001.

Barry BW. Breaching the skin's barrier to drugs. Nat Biotechnol 2004;22(2):165–167.

Baumann L. How to prevent photoaging? J Invest Dermatol 2005;125(4):xii–xiii.

Bazzano GS, Terezakis N, Galen W. Topical tretinoin for hair growth promotion. J Am Acad Dermatol 1986;15(4 Pt 2):880–883, 890–893.

Bedi MK, Shenefelt PD. Herbal therapy in dermatology. Arch Dermatol 2002;138(2):232–242.

Berardesca E, Distante F, Vignoli GP, et al. Alpha hydroxyacids modulate stratum corneum barrier function. Br J Dermatol 1997;137:934–938.

Berardesca E, Fluhr J, Maibach HI. Sensitive Skin Syndrome. New York: Taylor & Francis, 2006.

Bernstein EF, Lee J, Brown DB, et al. Glycolic acid increases type I collagen mRNA and hyaluronic acid content of human skin. Dermatol Surg 2001;27(5):429–433.

Bernstein EF, Brown DBM, Schwartz MD, et al. The polyhydroxyl acid gluonolactone protects against UV radiation in an in vitro model of cutaneous photoaging. Dermatol Surg 2004;30(2 Pt 1):189–195.

Biewenga GP, Haenen GR, Bast A. The pharmacology of the antioxidant lipoic acid. Gen Pharmacol 1997;29(3):315–331.

Bikowski J. The use of therapeutic moisturizers in various dermatologic disorders. Cutis 2001;68(5 Suppl):3–11.

Bissett D. Topical niacinamide and barrier enhancement. Cutis 2002;70(6 Suppl):8–12.

Bissett DL, Chatterjee R, Hannon DP. Photoprotective effect of superoxide-scavenging antioxidants against ultraviolet radiation-induced chronic skin damage in the hairless mouse. Photodermatol Photoimmunol Photomed 1990;7(2):56–62.

Bissett DL, Oblong JE, Berge CA. Niacinamide: a B vitamin that improves aging facial skin appearance. Dermatol Surg 2005;31(7 Pt 2):860–865.

Bissett DL, Robinson LR, Raleigh PS, et al. Reduction in the appearance of facial hyperpigmentation by topical N-acetyl glucosamine. J Cosmet Dermatol 2007;6(1):20–26.

Blank IH. Factors which influence the water content of the stratum corneum. J Invest Dermatol 1952;18(6):433–440.

Brennan M, Bhatti H, Nerusu KC, et al. Matrix metalloproteinase-1 is the major collagenolytic enzyme responsible for collagen damage in UV-irradiated human skin. Photochem Photobiol 2003;78(1):43–48.

Briganti S, Camera E, Picardo M. Chemical and instrumental approaches to treat hyperpigmentation. Pigment Cell Res 2003;16(2):101–110.

Brody HJ. Latest ways to rejuvenate sun-damaged skin. Skin Cancer Found J 1999;17:28–29.

Bronaugh RL, Maibach HI. In Vitro Percutaneous Absorption: Principles, Fundamentals, and Applications. Boca Raton: CRC Press, 1991.

Burgess CM, ed. Cosmetic Dermatology. Berlin: Springer, 2005.

Burke KE, Clive J, Combs GF Jr, et al. Effects of topical and oral vitamin E on pigmentation and skin cancer induced by ultraviolet irradiation in Skh:2 hairless mice. Nutr Cancer 2000;38(1):87–97.

Carcamo JM, Pedraza A, Borquez-Ojeda O, Golde DW. Vitamin C suppresses TNF alpha-induced NF kappa B activation by inhibiting I kappa B alpha phosphorylation. Biochemistry 2002;41:12995–13002.

Casado FJ, Nusimovich AD. LMW hyaluronic acid to induce epidermal regeneration. Drug Cosm Ind 1991;148:30–34.

Chakraborty AK, Funasaka Y, Komoto M, Ichihashi M. Effect of arbutin on melanogenic proteins in human melanocytes. Pigment Cell Res 1998;11(4):206–212.

Chamlin SL, Kao J, Frieden IJ, et al. Ceramide-dominant barrier repair lipids alleviate childhood atopic dermatitis: changes in barrier function provide a sensitive indicator of disease activity. J Am Acad Dermatol 2002;47(2):198–208.

Chan AC. Partners in defense, vitamin E and vitamin C. Can J Physiol Pharmacol 1993;71(9):725–731.

Chiu AE, Chan JL, Kern DG, et al. Double-blinded, placebo-controlled trial of green tea extracts in the clinical and histologic appearance of photoaging skin. Dermatol Surg 2005;31(7 Pt 2):855–860.

Cocera M, Lopez O, Coderch L, et al. Influence of the level of ceramides on the permeability of stratum corneum lipid liposomes caused by a C12-betaine/sodium dodecyl sulfate mixture. Int J Pharm 1999;183(2):165–173.

Coderch L, De Pera M, Fonollosa J, et al. Efficacy of stratum corneum lipid supplementation on human skin. Contact Derm 2002;47:139–146.

Coleman WP 3rd. Dermal peels. Dermatol Clin 2001;19:405–411.

Crane FL. Biochemical functions of coenzyme Q10. J Am Coll Nutr 2001;20(6):591–598.

Creidi P, Humbert P. Clinical use of topical retinaldehyde on photoaged skin. Dermatology 1999;199(Suppl 1):49–52.

Cusan L, Dupont A, Balanger A, et al. Treatment of hirsutism with the pure antiandrogen flutamide. J Am Acad Dermatol 1990;23(3 Pt 1):462–469.

Del Rosso JQ. Cosmeceutical moisturizers. In: Draelos ZD, ed. Procedures in Cosmetic Dermatology Series: Cosmeceuticals. Philadelphia: Elsevier, 2005:97–102.

Del Rosso JQ, Baum EW, Draelos ZD, et al. Azelaic acid gel 15%: clinical versatility in the treatment of rosacea. Cutis 2006;78:6–19.

DeLeo V. Irritant, allergenic and photocontact dermatitis potential of new cosmetic components. Cosmet Dermatol 1996; Suppl:20–21.

Devaraj S, Vega-Lopez S, Kaul N, et al. Supplementation with a pine bark extract rich in polyphenols increases plasma antioxidant capacity and alters the plasma lipoprotein profile. Lipids 2002;37(10):931–934.

Ditre CM, Griffin TD, Murphy GF, et al. Effects of alpha-hydroxy acids on photoaged skin: a pilot clinical, histologic, and ultrastructural study. J Am Acad Dermatol 1996;34:187–195.

Draelos ZD. New developments in cosmetics and skin care products. Adv Dermatol 1997;12:3–18.

Draelos ZD. Hydroxy acids for the treatment of aging skin. J Geriatr Dermatol 1997;5:236–240.

Draelos ZD. Sensitive skin: perceptions, evaluation, and treatment. Am J Contact Dermat 1997;8:67–78.

Draelos ZD. The development of cosmeceuticals. Cosmet Dermatol 1998;Oct:15–16.

Draelos ZD. Hydroxy acid update. Cosmet Dermatol 1998;11:27–29.

Draelos ZD. Cosmetics and skin care products. A historical perspective. Dermatol Clin 2000;18: 557–559.

Draelos ZD. Therapeutic moisturizers. Dermatol Clin 2000;18(4):597–607.

Draelos ZD. The biology of hair care. Dermatol Clin 2000;18:651–658.

Draelos ZD. Treating the patient with multiple cosmetic product allergies. A problem-oriented approach to sensitive skin. Postgrad Med 2000;107:70–72, 75–77.

Draelos ZD. Botanicals as topical agents. Clin Dermatol 2001;19:474–477.

Draelos ZD. Cosmetics in acne and rosacea. Semin Cutan Med Surg 2001;20:209–214.

Draelos ZD. Concepts in skin care maintenance. Cutis 2005;76:19–25.

Draelos ZD. The disease of cellulite. J Cosmet Dermatol 2005;4:221–222.

Draelos ZD. Novel approach to the treatment of hyperpigmented photodamaged skin: 4% hydroquinone/0.3% retinol versus tretinoin 0.05% emollient cream. Dermatol Surg 2005;31: 799–804.

Draelos ZD. Topical and oral estrogens revisited for antiaging purposes. Fertil Steril 2005;84:291–292.

Draelos ZK. Cosmeceuticals. Philadelphia: Elsevier Saunders, 2005.

Draelos ZD. The effect of a daily facial cleanser for normal to oily skin on the skin barrier of subjects with acne. Cutis 2006;78:34–40.

Draelos ZD, DiNardo JC. A re-evaluation of the comedogenicity concept. J Am Acad Dermatol 2006;54:507–512.

Draelos ZD, Fuller BB. Efficacy of 1% 4-ethoxybenzaldehyde in reducing facial erythema. Dermatol Surg 2005;31:881–885.

Draelos ZD, Marenus KD. Cellulite. Etiology and purported treatment. Dermatol Surg 1997;23:1177–1181.

Draelos ZD, Rietschel RL. Hypoallergenicity and the dermatologist's perception. J Am Acad Dermatol 1996;35:248–251.

Draelos ZD, Tanghetti EA. Optimizing the use of tazarotene for the treatment of facial acne vulgaris through combination therapy. Cutis 2002;69: 20–29.

Draelos ZD, Ertel K, Hartwig P, Rains G. The effect of two skin cleansing systems on moderate xerotic eczema. J Am Acad Dermatol 2004;50:883–888.

Draelos ZD, Ertel K, Berge C. Niacinamide-containing facial moisturizer improves skin barrier and benefits subjects with rosacea. Cutis 2005;76:135–141.

Draelos ZD, Ertel KD, Berge CA. Facilitating facial retinization through barrier improvement. Cutis 2006;78:275–281.

Draelos ZD, Green BA, Edison BL. An evaluation of a polyhydroxy acid skin care regimen in combination with azelaic acid 15% gel in rosacea patients. J Cosmet Dermatol 2006;5:23–29.

Duell EA, Kang S, Voorhees JJ. Unoccluded retinol penetrates human skin in vivo more effectively than unoccluded retinyl palmitate or retinoic acid. J Invest Dermatol 1997;109:301–305.

Edison BL, Green BA, Wildnauer RH, Sigler ML. A polyhydroxy acid skin care regimen provides antiaging effects comparable to an alpha-hydroxy-acid regimen. Cutis 2002;73:14–17.

Edwards CR, Teelucksingh S. Glycyrrhetinic acid and potentiation of hydrocortisone activity in skin. Lancet 1990;336:322–323.

Effendy I, Kwangsukstith C, Lee JY, Maibach HI. Functional changes in human stratum corneum induced by topical glycolic acid: comparison with all-trans retinoic acid. Acta Derm Venereol 1995;75:455–458.

El Gammal C, Pagnoni A, Kligman AM, el Gammal S. A model to assess the efficacy of moisturizers – the quantification of soap-induced xerosis by image analysis of adhesive-coated discs (D-Squames). Clin Exp Dermatol 1996;21(5):338–343.

Elias PM, Feingold KR. Coordinate regulation of epidermal differentiation and barrier homeostasis. Skin Pharmacol Appl Skin Physiol 2001:14(Suppl 1):28–34.

Elias PM, Feingold KR. Does the tail wag the dog? Role of the barrier in the pathogenesis of inflammatory dermatoses and therapeutic implications. Arch Dermatol 2001;137(8):1079–1081.

Elias PM, Feingold KR. Skin Barrier. New York: Taylor & Francis, 2006.

Elias PM, Menon GK. Structural and lipid biochemical correlates of the epidermal permeability barrier. Adv Lipid Res 1991;24:1–26.

Elias PM, Crumrine D, Rassner U, et al. Basis for abnormal desquamation and permeability barrier dysfunction in RXLI. J Invest Dermatol 2004;122(2):314–319.

Elsner P, Maibach HI. Cosmeceuticals and Active Cosmetics: Drugs Versus Cosmetics, 2nd edn. Boca Raton: Taylor & Francis, 2005.

Elsner P, Berardesca E, Maibach HI. Bioengineering of the Skin: Water and the Stratum Corneum. Boca Raton: CRC Press, 1994.

Elsner P, Merk HF, Maibach HI. Cosmetics: controlled efficacy studies and regulation. Berlin: Springer, 1999.

Farris PK. Cosmeceuticals: a review of the science behind the claims. Cosmet Dermatol 2003;16: 59–68.

Farris PK. Topical vitamin C: a useful agent for treating photoaging and other dermatologic conditions. Dermatol Surg 2005;31(7 Pt 2):814–817.

Feingold KR, Schmuth M, Elias PM. The regulation of permeability barrier homeostasis. J Invest Dermatol 2007;127(7):1574–1576.

Fischer T, Bangha E, Elsner P, Kistler GS. Suppression of UV-induced erythema by topical treatment with melatonin. Influence of the application time point. Biol Signals Recept 1999;8:132–135.

Fisher GJ, Wang ZQ, Datta SC, et al. Pathophysiology of premature skin aging induced by ultraviolet light. N Engl J Med 1997;337:1419–1428.

Fisher GJ, Kang S, Varani J, et al. Mechanisms of photoaging and chronological skin aging. Arch Dermatol 2002;138:1462–1470.

Fitzpatrick RE. Endogenous growth factors as cosmeceuticals. Dermatol Surg 2005;31(7 Pt 2):827–831.

Fitzpatrick RE, Rostan EF. Reversal of photodamage with topical growth factors: a pilot study. J Cosmet Laser Ther 2003;5(1):25–34.

Fluhr JW, Vienne MP, Lauze C, et al. Tolerance profile of retinol, retinaldehyde and retinoic acid under maximized and long-term clinical conditions. Dermatology 1999;199(Suppl 1):57–60.

Fluhr JW, Feingold KR, Elias PM. Transepidermal water loss reflects permeability barrier status: validation in human and rodent in vivo and ex vivo models. Exp Dermatol 2006;15(7):483–492.

Flynn TC, Petros J, Clark RE, Viehman GE. Dry skin and moisturizers. Clin Dermatol 2001;19(4): 387–392.

Froebe CL, Simion FA, Rhein LD, et al. Stratum corneum lipid removal by surfactants: relation to in vivo irritation. Dermatologica 1990;181:277–283.

Garmyn M, Yaar M, Boileau N, et al. Effect of aging and habitual sun exposure on the genetic response of cultured human keratinocytes to solar-simulated irradiation. J Invest Dermatol 1992;99: 743–748.

Gendler EC. Topical treatment of the aging face. Dermatol Clin 1997;15(4):561–567.

Gensler HL. Prevention of photoimmunosuppression and photocarcinogenesis by topical nicotinamide. Nutr Cancer 1997;29(2):157–162.

Ghadially R, Halkier-Sorensen L, Elias PM. Effects of petrolatum on stratum corneum structure and function. J Amer Acad Dermatol 1992;26(3 Pt 2):387–396.

Ghadially R, Brown BE, Sequeira-Martin SM, et al. The aged epidermal permeability barrier. Structural, functional, and lipid biochemical abnormalities in humans and a senescent murine model. J Clin Invest 1995;95(5):2281–2290.

Ghadially R, Brown BE, Hanley K, et al. Decreased epidermal lipid synthesis accounts for altered barrier function in aged mice. J Invest Dermatol 1996;106(5):1064–1069.

Ghersetich I, Lotti T, Campanile G, et al. Hyaluronic acid in cutaneous intrinsic aging. Int J Dermatol 1994;33(2):119–122.

Gilchrest BA, Garmyn M, Yaar M. Aging and photoaging affect gene expression in cultured human keratinocytes. Arch Dermatol 1994;130:82–86.

Glaser DA. Anti-aging products and cosmeceuticals. Facial Plast Surg Clin North Am 2004;12(3): 363–372.

Glaser DA, Rogers C. Topical and systemic therapies for the aging face. Facial Plast Surg Clin North Am 2001;9(2):189–196.

Glazier MG, Bowman MA. A review of the evidence for the use of phytoestrogens as a replacement for traditional estrogen replacement therapy. Arch Intern Med 2001;161(9):1161–1172.

Goodman DS. Retinoid-binding proteins. J Am Acad Dermatol 1982;6:583–590.

Goodman DS. Vitamin A and retinoids in health and disease. N Engl J Med 1984;310(16):1023–1031.

Goukassian D, Gad F, Yaar M, et al. Mechanisms and implications of the age-associated decrease in DNA repair capacity. FASEB J 2000;14:1325–1334.

Green B, Edison B, Wildnauer RH, Sigler ML. Lacto-bionic acid and gluconolactone: PHAs for photo-aged skin. Cosmet Dermatol 2001;14:24–28.

Greenway FL, Bray GA. Regional fat loss from the thigh in obese women after adrenergic modulation. Clin Ther 1987;9(6):663–669.

Griffiths CE. Drug treatment of photoaged skin. Drugs Aging 1999;14(4):289–301.

Grimes PE, Green BA, Wildnauer RH, Edison BL. The use of polyhydroxy acids (PHAs) in photo-aged skin. Cutis 2004;73(2 Suppl):3–13.

Grove GL, Grove MJ, Leyden JJ, et al. Skin replica analysis of photodamaged skin after therapy with tretinoin emollient cream. J Am Acad Dermatol 1991;25(2 Pt 1):231–237.

Grubauer G, Feingold KR, Harris RM, Elias PM. Lipid content and lipid type as determinants of the epidermal permeability barrier. J Lipid Res 1989;30(1):89–96.

Grubauer G, Elias PM, Feingold KR. Transepidermal water loss: the signal for recovery of barrier structure and function. J Lipid Res 1989;30(3):323–333.

Hakozaki T, Minwalla L, Zhuang J, et al. The effect of niacinamide on reducing cutaneous pigmentation and suppression of melanosome transfer. Br J Dermatol 2002;147(1):20–31.

Hamaoka H, Minakuchi K, Miyoshi H, et al. Effect of K+ channel openers on K+ channel in cultured human dermal papilla cells. J Med Invest 1997;44(1–2):73–77.

Harding CR, Long S, Richardson J, et al. The corni-fied cell envelope: an important marker of stratum corneum maturation in healthy and dry skin. Int J Cosmet Sci 2003;25(4):157–168.

Hensley K, Floyd RA. Reactive oxygen species and protein oxidation in aging: a look back, a look ahead. Arch Biochem Biophys 2002;397:377–383.

Humbert P. Topical vitamin C in the treatment of photoaged skin. Eur J Dermatol 2001;11(2):172–173.

Humphreys TR, Werth V, Dzubow L, Kligman A. Treatment of photodamaged skin with trichloroacetic acid and topical tretinoin. J Am Acad Dermatol 1996;34(4):638–644.

Idson B. Vitamins of the skin. Cosmet Toilet 1993;108:79–92.

Jacobson EL, Kim H, Kim M, et al. A topical lipophilic niacin derivative increases NAD, epider-mal differentiation and barrier function in photo-damaged skin. Exp Dermatol 2007;16:490–499.

James WD, Kligman AM. Back to basics: local care for skin disease. Cutis 2006;78:389–390.

Johnson AW. The skin moisturizer marketplace. In: Leyden J, Rawlings A, eds. Skin Moisturization. New York: Marcel Dekker, 2002:1–30.

Johnson AW. Cosmeceuticals: function and the skin barrier. In: Draelos ZD, ed. Procedures in Cosmetic Dermatology Series: Cosmeceuticals. Philadelphia: Elsevier, 2005:97–102.

Joyeux M, Lobstein A, Anton R, Mortier F. Com-parative antilipoperoxidant, antinecrotic and scavenging properties of terpenes and biflavones from Ginkgo and some flavonoids. Planta Med 1995;61(2):126–129.

Kagan VE, Serbinova EA, Forte T, et al. Recycling of vitamin E in human low density lipoproteins. J Lipid Res 1992;33(3):385–397.

Kagan VE, Serbinova EA, Safadi A, et al. NADPH-dependent inhibition of lipid peroxidation in rat liver microsomes. Biochem Biophys Res Commun 1992;186(1):74–80.

Kang S, Fisher GJ, Voorhees JJ. Photoaging and topi-cal tretinoin: therapy, pathogenesis, and prevention. Arch Dermatol 1997;133(10):1280–1284.

Kang S, Li XY, Duell EA, Voorhees JJ. The retinoid X receptor agonist 9-*cis*-retinoic acid and the 24-hydroxylase inhibitor ketoconazole increase activity of 1,25-dihydroxyvitamin D3 in human skin in vivo. J Invest Dermatol 1997;108:513–518.

Kang S, Fisher GJ, Voorhees JJ. Photoaging: patho-genesis, prevention, and treatment. Clin Geriatr Med 2001;17(4):643–659, v–vi.

Kang S, Leyden JJ, Lowe NJ, et al. Tazarotene cream for the treatment of facial photodam-age: a multicenter, investigator-masked, rand-omized, vehicle-controlled, parallel comparison of 0.01%, 0.025%, 0.05%, and 0.1% tazarotene creams with 0.05% tretinoin emollient cream applied once daily for 24 weeks. Arch Dermatol 2001;137:1597–1604.

Katayama K, Armendariz-Borunda J, Raghow R, et al. A pentapeptide from type I procollagen promotes extracellular matrix production. J Biol Chem 1993;268(14):9941–9944.

Katiyar SK, Elmets CA. Green tea polyphenolic anti-oxidants and skin photoprotection (review). Int J Oncol 2001;18(6):1307–1313.

Katiyar SK, Korman NJ, Mukhtar H, Agarwal R. Protective effects of silymarin against photocar-cinogenesis in a mouse skin model. J Natl Cancer Inst 1997;89(8):556–566.

Kligman AM. Skin permeability: dermatologic aspects of transdermal drug delivery. Am Heart J 1984;108:200–206.

Kligman AM. Tretinoin (Retin-A) therapy of photo-aged skin. Compr Ther 1992;18:10–13.

Kligman AM. Why cosmeceuticals? Cosmet Toilet 1993;108:37–38.

Kligman AM. The growing importance of topical retinoids in clinical dermatology: a retrospective and prospective analysis. J Am Acad Dermatol 1998;39:S2–S7.

Kligman AM. Cosmeceuticals as a third category. Cosmet Toilet 1998;113:33.

Kligman AM, Leyden JJ. Treatment of photo-aged skin with topical tretinoin. Skin Pharmacol 1993;6(Suppl 1):78–82.

Kligman AM, Fulton JE Jr, Plewig G. Topical vitamin A acid in acne vulgaris. Arch Dermatol 1969;99(4):469–476.

Kligman AM, Zheng P, Lavker RM. The anatomy and pathogenesis of wrinkles. Br J Dermatol 1985;113:37–42.

Kligman AM, Grove GL, Hirose R, Leyden JJ. Topical tretinoin for photoaged skin. J Am Acad Dermatol 1986;15:836–859.

Kligman D, Kligman AM. Salicylic acid peels for the treatment of photoaging. Dermatol Surg 1998;24:325–328.

Kligman DE, Draelos ZD. High-strength tretinoin for rapid retinization of photoaged facial skin. Dermatol Surg 2004;30:864–866.

Kligman LH, Kligman AM. The nature of photoaging: its prevention and repair. Photodermatol 1986;3:215–227.

Kligman LH, Kligman AM. Petrolatum and other hydrophobic emollients reduce UV-A-induced damage. J Dermatolog Treat 1992;3:3.

Kulkarni AP, Chaudhuri J, Mitra A, Richards IS. Dioxygenase and peroxidase activities of soybean lipoxygenase: synergistic interaction between linoleic acid and hydrogen peroxide. Res Commun Chem Pathol Pharmacol 1989;66(2):287–296.

Kumar CA, Das UN. Effect of melatonin on two stage skin carcinogenesis in Swiss mice. Med Sci Monit 2000;6(3):471–475.

Lahiri-Chatterjee M, Katiyar SK, Mohan RR, Agarwal R. A flavonoid antioxidant, silymarin, affords exceptionally high protection against tumor promotion in the SENCAR mouse skin tumorigenesis model. Cancer Res 1999;59(3):622–632.

Lamberg L. "Treatment" cosmetics: hype or help? JAMA 1998;279:1595–1596.

Lazar AP, Lazar P. Dry skin, water, and lubrication. Dermatol Clin 1991;9(1):45–51.

Lazarus M, Bumann L. Miscellaneous cosmetic products and procedures, In: Baumann L, ed. Cosmetic Dermatology: Principles and Practice. New York: Tata McGraw Hill, 2003:117–124.

Leung AY, Foster S. Encyclopedia of Common Ingredients Used in Food, Drugs and Cosmetics, 2nd edn. New York: John Wiley, 1996.

Levin C, Maibach H. Exploration of "alternative" and "natural" drugs in dermatology. Arch Dermatol 2002;138(2):207–211.

Levitt J. The safety of hydroquinone: a dermatologist's response to the 2006 Federal Register. J Am Acad Dermatol 2007;57(5):854–872.

Leyden JJ, Grove GL, Grove MJ, et al. Treatment of photodamaged facial skin with topical tretinoin. J Am Acad Dermatol 1989;21(3 Pt 2):638–644.

Leyden J, Dunlap F, Miller B, et al. Finasteride in the treatment of men with frontal male pattern hair loss. J Am Acad Dermatol 1999;40:930–937.

Leyden JJ, Lavker RM, Grove G, Kaidbey K. Alpha hydroxyl acids are more than moisturizers. Issues and perspectives of AHAs. Cosmet Dermat 1994;Suppl:33A–37A.

Li D, Yee JA, McGuire MH, et al. Soybean isoflavones reduce experimental metastasis in mice. J Nutr 1999;129(5):1075–1078.

Lin JY, Selim MA, Shea CR, et al. UV photoprotection by combination topical antioxidants vitamin C and vitamin E. J Am Acad Dermatol 2003;48(6):866–874.

Lin SY, Chang HP. Induction of superoxide dismutase and catalase activity in different rat tissues and protection from UVB irradiation after topical application of Ginkgo biloba extracts. Methods Find Exp Clin Pharmacol 1997;19(6):367–371.

Lodâen M, Maibach HI. Dry Skin and Moisturizers: Chemistry and Function. Boca Raton: CRC/Taylor & Francis, 2006.

Loden M, Andersson AC. Effect of topically applied lipids on surfactant-irritated skin. Br J Dermatol 1996;134(2):215–220.

Loden M. Barrier recovery and influence of irritant stimuli in skin treated with a moisturizing cream. Contact Derm 1997;36(5):256–260.

Loden M. Role of topical emollients and moisturizers in the treatment of dry skin barrier disorders. Am J Clin Dermatol 2003;4(11):771–788.

Loden M, Barany E. Skin-identical lipids versus petrolatum in the treatment of tape-stripped and detergent-perturbed human skin. Acta Derm Venereol 2000;80(6):412–415.

Lopez-Torres M, Shindo Y, Packer L. Effect of age on antioxidants and molecular markers of oxidative damage in murine epidermis and dermis. J Invest Dermatol 1994;102:476–480.

Lowe N, Horwitz S, Tanghetti E, et al. Tazarotene versus tazarotene plus hydroquinone in the treatment of photodamaged facial skin: a multicenter, double-blind, randomized study. J Cosmet Laser Ther 2006;8:121–127.

Ludwig A, Dietel M, Schafer G, et al. Nicotinamide and nicotinamide analogues as antitumor promoters in mouse skin. Cancer Res 1990;50(8):2470–2475.

Lynde CW. Moisturizers: what they are and how they work. Skin Ther Lett 2001;6(13):3–5.

Maguire JJ, Kagan V, Ackrell BA, et al. Succinate–ubiquinone reductase linked recycling of alpha-tocopherol in reconstituted systems and mitochondria: requirement for reduced ubiquinone. Arch Biochem Biophys 1992;292(1):47–53.

Man MQ, Feingold KR, Thornfeldt CR, Elias PM. Optimization of physiological lipid mixtures for barrier repair. J Invest Dermatol 1996;106(5):1096–1101.

Man MQ, Wood L, Elias PM, Feingold KR. Cutaneous barrier repair and pathophysiology following barrier disruption in IL-1 and TNF type I receptor deficient mice. Exp Dermatol 1999;8(4):261–266.

Mao-Qiang M, Brown BE, Wu-Pong S, et al. Exogenous non-physiologic vs physiologic lipids. Divergent mechanisms for correction of permeability barrier dysfunction. Arch Dermatol 1995;131(7):809–816.

Marks R, Pearse AD, Walker AP. The effects of a shampoo containing zinc pyrithione on the control of dandruff. Br J Dermatol 1985;112(4):415–422.

McNamara SH. Cosmeceuticals. Cosmet Dermatol 1994;7:28–29.

Menon GK, Feingold KR, Elias PM. Lamellar body secretory response to barrier disruption. J Invest Dermatol 1992;98(3):279–289.

Merfort I, Heilmann J, Hagedorn-Leweke U, Lippold BC. In vivo skin penetration studies of camomile flavones. Pharmazie 1994;49(7):509–511.

Meyer M, Pahl HL, Baeuerle PA. Regulation of the transcription factors NF-kappa B and AP-1 by redox changes. Chem Biol Interact 1994;91 (2–3):91–100.

Millikan LE. Cosmetology, cosmetics, cosmeceuticals: definitions and regulations. Clin Dermatol 2002;19(4):371–374.

Mukhtar H, Katiyar SK, Agarwal R. Green tea and skin – anticarcinogenic effects. J Invest Dermatol 1994;102(1):3–7.

Olsen EA, Katz HI, Levine N, et al. Tretinoin emollient cream for photodamaged skin: results of 48-week, multicenter, double-blind studies. J Am Acad Dermatol 1997;37:217–226.

Packer L, Colman C. The Antioxidant Miracle. New York: John Wiley, 1999.

Palumbo A, d'Ischia M, Misuraca G, Prota G. Mechanism of inhibition of melanogenesis by hydroquinone. Biochim Biophys Acta 1991;1073(1):85–90.

Pelle E, Muizzuddin N, Mammone T, et al. Protection against endogenous and UVB-induced oxidative damage in stratum corneum lipids by an antioxidant-containing cosmetic formulation. Photodermatol Photoimmunol Photomed 1999;15(3–4):115–119.

Phillips TJ, Gottlieb AB, Leyden JJ, et al. Efficacy of 0.1% tazarotene cream for the treatment of photodamage: a 12-month multicenter, randomized trial. Arch Dermatol 2002;138:1486–1493.

Piacquadio D, Kligman A. The critical role of the vehicle to therapeutic efficacy and patient compliance. J Am Acad Dermatol 1998;39:567–573.

Pierard GE. Instrumental evaluation of antiwrinkle activity of cosmetic products: what's new? J Eur Acad Dermatol Venereol 2001;15:194–195.

Pierard-Franchimont C, Pierard GE, Saint-Leger D, et al. Comparison of the kinetics of sebum secretion in young women with and without acne. Dermatologica 1991;183:120–122.

Pinnagoda J, Tupker RA, Agner T, Serup J. Guidelines for transepidermal water loss (TEWL) measurement. A report from the Standardization Group of the European Society of Contact Dermatitis. Contact Derm 1990;22:164–178.

Pinnell SR. Cutaneous photodamage, oxidative stress, and topical antioxidant protection. J Am Acad Dermatol 2003;48(1):1–19.

Pinnell SR, Yang H, Omar M, et al. Topical L-ascorbic acid: percutaneous absorption studies. Dermatol Surg 2001;27:137–142.

Rattan SI, Clark BF. Kinetin delays the onset of ageing characteristics in human fibroblasts. Biochem Biophys Res Commun 1994;201(2):665–672.

Rawlings AV, Canestrari DA, Dobkowski B. Moisturizer technology versus clinical performance. Dermatol Ther 2004;17(Suppl 1):49–56.

Reed JT, Ghadially R, Elias PM. Skin type, but neither race nor gender, influence epidermal permeability barrier function. Arch Dermatol 1995;131(10):1134–1138.

Sadick NS. Cosmeceuticals. Their role in dermatology practice. J Drugs Dermatol 2003;2:529–537.

Saint Leger D, Francois AM, Leveque JL, et al. Age-associated changes in stratum corneum lipids and their relation to dryness. Dermatologica 1988;177:159–164.

Scharffetter-Kochanek K, Wlaschek M, Brenneisen P. UV-induced reactive oxygen species in photocarcinogenesis and photoaging. Biol Chem 1997;378:1247–1257.

Scheinman PL. Exposing covert fragrance chemicals. Am J Contact Dermat 2001;12(4):225–228.

Scheman A. Adverse reactions to cosmetic ingredients. Dermatol Clin 2000;18(4):685–698.

Schmidt JB, Binder M, Demschik G, et al. Treatment of skin aging with topical estrogens. Int J Dermatol 1996;35(9):669–674.

Schwartz E, Cruickshank FA, Mezick JA, Kligman LH. Topical all-*trans* retinoic acid stimulates collagen synthesis in vivo. J Invest Dermatol 1991;96: 975–1991.

Schwartz JR, Marsh RG, Draelos ZD. Zinc and skin health: overview of physiology and pharmacology. Dermatol Surg 2005;31:837–847.

Seiberg M, Paine C, Sharlow E, et al. Inhibition of melanosome transfer results in skin lightening. J Invest Dermatol 2000;115(2):162–167.

Shindo Y, Witt E, Han D, et al. Enzymic and non-enzymic antioxidants in epidermis and dermis of human skin. J Invest Dermatol 1994;102(1): 122–124.

Shukuwa T, Kligman AM, Stoudemayer TJ. A new model for assessing the damaging effects of soaps and surfactants on human stratum corneum. Acta Derm Venereol 1997;77:29–34.

Simion FA, Rhein LD, Morrison BM Jr, et al. Self-perceived sensory responses to soap and synthetic detergent bars correlate with clinical signs of irritation. J Am Acad Dermatol 1995;32(2 Pt 1): 205–211.

Simion FA, Abrutyn ES, Draelos ZD. Ability of moisturizers to reduce dry skin and irritation and to prevent their return. J Cosmet Sci 2005;56: 427–444.

Smith EW, Maibach HI. Percutaneous Penetration Enhancers, 2nd edn. Boca Raton: CRC/Taylor & Francis, 2006.

Smith WP. Hydroxy acids and skin aging. Cosmet Toilet 1994;109:41–48.

Steenvoorden DP, van Henegouwen GM. The use of endogenous antioxidants to improve photoprotection. J Photochem Photobiol B 1997;41(1–2):1–10.

Stiler MJ, Bartolone J, Stern R, et al. Topical 8% glycolic and 8% lactic acid creams for the treatment of photodamaged skin. Arch Dermatol 1996;132:631–636.

Stratigos AJ, Katsambas AD. The role of topical retinoids in the treatment of photoaging. Drugs 2005;65(8):1061–1072.

Summers RS, Summers B, Chandar P, et al. The effect of lipids with and without humectant on skin xerosis. J Soc Cosmet Chem 1996;47:39.

Tabata N, Tagami H, Kligman AM. A twenty-four-hour occlusive exposure to 1% sodium lauryl sulfate induces a unique histopathologic inflammatory response in the xerotic skin of atopic dermatitis patients. Acta Derm Venereol 1998;78(4):244–247.

Terezakis N. Cosmeceuticals: a new breed of cosmetic products. Cosmet Dermatol 1993;6:40–41.

Thiele JJ, Weber SU, Packer L. Sebaceous gland secretion is a major physiologic route of vitamin E delivery to skin. J Invest Dermatol 1999;113(6):1006–1010.

Thiele JJ, Schroeter C, Hsieh SN, et al. The antioxidant network of the stratum corneum. Curr Probl Dermatol 2001;29:26–42.

Thornfeldt C. Cosmeceuticals containing herbs: fact, fiction, and future. Dermatol Surg 2005;31(7 Pt 2):873–880.

Urbach W. Cosmeceuticals – the future of cosmetics? Cosmet Toilet 1995;110:33.

US Food and Drug Administration Center for Food Safety and Applied Nutrition. CFSAN/Office of Cosmetics and Colors Fact Sheet: Is it a cosmetic, a drug, or both? (or is it soap?), 2002. Available at: http://www.cfsan.fda.gov/~dms/cos-218.html

Usuki A, Ohashi A, Sato H, et al. The inhibitory effect of GA and LA on melanin synthesis in melanoma cells. Exp Dermatol 2003;12(Suppl 2):43–50.

Van Scott EJ, Yu RJ. Hyperkeratinization, corneocyte cohesion, and alpha hydroxy acids. J Am Acad Dermatol 1984;11(5 Pt 1):867–879.

Van Scott EJ, Yu RJ. Alpha hydroxy acids: procedures for use in clinical practice. Cutis 1989;43:222–228.

Van Vliet M, Ortiz A, Avram MM, Yamauchi PS. An assessment of traditional and novel therapies for cellulite. J Cosmet Laser Ther 2005;7:7–10.

Varani J, Fisher GJ, Kang S, Voorhees JJ. Molecular mechanisms of intrinsic skin aging and retinoid-induced repair and reversal. J Investig Dermatol Symp Proc 1998;3(1):57–60.

Vermeer B, Gilchrest BA. Cosmeceutieals. A proposal for rational definition, evaluation, and regulation. Arch Dermatol 1996;132(3):337–340.

Wang Z, Boudjelal M, Kang S, et al. Ultraviolet irradiation of human skin causes functional vitamin A deficiency, preventable by all-*trans* retinoic acid pre-treatment. Nat Med 1999;5:418–422.

Weber SU, Thiele JJ, Cross CE, Packer L. Vitamin C, uric acid, and glutathione gradients in murine stratum corneum and their susceptibility to ozone exposure. J Invest Dermatol 1999;113(6): 1128–1132.

Wehr RF, Krochmal L. Considerations in selecting a moisturizer. Cutis 1987;39(6):512–515.

Wei H, Bowen R, Cai Q, et al. Antioxidant and antipromotional effects of the soybean iso-flavone genistein. Proc Soc Exp Biol Med 1995;208(1):124–130.

Weiss JS, Ellis CN, Headington JT, Voorhees JJ. Topical tretinoin in the treatment of aging skin. J Am Acad Dermatol 1988;19:169–175.

Weiss JS, Ellis CN, Headington JT, et al. Topical tretinoin improves photoaged skin. A double-blind vehicle- controlled study. JAMA 1988;259(4):527–532.

Yaar M, Gilchrest BA. Aging versus photoaging: postulated mechanisms and effectors. J Investig Dermatol Symp Proc 1998;3:47–51.

Yaar M, Gilchrest BA. Ageing and photoageing of keratinocytes and melanocytes. Clin Exp Dermatol 2001;26(7):583–591.

Yaar M, Arora J, Garmyn M, et al. Influence of aging and malignant transformation on keratinocyte gene expression. Rec Res Cancer Res 1993;128:205–214.

Yaar M, Eller MS, Gilchrest BA. Fifty years of skin aging. J Invest Dermatol Symp Proc 2002;7:51–58.

Zettersten EM, Ghadially R, Feingold KR, et al. Optimal ratios of topical stratum corneum lipids improve barrier recovery in chronologically aged skin. J Am Acad Dermatol 1997;37(3 Pt 1):403–408.

Botulinum toxin for cosmetic use

3

Rajeev Mallipeddi and Sarah Weitzul

Key Points

- Botulinum toxin is a derived from the bacterium *Clostridium botulinum* and has important medical and cosmetic uses.
- Botulinum toxin is an effective treatment for dynamic rhytides.
- There are several different serotypes of botulinum toxin. BTX-A is approved by the Food and Drug Administration for cosmetic use in the USA, and is used most commonly. Dosage is reported in units, and is not interchangeable between serotypes or even between brands of the same serotype.
- Botulinum toxin cleaves the SNARE protein, preventing acetylcholine release at the neuromuscular junction.
- Botulinum toxin activity for dynamic rhytides lasts for 2–6 months, the average being 3 months.
- An understanding of facial anatomy is critical for successful use of botulinum toxin.
- The facial musculature and hence dosage of botulinum toxin varies between patients. Males tend to need higher doses, as do those with strong musculature.
- After injecting botulinum toxin, see the patient back in 2 weeks for an office visit. Some patients, especially those who have never undergone treatment, may need additional drug injected.
- Patients with deep, etched, dynamic rhytides present at rest may not respond as well as patients with rhytides present only upon facial expression. Patient expectations should be managed proactively.
- Complications may occur with botulinum toxin injection, including eyebrow or eyelid ptosis as well as diplopia. Physicians must avoid danger areas and know how to manage complications should they occur.

Introduction

Clostridium botulinum is a rod-shaped, Gram-positive, anaerobic bacterium with seven serotypes: A, B, C, D, E, F, and G. Each produces a unique form of neurotoxin, and types A, B, and E are commonly found in human botulism, a flaccid paralytic disease that can be fatal. Botulinum toxin was first used to treat human disease in the 1960s by Alan Scott and Edward Schantz of the Smith-Kettlewell Eye Research Foundation in San Francisco, who were attempting to alleviate strabismus nonsurgically. Scott was given US Food and Drug Administration (FDA) approval to inject botulinum toxin A (BTX-A) into human volunteers for strabismus in 1978. Its use in ophthalmology now includes blepharospasm, strabismus, and other conditions of hyperactive extraocular muscles.

In 1987, Jean and Alistair Carruthers observed the improvement of glabellar rhytides in patients treated for blepharospasm, and 5 years later published the first dermatological use of BTX-A in the treatment of glabellar lines. Since then, the use of botulinum toxin for facial rejuvenation has increased so tremendously that it is now by far the most commonly performed cosmetic procedure in North America. To put this into context, according to figures from the American Society for Aesthetic Plastic Surgery it was used 3,181,592 times in 2006 and is performed approximately twice as frequently as administration of hyaluronic acid-based fillers, the next most common procedure. It is therefore important for any dermatologist to understand fully the therapeutic potential of botulinum toxin, and this chapter aims to provide the necessary information on how to use this drug for the purposes of facial rejuvenation. Patient evaluation, relevant anatomy, injection technique, the management of adverse events, and future directions will be discussed.

Botulinum toxin formulations and pharmacology

BTX-A, available as Botox® Cosmetic (Allergan, Irvine, CA, USA), was approved by the FDA in 2002 for the temporary improvement in the appearance of moderate to severe glabellar lines associated with corrugator and/or procerus muscle activity in adult patients less than 65 years of age. Although at the time of writing Botox® is the only licenced form of BTX-A in the USA, another formulation, Dysport® (Reloxin®/BoNT-A; Ipsen, Slough, UK), is commonly used in Europe and awaits FDA approval. Other BTX-A formulations available globally include Xeomin® (Merz Pharmaceuticals, Frankfurt am Main, Germany), Neuronox® (Medy-Tox, Seoul, Korea), and Chinese BTX-A (Lanzhou Biological Products Institute, Lanzhou, China).

BTX-B is available as Myobloc® (Solstice Neurosciences, South San Francisco, CA, USA) and was approved by the FDA in 2000 for the treatment of cervical dystonia to reduce the severity of abnormal head position and neck pain.

Although each toxin is produced by a different strain of C. botulinum, all are zinc metalloproteases. The toxins are initially synthesized as a single-chain polypeptide pro-toxin before being cleaved into the active toxin with a light chain of about 50 kDa and a heavy chain of about 100 kDa, linked by a disulfide bridge and noncovalent interactions. All bind to specific receptors on cholinergic presynaptic terminals and are taken up by endocytosis, forming pores in the endocytic vesicle membrane through which the light chain translocates into the cytosol.

Once in the cytosol, the protease toxin is active, and each type of toxin cleaves a specific synaptic terminal protein or SNARE (soluble N-ethylmaleimide-sensitive fusion attachment protein receptor) protein. Botulinum toxins A and E cleave SNAP-25 (synaptosome-associated protein of 25 000 Da), toxins B, D, F and G cleave VAMP (vesicle-associated membrane protein, or synaptobrevin), and toxin C cleaves syntaxin (Table 3-1). By cleaving the SNARE protein, which is necessary for acetylcholine vesicle exocytosis, there is a loss of acetylcholine transmission at the neuromuscular junction. A state of functional denervation results, but the nerve persists. Gradually, new nerve terminals arise, forming new neuromuscular junctions with muscle fibers over

a period of months. However, research also shows these new nerve terminals to be transient, and that neurotransmission is, in fact, restored at the original nerve terminals. More work is required for further elucidation of these details.

Comparison of botulinum formulations

The potency of botulinum toxin is measured by a mouse lethality assay (MLA); 1 unit is defined as the murine lethal dose $(LD)_{50}$ which is the amount of toxin required to kill 50% of a group of 18–22-g Swiss–Webster mice, following intraperitoneal injection. In clinical use, there is a marked variation between the equivalent unit dosing among the different botulinum toxin products. This may be due, in part, to variability in potency assays among manufacturers. Furthermore, there is variability between each toxin serotype in terms of affinity for the respective presynaptic terminal receptor, as well as the consequent molecular interactions.

Studies have shown that 1 unit of Botox® may be equivalent to between 2 and 6 units of Dysport®, and to between 50 and 100 units of Myobloc®. However, the inherent differences between the formulations in terms of diffusion and electrophysiologic characteristics make a single reliable dose conversion ratio impossible. Currently, the authors use only Botox® in their practice; therefore, all references to BTX-A in this chapter relate to Botox® unless otherwise specified.

Evidence base for the use of botulinum toxin in facial rejuvenation

Botulinum toxin A

Botox®

Botox® has been well studied and there is now a wealth of data regarding its use, including numerous randomized controlled trials. Two multicenter placebo-controlled studies in patients confirmed that a total of 20 units of Botox® injected into five glabellar sites was a safe and effective treatment for glabellar lines when compared with placebo. The benefit could be seen for up to 120 days in many patients. More recently, patient-reported outcomes with Botox® treatment for upper face rhytides have been assessed with the Facial Line Outcomes (FLO) questionnaire in randomized controlled trials. Specifically, patients report that, by reducing facial lines, issues that concern them such as the desire to improve facial appearance, not to look beyond their years, and avoid appearing tired, stressed, or angry when this was not the

Table 3-1 Various botulinum toxin subtypes and their respective SNARE proteins

Botulinum toxin subtype	SNARE protein cleaved
A	SNAP-25
B	VAMP
C	Syntaxin, but also SNAP-25
D	VAMP
E	SNAP-25
F	VAMP
G	VAMP

case, were all significantly improved. A prospective, randomized, double-blinded, parallel-group study showed Botox® to be safe and effective in treating horizontal forehead rhytides in a dose-dependent manner in women (doses of 16, 32, or 48 units). For periorbital rhytides, randomized controlled trials have also shown Botox® to be safe and effective in a dose-dependent manner, with 12 units per side appearing to be optimal. Furthermore, there is evidence that 2 units of Botox® can be injected into the central lower eyelid to widen the eye, particularly when used in conjunction with lateral orbital injections. The literature also provides a rationale for using Botox® in many other cosmetic applications, including nasal wrinkles on the dorsum of the nose ('bunny lines'), fine wrinkles around the lips, chin dimpling, and platysmal bands.

Dysport® (Reloxin®)

Compared with Botox® there is a relative paucity of literature regarding Dysport® for cosmetic use, but data are accumulating. Two separate multicenter, randomized, double-blind, placebo-controlled trials from Europe in 2004 (with 119 patients) and from North America in 2007 (with 373 patients) tested 25, 50, and 75 units (with five injection sites), and showed Dysport® to be a safe and effective treatment of glabellar lines, with 50 units considered to be the optimal dose. Another European multicenter, randomized, double-blind, placebo-controlled trial of 110 patients again showed Dysport® to be safe and effective in the treatment of the glabellar lines, but found 30 units injected in three glabellar sites to be as effective as 50 units injected into five sites (the two additional sites were in the central forehead, targeting the frontalis). A retrospective cross-sectional patient chart review of 945 patients who had received at least three treatment cycles of Dysport® in various facial sites showed no loss of effectiveness or cumulative adverse effects with repeated injections over time (median injection interval 5.9–6.5 months).

Few studies have directly compared Botox® and Dysport®. Of note is a randomized controlled trial in which 62 patients with moderate or severe glabellar lines at maximal contraction were randomly assigned to receive either 20 units of Botox® or 50 units of Dysport®. With this dose ratio, Botox® had a more prolonged efficacy at 16-week follow-up.

Botulinum toxin B

Myobloc®

Evidence shows that Myobloc® is a safe and effective treatment for glabellar rhytides in doses of up to 3000 units, including one multicenter, randomized, double-blind, placebo-controlled trial of 139 patients. An open-label study showed safety and efficacy of up to 3125 units in the glabella (26 patients) and 3750 units in the frontalis (18 patients). Another randomized, double-blind, controlled pilot study enrolling 20 patients revealed its efficacy and safety in the treatment of crow's feet.

Few studies have compared Myobloc® directly with Botox®. One randomized, double-blind trial enrolled 10 patients to have Botox® (total of 15 units) injected into one set of lateral canthal rhytides (crow's feet) and Myobloc® (total of 750 units) into the contralateral side. Myobloc® was found to have a more rapid onset of action but a shorter duration of effect, as well as more pain upon injection. Another study randomized eight patients to receive 5 units Botox® and 500 units Myobloc® in either the left or right side of the forehead, and showed Myobloc® to have a more rapid onset of action and greater area of diffusion.

One potentially important use of Myobloc® may be when patients become refractory to the effects of BTX-A, and indeed one study has confirmed this. Twenty women with glabellar rhytides who had developed a negligible or decreased clinical effect to BTX-A were treated with a total of 2500 units of Myobloc®; all patients showed improvement of glabellar rhytides, with a peak benefit at 1 month.

Dilution and storage

Botox® is supplied in a vial containing 100 units of vacuum-dried C. botulinum type A neurotoxin powder. During preparation, it is dissolved in sterile sodium chloride solution containing human albumin, and is sterile filtered prior to filling and vacuum drying. It can be stored unopened in a refrigerator between 2 and 8°C for up to 36 months. The prescribing information also recommends that the powder in each vial should be reconstituted with 2.5 mL of 0.9% preservative-free saline to make a concentration of 4.0 units per 0.1 mL. This is the concentration that the authors use, and a previous review of the literature suggested that most clinicians use a dilution of 2.5–3.0 mL per vial. A recent randomized, controlled, double-blind, parallel-group study, specifically designed to address the issue of whether dilution made a difference in the treatment of glabellar rhytides, suggested that it did not, when dilutions of 100, 33.3, 20, and 10 units/mL were compared. This reinforced the findings of an earlier study. However, another prospective randomized controlled study of 10 patients showed that a concentration of 2 units/0.1 mL, compared with 2 units/0.02 mL, resulted in a greater diffusion and larger area of effect when treating horizontal forehead rhytides.

A two-center, randomized, evaluator-blinded study compared 5 units/0.05 mL with 5 units/0.25 mL in the treatment of lateral canthal rhytides, as a single injection had shown that the higher concentration may be more effective, but the study population was too small for the authors to draw definitive conclusions. It may be that a greater volume of dilution results in a shorter duration of effect. Clearly, various dilutions can be used with benefit and it is important to choose one that minimizes the risk of diffusion into neighboring muscle groups. Particularly for the novice, it would be wise to gain experience with one dilution before experimenting with others.

Manufacturer guidelines also recommend that, once reconstituted with nonpreserved 0.9% saline, the vial be stored in a refrigerator between 2 and 8°C, and disposed of within 4 hours. However, it is well known that the product retains efficacy for up to 6 weeks and it is likely that most practitioners store their vials for more than 4 hours. The drug should not be frozen again once reconstituted, however. The authors use preserved saline, which can be used for reconstitution without compromising the efficacy of the product and may reduce the pain upon injection due to the benzyl alcohol component of the saline.

Dysport® vials contain 500 units of C. botulinum type A toxin–hemagglutinin complex in addition to human serum albumin and lactose. Guidelines for reconstitution and storage are similar to those for Botox®, except that once reconstituted it can be kept at the same temperature for up to 8 hours. No data are available to suggest that it can be stored for longer.

Myobloc® is provided as a ready-to-inject solution of 5000 units/mL BTX-B, human serum albumin, sodium succinate, and sodium chloride at approximately pH 5.6. Three different vial volumes are available, 0.5 mL (2500 units), 1 mL (5000 units), and 2 mL (10 000 units), but can be further diluted with normal saline (best done in a syringe). Vials should be stored between 2 and 8°C, and once opened or diluted should used within 4 hours. As for Dysport®, data are not available regarding the possibility of longer storage.

Patient evaluation and education

As with any cosmetic procedure, assessing and understanding the patient's desires and expectations are crucial to success. It should be clearly explained that the botulinum toxin is best at reducing dynamic facial wrinkles or lines caused by underlying muscle contraction, but will not in isolation improve the loss of dermal elasticity or the volumetric changes secondary to collagen degeneration, such as deep wrinkles present at rest. In addition, botulinum toxin chemodenervation does not specifically address other changes related to photo-damage such as pigmented lesions (ephelids and lentigines), telangiectasias, and loss of skin texture. Therefore, during the cosmetic consultation, it is vital to establish what specifically bothers the patient in order to develop an effective treatment plan. To address the different facets of aging, a multifarious approach may ultimately be necessary, including interventions such as soft tissue augmentation and lasers in addition to botulinum toxin.

The patient should be made aware that BTX-A is approved only for glabellar frown-lines and that use for other cosmetic purposes is considered off-label. Obviously, the procedure should be explained carefully, including potential side-effects, which are generally mild or transient. It is helpful to advise patients to stop elective anticoagulants such as aspirin, nonsteroidal anti-inflammatory drugs, and vitamin E for at least 10 days before treatment to minimize bruising post-injection, if other health issues do not preclude this. The patient should be warned that the onset of BTX-A action may not be seen for up to 1 week and that the effect will wane within 3–6 months, necessitating repeated treatments as desired.

Photographing the patient before treatment and at follow-up, with pictures showing muscles at rest and during maximal contraction, will help to plan touch-ups and retreatments. The authors recommend digital photography for ease of use and the ability to archive and access images rapidly.

Contraindications and cautions

BTX-A is contraindicated in the presence of infection at the proposed injection site(s) and in individuals with known hypersensitivity to any ingredient in the formulation including albumin. Caution should also be exercised when treating patients with peripheral neuropathic diseases or neuromuscular junctional disorders such as myasthenia gravis. Concomitant aminoglycosides such as gentamicin, streptomycin, and/or other agents such as quinidine may interfere with neuromuscular transmission and potentiate the effects of BTX-A. Pregnancy (category C) and lactation are cautions, but no human data are available to define the degree of risk if used in these situations. However, pregnant women who have inadvertently been injected with botulinum toxin have had uneventful deliveries. A previous history of (cutaneous) surgery is another context in which caution should be exercised, as the underling anatomy can be altered.

General injection technique and considerations

A variety of syringes are available for injection of botulinum toxin. The authors have found the 1-mL Injekt™ - F Low Waste Syringe (B. Braun Medical, Bethlehem, PA, USA) to be both economical and effective (Fig. 3-1). It provides accurate dosing to 0.01 mL and the plunger design enables ejection of virtually all the solution from the syringe owing to extension of the plunger portion of the syringe which expels all of the solution through the hub. A 30-gauge ½-inch needle is attached, which can be changed easily as necessary. In contrast to the Inject™ syringe, most other syringes have a flat plunger which, even when fully compressed, leaves costly botulinum toxin in the hub of the needle. Others have used tuberculin syringes with fixed needles, but the authors have found these to be more painful when used in botulinum toxin injection due to a more rapid dulling of the attached needle.

The authors have the patient only slightly reclined and ask them to animate the area(s) concerned in order to illustrate the functional anatomy. This highlights the characteristics, strength, and mass of the involved muscles, which will influence the number of units to be injected. Generally, men require higher doses of BTX-A owing to increased muscle mass. In addition, despite injections being intramuscular, thicker skin (e.g. Asian skin compared with Caucasian skin) may require higher doses.

The injections should be angled perpendicular to the skin into the belly of the muscle wherever possible. However, when skin is thin, such as around the eyes and lips, injections should be made superficially in the subcutaneous plane.

Assessing the overall facial symmetry and being acutely aware that all muscles of facial expression have intricate interactions is important, because the aim is not to remove wrinkles in isolation but to create balance. For example, treating any region of the upper face (glabellar, periorbital, or forehead lines) can alter eyebrow shape and/or position, and treatment of the perioral area or chin may alter the position of the mouth or affect the smile. Other considerations to consider include that of gender. Women tend to have a higher, more arched, brow than the lower, more horizontal, brow in men. These potential effects should be taken into account before injecting.

Common treatment areas by anatomic site

A thorough knowledge of facial anatomy is essential if the best outcomes are to be achieved with the fewest complications. Understanding the effect of paralyzing a particular muscle is key to achieving the exact result intended. Figure 3-2 illustrates the main muscles of facial expression relevant to chemodenervation with botulinum toxin. Each treatment area is discussed separately.

The glabellar complex

Anatomy

The muscles to be targeted here are the procerus, corrugator supercilii, and depressor supercilii (Fig. 3-3). All of these muscles act mainly as brow depressors, but more specifically the corrugator acts as a brow adductor moving the eyebrow downward and medial, whereas the procerus depresses the medial head of the eyebrows producing transverse lines on the nasal dorsum. However, medial fibers of the orbicularis oculi and frontalis may interdigitate with the corrugator.

Injection technique

The authors typically use five injection points, as recommended in the prescribing information (Fig. 3-4), but would point out that additional points above the superior orbital rim may be injected (making a total of seven). This may be required where a larger muscle mass is being treated, particularly in men. We like to grasp the corrugator supercilii between the thumb and index finger with the nondominant hand, as this helps to isolate the muscle belly and allows concurrent palpation of the bony supraorbital ridge, an important landmark in this area (Fig. 3-5). It is important to inject 1 cm above this rim. Grasping the procerus in a similar manner at the upper nasal bridge is also helpful; another key benefit is that it minimizes toxin diffusion into the orbit.

Dose

With five injection points, we generally start with a total of 20 units for women and 40 units for men, divided equally between the injection sites, but may need to use up to 40 units in women and up to 80 units in men, as indicated in studies. It is prudent to halve the volume of saline used to reconstitute the vial when preparing for a man, to maintain the volume injected and limit unwanted diffusion. Finally, the total dose not always need to be divided equally among the injection points

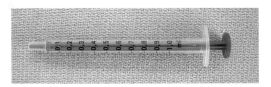

Figure 3-1 Photograph of the Injekt™ - F Low Waste Syringe

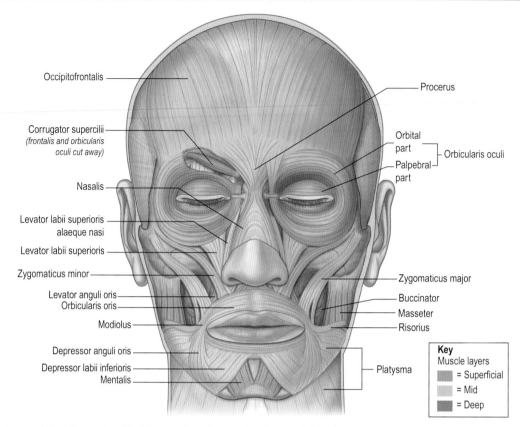

Figure 3-2 Main muscles of facial expression relevant to botulinum toxin injection

and should be tailored to the individual patient's muscle function and aesthetic desires.

Horizontal forehead lines

Anatomy

The frontalis is a large, vertically oriented muscle in the forehead that interacts with the procerus, corrugators, and orbicularis oculi; its primary function is to raise the eyebrows (Fig. 3-6). Individual differences in forehead shape, furrow sizes, and eyebrow shape should be carefully scrutinized before commencing treatment.

Injection technique

Usually four to five injections are needed, as illustrated (Fig. 3-7), but the exact sites are guided by observing the individual patient's animation and muscle function. We avoid the first horizontal line above the brow and try to stay in the upper two thirds of the forehead in order to avoid brow ptosis. This is particularly relevant at the lateral aspects of the forehead (i.e. lateral to the midpupillary line) in order to avoid a questioning or quizzical eyebrow appearance, which can occur with lower lateral forehead injections. It is particularly important to have the patient raise their eyebrows fully to see how far laterally the horizontal rhytides extend. Many patients have rhytides extending into the hairline; these must be treated for optimal results.

There are significant differences in injection technique for the forehead between men and women. Men generally have flatter, less arched, brows and so we tend to inject horizontally across the forehead in men (Fig. 3-8) and in a "V" shape in women.

Dose

We start with a total dose of 16–20 units in women and 30 units in men. We typically used 2–4-unit aliquots at each injection site.

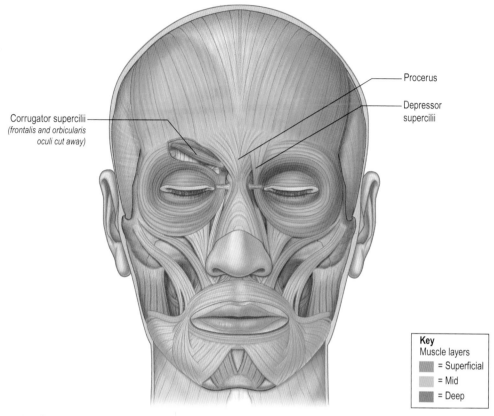

Procerus

Depressor
supercilii

Corrugator supercilii
*(frontalis and orbicularis
oculi cut away)*

Key
Muscle layers
■ = Superficial
■ = Mid
■ = Deep

Figure 3-3 Procerus, corrugator supercilii, and depressor supercilii muscles

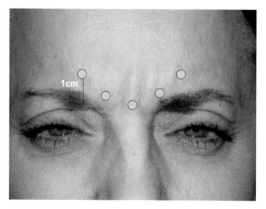

1cm

Figure 3-4 Injection points for treatment of the glabellar complex

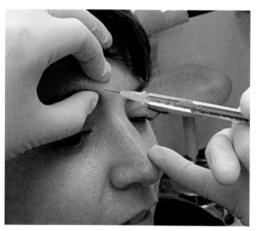

Figure 3-5 Grasping the corrugator supercilii muscle during injection

PEARLS

To minimize the risk of brow ptosis, inject at least 2.5 cm above the orbital rim when injecting lateral to the pupil.

Avoid paralyzing the muscle to prevent a 'frozen' appearance with lack of expression.

Excessive weakening of the frontalis without treating the brow depressors (glabellar complex)

will lower the brow, producing a stern or angry appearance. This can be undertaken at the same time or separately. If the latter, treat the depressors first, then treat the frontalis at a 2-week re-evaluation. This may also reduce the amount of botulinum toxin required, owing to overlap from diffusion.

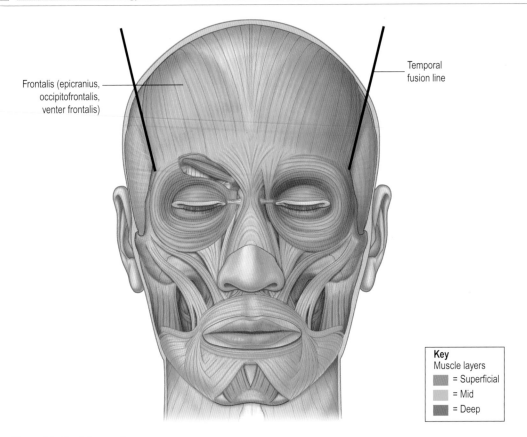

Frontalis (epicranius, occipitofrontalis, venter frontalis)

Temporal fusion line

Key
Muscle layers
■ = Superficial
□ = Mid
■ = Deep

Figure 3-6 Frontalis muscle

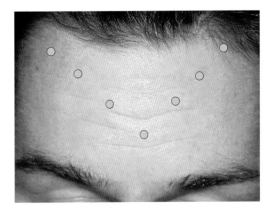

Figure 3-7 Injection points for treatment of the frontalis in women

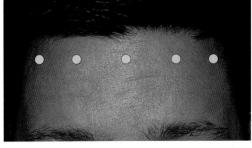

Figure 3-8 Injection points for treatment of the frontalis in men

Re-evaluation in 2 weeks is also important for potentially adjusting eyebrow position, if necessary with additional injections. Some 1–3 units injected into the lateral orbicularis (outside of the orbital rim) may allow eyebrow elevation if needed (see Fig. 3-10).

Some older patients use the frontalis function to enhance their visual field and this should be considered, as lower treatment doses or avoiding treatment altogether may be appropriate.

Periorbital (Lateral Canthal) rhytides (Crow's Feet)

Anatomy

The target muscle when treating crow's feet is the orbicularis oculi, which has a sphincteric action (Fig. 3-9). There are three components: the palpebral portion covering the eyelid, the orbital portion surrounding the orbit from forehead to cheek, and a small, lacrimal portion at the medial aspect of the orbit. All portions interact with one another with the main function

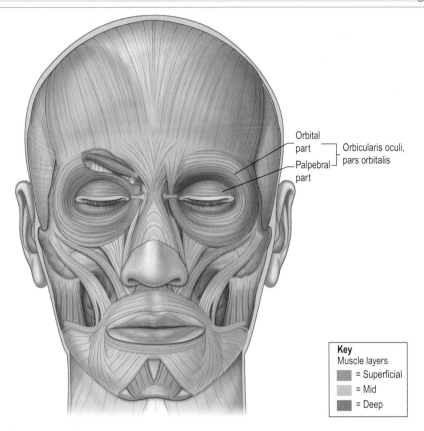

Figure 3-9 Orbicularis oculi muscle

Key
Muscle layers
= Superficial
= Mid
= Deep

of closing the eye; however, the palpebral portion acts involuntarily, as during blinking, but the orbital portion is under voluntary control and also serves to move the eyebrow medially. Injections are targeted to the lateral orbital portions of the muscle, which cause the visible rhytides.

Injection technique

It is important to ask the patient to smile first, in order to define the individual wrinkle pattern in this area, which can vary significantly between people. For most patients, three injection points are sufficient (Fig. 3-10), but up to five points have been reported in selected individuals. Injection sites should be 1–1.5 cm lateral to the orbital rim, and placed superficially as intradermal blebs. Orient the needle away from the eyeball to avoid injury if the patient moves unexpectedly. To treat the rolled appearance of hypertrophic orbicularis oculi on the lower lid, a small amount of botulinum toxin can be injected in the midpupillary line 3–5 mm inferior to the eyelash line. This should not be done in patients with lax lower eyelids, though, as this could cause ectropion. The snap test should be performed prior to injecting in the lower eyelid.

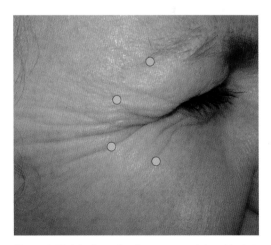

Figure 3-10 Injection points for treatment of the orbicularis muscle. The injection point at the superolateral aspect used to elevate the lateral brow is also shown

Dose

The literature reports a variety of doses from 2.5 to 18 units per side. One single-center, prospective, double-blind, randomized, controlled trial (60 patients) reported no significant efficacy difference between 6 units and 18 units per

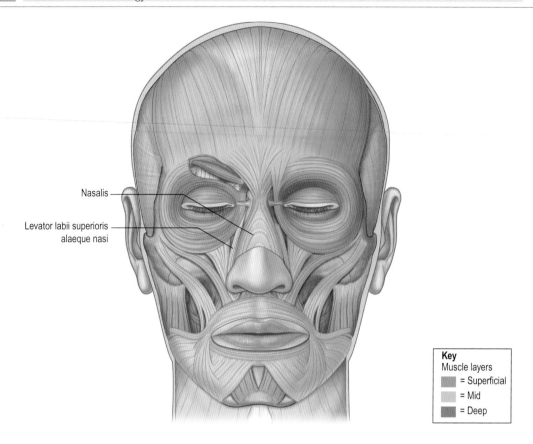

Nasalis

Levator labii superioris
alaeque nasi

Key
Muscle layers
▓▓ = Superficial
░░ = Mid
▓▓ = Deep

Figure 3-11 Nasalis muscle

side. However, another more recent, multicenter, prospective, double-blind, randomized, controlled dosing study (162 patients) showed a dose–response between 3 units and 18 units per side, with a plateau effect after 12 units. The authors most often use 10 or 12 units per side, delivered over three injection points. If 10 units are used, we distribute 2 units at the uppermost injection point and 4 units at the mid and lower injection points, but for 12 units the aliquots are all 4 units. As mentioned above, 1–3 units injected into the lateral orbicularis at the lateral brow can be used to elevate the brow. We recommend injecting at the junction of the eyebrow and the temporal suture line. For the hypertrophic orbicularis oculi of the lower eyelid, we recommend 1–2 units be injected very superficially.

PEARLS

Check lid laxity with a snap test, as laxity would make a lower injection risky for ectropion.

Do not inject below the zygomatic arches as this could affect the zygomaticus major muscle, causing cheek and upper lip ptosis.

To minimize bruising, avoid injecting around visible veins in this area.

Use pressure and ice to minimize ecchymoses.

Always direct the needle away from the globe, particularly when injecting below the lash line.

Nasal rhytides ('Bunny Lines')

Anatomy

The nasalis is the main target muscle when treating nasal rhytides (Fig. 3-11). This muscle originates from the maxilla, and its fibers cross over the nasal dorsum to decussate in the midline at an aponeurosis at the bridge of the nose that is continuous with the aponeurosis of the procerus. The nasalis is important for opening the nasal aperture and valve during exercise or deep inspiration. However, several other muscles also contribute to the formation of perinasal wrinkles in this region, for example the levator labii superioris alaeque nasi, a thin muscle that arises from the upper part of the frontal process of the maxilla and passes obliquely, lateral to the alar cartilage on the lateral nose, to insert on the upper lip, blending with the orbicularis oris. Contraction deepens the nasolabial fold, dilates nasal ala, and everts the upper lip. In addition, the zygomaticus major and minor, by moving the angle of the mouth and affecting perioral and nasolabial folds, can cause perinasal skin to wrinkle, and contraction of the orbicularis oculi produces nasociliary wrinkles.

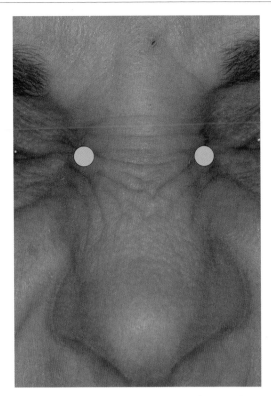

Figure 3-12 Injection points for treatment of the nasalis muscle

Injection technique

To treat the nasalis, the authors use two injection points, one into each side of the nasalis (Fig. 3-12). However, a midline injection is used by some authors, targeting more the transverse nasal portion of the procerus, either as the only injection point to soften the lines or in combination with the two side injections. One retrospective study of 250 patients found that, despite treating the nasalis, 60% had persistent wrinkles characterized as either naso-orbicular rhytides (when wrinkles were at the root of the nose due to the nasal portion of the orbicularis oculi muscle) or nasociliary rhytides (wrinkles from the root of the nose to the medial margin of the eyebrow and glabella) in conjunction with nasoalar wrinkles (around the alar groove due to contraction of the alar portion of the levator labii superioris alaeque nasi). When this occurred, the authors of the study found value in additionally treating these areas. The injection points were: for nasoalar rhytides, into the lower lateral nasal wall–cheek junction in the external groove of the nostril; for the naso-orbicular rhytides, into the lower medial portion of the orbicularis oculi muscle, a point located 0.5 cm below and medial to the inner palpebral margin; and for the nasociliary rhytides, into a point representing the upper medial portion of the orbicularis oculi muscle located 0.5 cm

above and medial to the inner palpebral margin and superior to the nasal root.

Dose

Inject 1–3 units bilaterally into the left and right portions of the upper nasalis. If a midline injection is to be used, 1 unit has been recommended. For the nasoalar, naso-orbicular, and nasociliary injections described above, 2 units were used.

PEARLS

Bunny lines are usually not treated in isolation and treating the glabellar complex in conjunction may help overall.

Avoidance of upper lip ptosis is extremely important; ensuring that injections do not affect the levator labii alaeque nasi and levator labii superioris will help achieve this.

Keep injections superficial to avoid bruising, in addition to pressure and ice.

Vertical perioral rhytides

Anatomy

Several factors contribute to the formation of these lines, including animation, aging, photodamage, and smoking. The main target muscle is the orbicularis oris, which serves to close and protrude the lips as well as assist in mastication and phonation.

The orbicularis oris consists of numerous muscular fibers surrounding the orifice of the mouth, but in different directions (Fig. 3-13). It consists partly of fibers derived from the other facial muscles that are inserted into the lips, the main one being the buccinator, which forms the deeper stratum of the orbicularis. More superficially is a second stratum, formed on either side by the caninus and triangularis, which cross each other at the angle of the mouth; however, fibers from the caninus pass to the lower lip, whereas those from the triangularis pass to the upper lip, to be inserted into the skin near the median line. In addition to these there are fibers from the levator labii superioris, the zygomaticus, and the levator labii inferioris; these intermingle with the transverse fibers described above and principally have an oblique direction. Finally, there are fibers by which the muscle is connected with the maxillae and the septum of the nose above and with the mandible below.

Injection technique

The upper lip needs treatment more often than the lower lip. Injections are placed symmetrically just above the vermilion border for the upper lip and just below the vermilion border for the lower lip, with four potential injection sites for the former and two for the latter (Fig. 3-14).

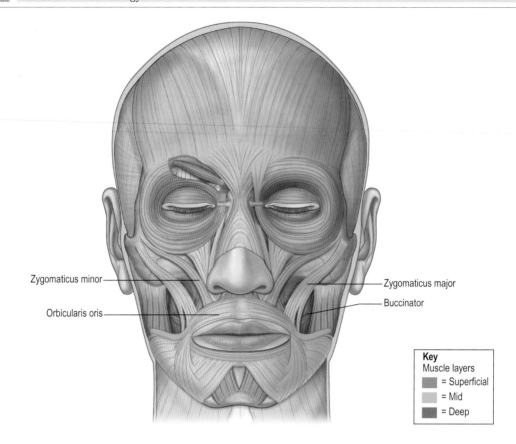

Zygomaticus minor

Zygomaticus major

Buccinator

Orbicularis oris

Key
Muscle layers
= Superficial
= Mid
= Deep

Figure 3-13 Orbicularis oris

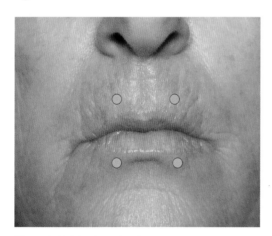

Figure 3-14 Injection points for treatment of the orbicularis oris

However, exact sites should be adjusted depending on the wrinkle pattern. The midline should be avoided to maintain the integrity of the cupid's bow. Should lines be persistent after the initial injections, one study found two additional injection points 7–10 mm above vermilion border lateral to the philtral columns helpful, when rhytides persisted at a 2–3-week follow-up. Injections should be superficial.

Dose

Typical doses used are 1–2 units per injection site. Some authors have suggested that, if more conservative treatment is preferred, as little as 0.5–0.75 units per injection site may be effective.

PEARLS

Initially treat conservatively, using as few injection points as possible, but keep them symmetrical. Additional injections can always be performed at a 2-week follow-up.

Lower lip injections are more likely to cause functional problems and so, when beginning, it may be best to avoid these.

Because even low doses can significantly weaken lips, be careful with individuals who depend on lip control for their livelihood, such as professional speakers, singers, and wind instrument musicians, in whom treatment may best be avoided.

Avoid the angle of the mouth as there is a higher risk of functional disturbance such as drooling.

For the perioral area, results are often significantly more satisfying when botulinum toxin treatment is combined with fillers and/or resurfacing.

Use pressure and ice to minimize bruising.

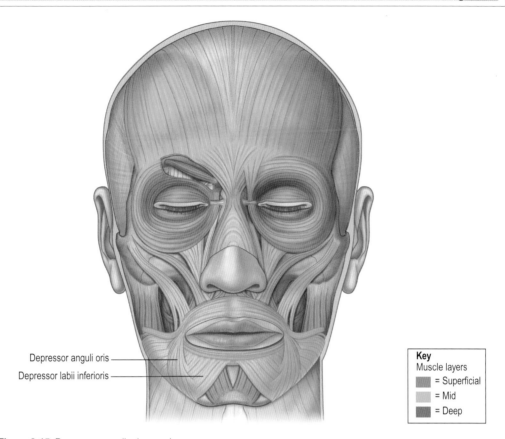

Depressor anguli oris
Depressor labii inferioris

Key
Muscle layers
■ = Superficial
□ = Mid
■ = Deep

Figure 3-15 Depressor anguli oris muscle

Marionette lines

Anatomy

These lines, which radiate down radially from the corner of the mouth, are formed by contraction of the depressor anguli oris (DAO) (Fig. 3-15). This muscle originates from the mental tubercle on the mandible, lateral to the mental foramen, and inserts onto the lower lip and modiolus (a dense, fibromuscular interface of the muscles contributing to oral commissure integrity and movement). Its contraction results in a downturn of the angle of the mouth and a sad appearance. Botulinum toxin treatment raises the corners of the mouth at rest and at full smile.

Injection technique

The injection point is around 1 cm lateral to the oral commissure at the level of the mandible (Fig. 3-16). This targets the posterior border of the muscle and avoids an effect on the depressor labii inferioris, which the DAO overlies. The depressor labii inferioris everts the lip, so inadvertently affecting this muscle will result in an asymmetrical smile.

Dose

The authors use 2–4 units per side. However, 3–5 units per side have also been recommended in the literature.

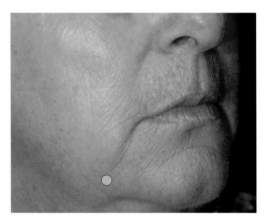

Figure 3-16 Injection point for treatment of the depressor anguli oris

---

PEARLS

It may be difficult for a patient to visualize what the effects of DAO injection may be. Therefore, showing the patient in the mirror exactly what the benefits with DAO injection could be, as well as possible side-effects such as an asymmetrical smile, can be informative.

Reassess in 2 weeks for response and potential side-effects.

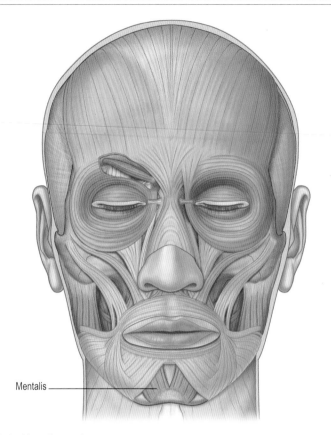

Mentalis

Key
Muscle layers
= Superficial
= Mid
= Deep

Figure 3-17 Mentalis muscle

Many individuals will need treatment of the mentalis (see below) in conjunction with the DAO for significant improvement of the mouth frown.

If the DAO is treated at the same time as perioral rhytides, fewer units may be required for the latter.

Mental crease and dimpled (Peau D'orange) chin

Anatomy

The mentalis is the target muscle when injecting this area (Fig. 3-17). It arises from the mandible and inserts into the skin of the chin below the lip. Contraction wrinkles the chin and protrudes the lower lip.

Injection technique

The authors use a single midline injection point just below the bony prominence of the chin into the mass of the muscle. Grasping the muscle between the thumb and index finger of the noninjecting hand can help guide the injection (Fig. 3-18). Note that two injection points on either side of the midline have also been suggested.

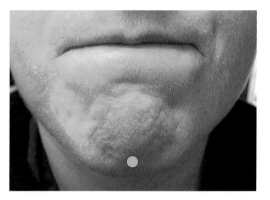

Figure 3-18 Injection technique for treatment of the mentalis

Dose

Generally a total of 5–10 units is sufficient, and the authors usually start with 5 units in both women and men.

PEARLS

Always inject below the level of the mental crease (and not at the level) to avoid weakening of the lip depressors and orbicularis oris leading to oral incompetence.

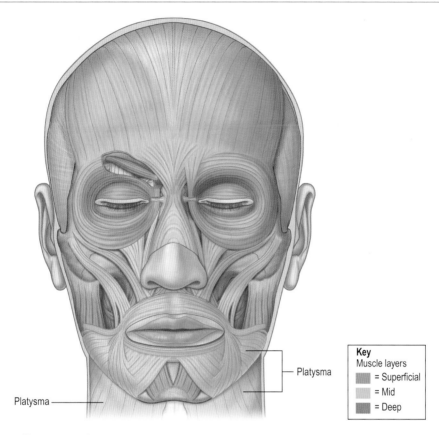

Figure 3-19 Platysma muscle

Key
Muscle layers
■ = Superficial
■ = Mid
■ = Deep

Massage laterally after injection.

A dimpled chin secondary to a hypertrophic mentalis muscle may be a sign of predisposition to oral incompetence. Be aware of this and avoid treating if suspected.

Platysmal bands and necklace lines

Anatomy

The platysma is a thin sheet of muscle arising from the fascia covering the pectoral and deltoid muscles to extend over the anterolateral neck; anterior fibers interlace with fibers from the other side at the lower chin margin (Fig. 3-19). Posterior fibers extend laterally over the mandible and attach to muscles of the angle and lower mouth, as well as to subdermal tissue of the lower face. Contraction of the platysma produces a slight wrinkling of the surface of the skin of the neck, in an oblique direction. The thickest anterior portion depresses the lower jaw and also serves to draw down the lower lip and angle of the mouth. Vertical bands become more obvious with age, owing to skin laxity and thinning of the subcutaneous tissue. These may be more pronounced during speaking or animation.

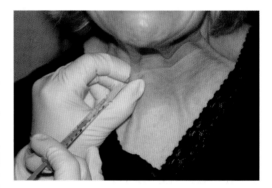

Figure 3-20 Grasping the platysmal band during injection

Horizontal necklace lines are skin indentations caused by subcutaneous muscular aponeurotic attachments.

Injection technique

For platysmal bands, the patient is asked to hyperextend and tense the neck to highlight the bands, and prior to injecting the band is grasped between the thumb and index finger to isolate it (Fig. 3-20). The authors use three to five injection points along each band, about 1 cm apart, and inject into the body of the band (Fig. 3-21).

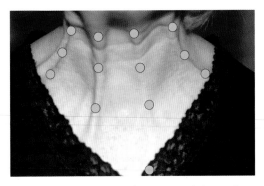

Figure 3-21 Injection points for treatment of platysmal bands

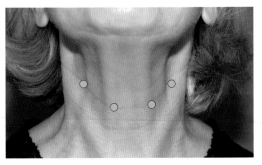

Figure 3-22 Injection points for treatment of horizontal necklace lines

For horizontal necklace lines, injections are place directly into the line intradermally, again approximately 1 cm apart (Fig. 3-22).

Dose

For platysmal bands, the authors generally do not use more than 15 units per band, so that the total dose is below 30 units per session, as has been recommended to avoid side-effects such as dysphagia.

For necklace lines, use 1–2 units per injection site and keep the total dose to less than 20 units per treatment session.

PEARLS

Counsel patients adequately about the potential benefits. This is not a substitute for surgical rhytidectomy and will obviously not correct skin laxity or fat descent. Patients with good skin elasticity as well as minimal fat descent are the best candidates.

It can be a useful adjunct 2–3 weeks before performing neck liposuction in individuals with prominent platysmal bands.

When injecting horizontal necklace lines, do not inject below the deep dermis, i.e. avoid the subcutaneous plane in order to avoid the venous perforators and the muscles of deglutition.

Other treatment areas and uses

This section discusses some of the other uses of botulinum toxin that have been reported in the literature. It is by no means an exhaustive list, but highlights the range of uses of botulinum toxin and a few nuances in the topic. Many of these applications require a detailed knowledge of facial anatomy and can result in devastating side-effects if performed improperly without the necessary experience. Injection under electromyographic guidance has been recommended if a physician has any doubt about the target anatomy.

Chemical brow lift

As discussed above, injections into the glabellar complex can lead to a brow lift as an additional benefit. However, a brow lift may also be the primary aim of botulinum toxin treatment. One study revealed that 7–10 units of BTX-A injected into three points at the superolateral orbicularis oculi bilaterally, but staying outside of the orbital rim, produced an average brow elevation from the midpupil of 1.0 mm and from the lateral canthus of 4.8 mm in 22 patients. Another study of 11 patients involved one 5-unit injection into each corrugator just medial to and above the brow, as well as a total of 10 units injected over four equally spaced sites along the lateral orbital rim below the brow. The mean elevations for the relaxed eye position were 3.1 and 1.9 mm, and for the elevated position 2.9 and 2.1 mm, for the left and right eyebrows respectively. It has recently been suggested that the eyebrow elevation seen after injection of the brow depressors is in fact due to partial inactivation of the inferomedial frontalis, resulting in increased tone throughout the rest of the muscle. This retrospective analysis of the photographs of 79 women who had been part of a previous parallel-group dosing study involving injections BTX-A into the glabella alone showed elevations of the lateral brow first (this area is unlikely to be affected by the glabellar injection points) followed by the rest of the brow with 20–40 units.

Widening the palpebral aperture

BTX-A injected into the lower eyelid orbicularis has been shown to widen the eye, with 2 units being the typical dose administered at one injection point. A dose-finding study involving 19 patients used two injection points 3 mm below the ciliary margin, one at the midpupillary line, and another halfway between the midpupillary line and the lateral canthus, to compare a total lower eyelid dose of 4 or 8 units, in conjunction with three 4-unit lateral orbital injections 1.5 cm from the lateral canthus. A plateau effect was seen with 8 units, along with increased side-effects such as excessive scleral show, photophobia, incomplete lid sphincter ability- and lower lid edema, so 2 or 4 units was recommended to increase the palpebral aperture.[8] This particular treatment may be more beneficial in Asian patients and should be avoided in those with dry eyes, lid laxity, and pre-existing scleral show. The present authors agree that a single 2-unit injection is usually an effective and safe dose for this purpose.

Repeated nasal flare

Repeated involuntary dilatation of the nostrils can be socially embarrassing. This is caused by contraction of the lower nasalis fibers; injection of 5–10 units of BTX-A bilaterally into this portion of the muscle, which covers the lateral nasal ala, has benefited some patients for 3–4 months.

Nasal tip droop

The depressor septi is a small muscle that inserts into the nasal septum and back part of the ala, and serves to antagonize the other muscles of the nose, drawing the ala downwards. It contributes to nasal tip ptosis seen with aging; injecting 2–3 units of BTX-A at the base of the columnella can help to elevate the tip slightly, although upper lip ptosis is a risk.

Nasolabial (Melolabial) folds

This skin crease extends from the lateral ala to a point lateral to the corner of the mouth and becomes more prominent with age. Although this is most commonly treated with soft tissue fillers, 1 unit of BTX-A injected into the lip elevator complex in the nasofacial groove has been reported to collapse the upper part of the fold whilst elongating the upper lip; this is helpful in some patients with a short upper lip. The effect may last for up to 6 months and thus patient selection is critical if attempting this.

Facial asymmetry

This may be due to neuromuscular causes such as hemifacial spasm, acquired as part of a pathophysiologic process, for example in facial nerve (Bell's) palsy, iatrogenic such as after deep surgical resection for cancer, or familial such that muscles on one side of the face are comparatively stronger or more hyperactive than the corresponding ones on the contralateral side. By neutralizing the hyperfunctional or unopposed side, symmetry can be restored, as in the case of unilateral facial nerve palsy with BTX-A injections (1–2 units) into the orbicularis oris, zygomaticus, and risorius, as well as the masseter (5–10 units). The same principle can be applied when the orbicularis oris or risorius muscle is traumatized and the mouth deviates to the contralateral (normal) side. By injecting into the risorius lateral to the angle of the mouth in the midpupillary line of the unopposed side, the mouth can become centralized. In addition, with congenital or acquired weakness of the depressor anguli oris, injecting the normal side can restore symmetry and balance.

More recently, asymmetrical smiles as a familial trait caused by unilateral hyperkinetic depressor labii inferioris muscles have been addressed. A study of five patients showed how 1–3 units of BTX-A injected into the offending depressor labii inferioris could restore symmetry, with the benefit lasting for at least 6 months in all patients.

Facial contouring

Prominence of the mandibular angle and masseter muscle hypertrophy can pose an aesthetic problem for certain individuals due to the masculine profile. Botulinum toxin treatment offers an alternative to surgical resection of the mandibular angle, as shown in a study of 45 patients who received injections of 25–30 units of BTX-A into the prominent portions of the mandible at five or six points. Over the next 3 months, masseter muscle thickness as measured by computed tomography and/or ultrasonography gradually decreased; the benefit lasted for 6–7 months, with 36 of the patients being satisfied and 1 being very satisfied with the results. Side-effects included mastication difficulty, speech disturbance, and muscle aching, but were transient, lasting between 1 and 4 weeks post-injection.

Scar improvement

Wound edge tension is an important factor in determining the appearance of scars. The aim is always to have as little tension as possible so as to achieve the most favorable cosmetic outcome. As muscle tension contributes to wound tension, botulinum toxin injections would seem a reasonable therapeutic intervention to reduce this. A single-center, prospective, randomized, placebo-controlled trial assessed 31 patients undergoing forehead wound closure for lacerations or post-tumor excision, and placebo or 15 units of BTX-A was injected into the adjacent wound musculature in a diameter of 1–3 cm from the wound edge. There were no significant adverse events and at 6-month follow-up two blinded physicians used a visual analogue scale to rate the scars. They found a statistically significant and clinically relevant improvement in cosmetic outcome in the BTX-A-immobilized group.

Another study used BTX-A in 40 patients undergoing scar revision for cosmetically unacceptable facial scars. Following excision and closure of the original scar, 1.5 units of BTX-A was injected along the length of the wound at 1-cm intervals, 3–4 mm from the wound edge. Thirty-six patients (90%) noticed a marked improvement in scar width, level, and color match. No patient developed complications from toxin diffusion, such as lid ptosis, cheek flaccidity, drooling, or mastication problems, but smile asymmetry was noted in those with cheek scars – although this was not a cause of complaint.

Postoperative care

The authors provide patients with verbal as well as written postoperative instructions. This gives them a clear idea of what to expect. Important information to include is the possibility of bruising and that the effect may take up to 10–14 days to become apparent. Patients are advised to remain upright for 4 hours, not to manipulate the treated area to minimize unwanted toxin diffusion, and to exercise the injected muscles as much as possible for 2–3 hours after injection to facilitate cellular uptake of the toxin. The latter can be inconvenient for the patient and, interestingly, it has been suggested that perhaps just 1 hour of muscle contraction is needed, on the basis that it takes only 32–64 minutes for binding of the toxin to cholinergic receptor sites in actively contracting muscles.

The authors routinely underake a 2–3-week follow-up after treatment to assess response, address any issues the patient may have, and provide touch-up treatments if necessary.

Complications

Key Points

- Systemic complications from botulinum toxin injection are very rare when appropriate doses and techniques are used.
- Site-specific complications may occur, particularly in less experienced hands. All physicians injecting botulinum toxin should know how to manage such complications.
- Eyelid ptosis can occur after glabellar injection. This may occur due to injection too close to the orbit. Apraclonidine or phenylephrine solution can be used to stimulate Mueller's muscle and mitigate this complication.
- Treating the frontalis too low lateral to the midpupillary line can lead to brow ptosis. Patients should be informed before surgery that the lateral, low forehead lines cannot be treated with botulinum toxin.
- A quizzical or "Spock" eyebrow may result after injection of the frontalis. Injecting a small amount of botulinum toxin along the temporal suture line 2–4 cm above the eyebrow on the affected side will treat this complication.
- Overtreatment of the neck can result in dysphagia. Lower initial doses, such as 30 units of Botox® are recommended, with reassessment at 2 weeks.

Although side-effects and complications are inevitable, proper patient selection, evaluation, and education will ensure the best possible outcome for both patient and doctor. Fortunately in the case of botulinum toxin therapy, side-effects are usually mild and resolve over time, as the effects of the drug are temporary. In fact, no cases of botulism and no deaths have ever resulted from botulinum toxin use for cosmetic purposes. Furthermore, serious adverse events are rare, particularly when compared to therapeutic (noncosmetic) use, in part due to the lower doses used. However, despite the excellent safety record, it is important to anticipate and manage complications when they arise; they can be categorized as injection site, anatomic specific, and generalized (idiosyncratic). Some of what is discussed has been covered in the treatment section, but is worth reinforcing.

Injection site reactions

Pain, edema, erythema, and bruising related to the area of injection are the most common local reactions that occur. Pain can be minimized by applying an ice pack over the injection site, both before and immediately after injection, as well injecting slowly with a small-gauge needle, such as 30 or 32 G. Topical anesthetics may be used prior to injection to minimize discomfort, but the authors do not find this to be necessary routinely. As mentioned previously, reconstituting the botulinum toxin with preserved saline may also result in less pain upon injection due to the benzyl alcohol acting as an anesthetic.

Bruising can be reduced by patients avoiding elective aspirin, nonsteroidal anti-inflammatory agents, vitamin E, and gingko biloba 7–10 days prior to treatment. Vigilant avoidance of injections around blood vessels, particularly around the orbit, will minimize ecchymoses. Limiting the number of injections and firm pressure immediately after injecting will be beneficial.

Mild headaches can occasionally occur after injection, particularly in the forehead, but typically require no treatment or can be alleviated with mild analgesics. In two large multicenter trials studying BTX-A for the treatment of glabellar lines, the frequency of headache was similar to placebo in one (15.3% for BTX-A groups versus 15.0% for the placebo group) and less than placebo in the other (11.4% for BTX groups versus 20.0% for the placebo group). Furthermore, they were usually mild and resolved without sequelae within a few hours. However, severe debilitating headaches following BTX-A injections for cosmetic purposes can occur, and a case series reported symptoms lasting up to 4 weeks. Although rare, this should be brought to the patient's attention.

Anatomic specific complications

Glabellar complex

Patients should be warned about the possibility of upper eyelid ptosis after treatment of the glabellar complex. This occurs due to diffusion of the toxin through the orbital septum so that the levator palpebrae superioris muscle is affected. Remember that botulinum toxin can diffuse up to 3 cm from the injection point.

The frequency of upper eyelid ptosis has been reported as 3% (of 405 subjects) in the Botox® cosmetic package insert, and in two separate multicenter trials assessing Botox® for glabellar lines 5.4% (of 203 patients treated with the drug) and 1% (202 patients treated). It may become apparent as early as 2 days and as late as 10 days postinjection, potentially persisting for 2–4 weeks.

The authors employ several maneuvers to limit unwanted diffusion during injection, such as keeping the needle perpendicular to the skin to ensure accurate placement, grasping the procerus or corrugator muscle, using smaller injection volumes, and avoiding massage inferiorly towards the infraorbit. Placing corrugator injections at least 1 cm above the orbital rim will also reduce the risk. It is important to remember that elderly patients may have a diminished orbital septum, thereby increasing the propensity for undesired diffusion, warranting a more conservative approach in these patients.

If upper lid ptosis does occur, apraclonidine 0.5% (Iopidine; Alcon Laboratories, Fort Worth, TX, USA) or phenylephrine 2.5% ophthalmic solution can be used as an α-adrenergic agent to stimulate Mueller's muscle (located beneath the levator palpebrae superioris muscle) and elevate the upper eyelid lashline by 1–2 mm. Two drops, two to three times daily, can be used until the symptoms resolve. Apraclonidine has a risk of contact allergy, but tends to affect the pupil less than phenylephrine.

Forehead

Treating the frontalis can lead to brow ptosis, which may be more pronounced when the brow depressors are left untreated. Brow ptosis after frontalis injections has been reported at a frequency of up to 5%; however, one study reported that, of 25 patients injected for forehead rhytides, 22 suffered with a degree of brow ptosis, varying from 1 to 6 mm. When evaluating patients, check for preexisting brow ptosis, which may preclude frontalis injections, and evaluate the shape of the forehead. The latter is important because the injection technique can be modified to optimize results and limit side-effects in those with narrow (short) versus wide (long) foreheads.

As the lower 2.5–4 cm of the frontalis raises the brow, keeping the injections at least 2.5 cm above the orbital rim will minimize the risk of both brow and upper eyelid ptosis. The frontalis tends to stop at the temporal fusion line (see Fig. 3-6), but in some individuals this line is shifted and there may be well developed, active, lateral frontalis fibers; if these are not injected, a lateral

eyebrow pull results. Often termed "Spock" or "Jack Nicholson" brows due to the quizzical appearance, this problem can be dealt with by injecting 1–3 units into the lateral frontalis fibers, 2 cm above the lateral aspect of the brow at or close to the temporal fusion plane. However, be aware that overcorrection can result in a hooded brow that partially covers the eye.

Overtreatment of the frontalis can also result in a frozen or mask-like appearance. Treating the glabellar complex at the same time as the frontalis naturally involves a higher overall dose of toxin and, owing to the potential for diffusion, can increase the risk of excessive muscle paralysis. Therefore, particularly for beginners, it may be wise to treat the glabella first and then the frontalis 2–3 weeks later.

Periorbital treatments

It is important to avoid ectropion, diplopia, strabismus, lateral brow ptosis, as well as lip and cheek ptosis when treating this area. Ectropion can be avoided by excluding lower lid laxity as determined by a snap test. To perform this, pull the lower lid downward and outwards, then allow the lid to snap back to apposition with the globe. Laxity is suggested if the lid does not snap back immediately and into full apposition. In addition, caution should be exercised if there is a history of lower eyelid blepharoplasty. Also ask about dry eyes and, if in doubt, perform a Schirmer's test as tear production can potentially be affected when treating the orbicularis oculi.

Keeping injection volumes small (i.e. 0.1–0.2 mL) and at least 1 cm outside the bony orbit or 1.5 cm lateral to the lateral canthus, should avoid affecting the lateral rectus muscle and diplopia or strabismus. In addition, by maintaining injections above the inferior margin of the zygomatic arch, the zygomaticus major muscle will not be affected; this is important, otherwise cheek and upper lip ptosis can occur resulting in a Bell's palsy-like appearance. Even so, zygomatic lines, which are associated with periorbital wrinkles, can become more prominent when only the crow's feet are treated. This produces a less desirable cosmetic outcome, and treatment modalities such skin resurfacing or fillers are better suited to treat this problem. Crow's feet injections can also be associated with lateral brow ptosis, due to the lateral frontalis being affected; this can be avoided by ensuring that injections are below the brow.

Lower eyelid injections can be used to widen the eye, but should be avoided in those with lower lid laxity, excessive scleral show, and a history of lower lid surgery. As stated previously, only 2 units of BTX-A is usually necessary to achieve the effect, but 1 unit can be tried if a more conservative approach is deemed appropriate. Preexisting fat herniations can become more prominent with infraorbital injections and so should also be avoided in this context. The target muscles in the periocular area are superficial, and by keeping injections intradermal for this purpose there should be less risk of toxin diffusion.

Perioral injections

As the orbicularis oris muscle is important for oral competence including eating and speech, excessive weakening during injection of radial lip rhytides can have disastrous consequences. These include symptoms resulting from oral incompetence, such as dribbling or drooling from the mouth, inability to form certain sounds, pucker the lips, drink from a straw, kiss as before, and apply lipstick, as well as mouth asymmetry. As would be expected for individuals who depend on nothing less than complete oral competence, such as musicians playing wind instruments, singers, actors, and scuba divers, the effects can be even more devastating, and therefore botulinum toxin injections in this location should be avoided in these patients. When performing the injections, the risks can be minimized by injecting superficially (subcutaneously) just above the vermilion border, spacing injections symmetrically across the midline, using small doses (1–2 units of BTX-A per injection), and not exceeding a total of 4 units per lip.

When treating the DAO to improve the downturn of the corners of the mouth or a frown-like appearance, it is also important to avoid oral incompetence and an asymmetric smile as side-effects. These occur if the depressor labii inferioris is weakened by injections being too medial or too close to the mouth, when the orbicularis oris may be affected inadvertently. Therefore, injecting at the level of the mandible, 1 cm lateral to the oral commissure, is critical for specific targeting of the DAO at its posterior margin.

When treating the mentalis muscle, ensure the injection point is at or just below the bony prominence of the chin in the midline. Injecting at the level of the mental crease can affect the orbicularis oris, and if too lateral the depressor labii muscle may be weakened. Again, oral incompetence or mouth asymmetry may result.

Treating the neck

Complications arise in this area mainly when injections are placed in too deep a plane, the doses of botulinum toxin used are high, or both. They include temporary dysphagia when laryngeal muscles of deglutition are affected, and neck weakness if the sternocleidomastoid muscle is compromised. Injections should be as superficial as possible; aiming for the deep dermis rather than the subcutaneous plane can also be helpful in avoiding other deeper cholinergic muscular structures. The suggested maximum dose of BTX-A when treating the neck varies in the literature, but there was a case of 60 units causing such profound dysphagia that the patient needed a nasogastric tube for 6 weeks until normal swallowing returned. Some authors have suggested not exceeding a total of 30 units per treatment session, which the present authors believe makes the procedure a very low risk for such complications, when accompanied by the appropriate injection technique. Patients can usually be scheduled for another visit 2 weeks later should more toxin be needed.

Generalized reactions

Electromyographic studies have shown that the effects of botulinum toxin can be at sites distant from the injection site, possibly due to small amounts of toxin diffusing into the circulation. Generalized muscular weakness (distant from injection sites) has been seen in three patients treated with BTX-A (Dysport®) for dystonia, as well as in two patients treated for neurogenic detrusor overactivity (one tetraplegic patient treated with Botox® and the other paraplegic with Dysport®). Other reported systemic idiosyncratic reactions include nausea, fatigue, and flu-like symptoms.

Immune tolerance

Repeated botulinum toxin injections can produce neutralizing antibodies, resulting in a diminished or lack of response to treatment. Higher doses and more frequent injections may lead to a greater risk for antibody formation; however, the minimum dose and injection schedule required to induce antibody formation is unknown. Owing to the relatively low doses used, resistance to BTX-A from cosmetic use is extremely rare, particularly with newer batches of BTX-A, but has been reported. Therefore, it worth notifying patients of this possibility; when resistance to BTX-A is suspected, BTX-B is an alternative.

Botulinum toxin as combination therapy

Botulinum toxin is often used in conjunction with other rejuvenation modalities that can address other aspects of aging, such deep wrinkles at rest, pigmented lesions (ephelides and lentigines), telangiectasias, and loss of skin texture. Soft tissue fillers improve volume loss and work well with botulinum toxin. A randomized prospective study of 38 patients showed that BTX-A in conjunction with non-animal stabilized hyaluronic acid (NASHA; Restylane®) produced a greater and longer lasting benefit in the treatment of moderate to severe glabellar rhytides than either treatment alone. The use of botulinum toxin may reduce the amount of filler substance required, and the authors find this particularly relevant in the lower face. For example, if the DAO muscle is treated with botulinum toxin first and then 2–3 weeks later the marionette lines are injected with a filler, there is a synergistic benefit on the patient's smile; other authors have also commented on this.

Lasers treatments can also be enhanced with adjunctive botulinum toxin therapy. One study of 20 patients showed that BTX-A for 1–3 months following carbon dioxide laser resurfacing for facial rhytides in the glabella, forehead, and/or lateral canthal rhytides prolonged the reduction of wrinkles when compared with laser resurfacing alone in 20 patients. Another randomized, prospective, placebo-controlled study of 33 patients found that BTX-A injected before and after erbium:Yag laser for periorbital resurfacing significantly improved the outcome. If BTX-A is to be used prior to laser resurfacing, it should be performed 2–3 weeks beforehand to ensure adequate muscle relaxation.

A randomized prospective study of 30 patients has also shown that BTX-A can enhance the effect of intense pulsed light (IPL – broadband light). Half of the patient group had bilateral periorbital rhytides injected with BTX-A in addition to IPL therapy, whereas the other half had IPL treatment alone. Interestingly it was not only a more profound improvement in the periorbital rhytides that was seen in the combination therapy group, but also a better outcome in terms of telangiectasias, lentigines, pore size, and facial skin texture.

Another piece of positive evidence is that neither nonablative lasers nor IPL seem to inactivate botulinum toxin. In a study of 19 subjects, one side of the face was treated with BTX-A (treatment areas included glabella, horizontal forehead lines, and periorbital rhytides), followed within 10 minutes by treatment with a nonablative rejuvenation device including a vascular laser, IPL, and a radiofrequency device. The other side was also treated with the same device but BTX-A was injected only until the nonablative rejuvenation procedure had been completed, and this side served as a control; all subjects displayed symmetrical chemodenervation 2–3 weeks later.

It has also been suggested that botulinum toxin used prior to chemical peeling may improve the collagen remodeling that takes place after a chemical peel, as immobilized skin can regenerate more effectively. Again, 2 weeks is the recommended interval between botulinum toxin therapy and the peel.

Future directions and conclusions

As has been discussed, botulinum toxin has proved to be an excellent treatment for dynamic facial rhytides and plays an important adjunctive role when used with other treatment modalities to address the various aspects of aging. Its use has expanded tremendously over the past two decades and novel applications will continually be discovered in the coming years. A recent randomized double-blind study of 14 patients, which showed that the addition of 1:100 000 epinephrine to BTX-A may accelerate its onset of action as well as improve short-term efficacy in the treatment of periorbital rhytides, is an illustration of the constant innovation with botulinum toxin therapy.

In the future we will see many more neurotoxins in the market, some of which are in development. Toxins will hopefully evolve so that clinicians and their patients can see a more rapid onset of action, fewer side-effects, longer lasting benefits, and effects specific to the muscles targeted, with limited but controlled diffusion. Newer toxins not yet licenced in the USA, such as Xeomin® and Purtox® (Mentor, Santa Barbara, CA, USA), which at the time of writing is undergoing clinical trials, are free of complexing proteins and it will be interesting to see whether this translates into a significant clinical benefit.

Whatever the future holds, diligence should always be paid to patient selection and evaluation. When this is combined with a sound knowledge of facial anatomy and meticulous injection technique, the outcome should be optimal.

Further reading

Ahn KY, Park MY, Park DH, Han DG. Botulinum toxin A for the treatment of facial hyperkinetic wrinkle lines in Koreans. Plast Reconstr Surg 2000;105:778–784.

Ahn MS, Catten M, Maas CS. Temporal brow lift using botulinum toxin A. Plast Reconstr Surg 2000;105:1129–1135.

Alam M, Arndt KA, Dover JS. Severe, intractable headache after injection with botulinum a exotoxin: report of 5 cases. J Am Acad Dermatol 2002;46:62–65.

Alam M, Dover JS, Arndt KA. Pain associated with injection of botulinum A exotoxin reconstituted using isotonic sodium chloride with and without preservative: a double-blind, randomized controlled trial. Arch Dermatol 2002;138:510–514.

Alam M, Dover JS, Klein AW, Arndt KA. Botulinum A exotoxin for hyperfunctional facial lines: where not to inject. Arch Dermatol 2002;138:1180–1185.

Allergan. Botox Cosmetic (Botulinum Toxin Type A) Purified Neurotoxin Complex (package insert). 2002. Irvine: Allergan, 2002.

Alster TS, Lupton JR. Botulinum toxin type B for dynamic glabellar rhytides refractory to botulinum toxin type A. Dermatol Surg 2003;29:516–518.

American Society for Aesthetic Plastic Surgery. 11.5 million cosmetic procedures in 2006. Available at: http://www.surgery.org/press/news-release.php?iid=465 (accessed 26 Feb 2008)

Aoki KR. Pharmacology and immunology of botulinum toxin serotypes. J Neurol 2001;248:3–10.

Ascher B, Zakine B, Kestemont P, Baspeyras M, Bougara A, Santini J. A multicenter, randomized, double-blind, placebo-controlled study of efficacy and safety of 3 doses of botulinum toxin A in the treatment of glabellar lines. J Am Acad Dermatol 2004;51:223–233.

Baek SM, Kim SS, Bindiger A. The prominent mandibular angle: preoperative management, operative technique, and results in 42 patients. Plast Reconstr Surg 1989;83:272–280.

Baumann L, Slezinger A, Vujevich J, et al. A double-blinded, randomized, placebo-controlled pilot study of the safety and efficacy of Myobloc (botulinum toxin type B)-purified neurotoxin complex for the treatment of crow's feet: a double-blinded, placebo-controlled trial. Dermatol Surg 2003;29:508–515.

Beer K, Yohn M, Closter J. A double-blinded, placebo-controlled study of Botox for the treatment of subjects with chin rhytids. J Drugs Dermatol 2005;4:417–422.

Benedetto A. Cosmetic uses of botulinum toxin a in the mid face. In: Benedetto AV, ed. Botulinum Toxin in Clinical Dermatology. London: Taylor & Francis, 2005:156–161.

Benedetto AV. Asymmetrical smiles corrected by botulinum toxin serotype A. Dermatol Surg 2007;33:S32–S36.

Bentsianov B, Blitzer A. Facial anatomy. Clin Dermatol 2004;22:3–13.

Bhatia KP, Munchau A, Thompson PD, et al. Generalised muscular weakness after botulinum toxin injections for dystonia: a report of three cases. J Neurol Neurosurg Psychiatry 1999;67:90–93.

Blitzer A, Binder WJ, Aviv JE, Keen MS, Brin MF. The management of hyperfunctional facial lines with botulinum toxin. A collaborative study of 210 injection sites in 162 patients. Arch Otolaryngol Head Neck Surg 1997;123:389–392.

Borodic G. Immunologic resistance after repeated botulinum toxin type a injections for facial rhytides. Ophthal Plast Reconstr Surg 2006;22:239–240.

Brandt FS, Boker A. Botulinum toxin for the treatment of neck lines and neck bands. Dermatol Clin 2004;22:159–166.

Brashear A, Lew MF, Dykstra DD, et al. Safety and efficacy of NeuroBloc (botulinum toxin type B) in type A-responsive cervical dystonia. Neurology 1999;53:1439–1446.

Bulstrode NW, Grobbelaar AO. Long-term prospective follow-up of botulinum toxin treatment for facial rhytides. Aesthetic Plast Surg 2002;26:356–359.

Carruthers A, Carruthers J. Botulinum toxin type A: history and current cosmetic use in the upper face. Semin Cutan Med Surg 2001;20:71–84.

Carruthers A, Carruthers J. Prospective, double-blind, randomized, parallel-group, dose-ranging study of botulinum toxin type A in men with glabellar rhytids. Dermatol Surg 2005;31:1297–1303.

Carruthers A, Carruthers J. Single-center, double-blind, randomized study to evaluate the efficacy of 4% lidocaine cream versus vehicle cream during botulinum toxin type A treatments. Dermatol Surg 2005;31:1655–1659.

Carruthers A, Carruthers J. Eyebrow height after botulinum toxin type A to the glabella. Dermatol Surg 2007;33:S26–S31.

Carruthers J, Carruthers A. Aesthetic botulinum A toxin in the mid and lower face and neck. Dermatol Surg 2003;29:468–476.

Carruthers J, Carruthers A. A prospective, randomized, parallel group study analyzing the effect of BTX-A (Botox) and nonanimal sourced hyaluronic acid (NASHA, Restylane) in combination compared with NASHA (Restylane) alone in severe glabellar rhytides in adult female subjects: treatment of severe glabellar rhytides with a hyaluronic acid derivative compared with the derivative and BTX-A. Dermatol Surg 2003;29:802–809.

Carruthers J, Carruthers A. The effect of full-face broadband light treatments alone and in combination with bilateral crow's feet Botulinum toxin type A chemodenervation. Dermatol Surg 2004;30:355–366.

Carruthers J, Carruthers A. Botulinum toxin type A treatment of multiple upper facial sites: patient-reported outcomes. Dermatol Surg 2007;33: S10–S17.

Carruthers JD, Carruthers A. Treatment of glabellar frown lines with C. botulinum-A exotoxin. J Dermatol Surg Oncol 1992;18:17–21.

Carruthers JD, Carruthers A. Botulinum A exotoxin in clinical ophthalmology. Can J Ophthalmol 1996;31:389–400.

Carruthers A, Bogle M, Carruthers JD, et al. A randomized, evaluator-blinded, two-center study of the safety and effect of volume on the diffusion and efficacy of botulinum toxin type a in the treatment of lateral orbital rhytides. Dermatol Surg 2007;33:567–571.

Carruthers A, Carruthers J, Cohen J. A prospective, double-blind, randomized, parallel-group, dose-ranging study of botulinum toxin type a in female subjects with horizontal forehead rhytides. Dermatol Surg 2003;29:461–467.

Carruthers A, Carruthers J, Cohen J. Dilution volume of botulinum toxin type A for the treatment of glabellar rhytides: does it matter? Dermatol Surg 2007;33:S97–S104.

Carruthers A, Carruthers J, Flynn TC, Leong MS. Dose-finding, safety, and tolerability study of botulinum toxin type B for the treatment of hyperfunctional glabellar lines. Dermatol Surg 2007;33:S60–S68.

Carruthers A, Carruthers J, Said S. Dose-ranging study of botulinum toxin type A in the treatment of glabellar rhytids in females. Dermatol Surg 2005;31:414–422.

Carruthers J, Fagien S, Matarasso SL. Consensus recommendations on the use of botulinum toxin type a in facial aesthetics. Plast Reconstr Surg 2004;114(Suppl):1S–22S.

Carruthers JA, Lowe NJ, Menter MA, et al. A multi-center, double-blind, randomized, placebo-controlled study of the efficacy and safety of botulinum toxin type A in the treatment of glabellar lines. J Am Acad Dermatol 2002;46:840–849.

Carruthers JD, Lowe NJ, Menter MA, Gibson J, Eadie N. Double-blind, placebo-controlled study of the safety and efficacy of botulinum toxin type A for patients with glabellar lines. Plast Reconstr Surg 2003;112:1089–1098.

Cote TR, Mohan AK, Polder JA, Walton MK, Braun MM. Botulinum toxin type A injections: adverse events reported to the US Food and Drug Administration in therapeutic and cosmetic cases. J Am Acad Dermatol 2005;53:407–415.

Fagien S. Botulinum toxin type A for facial aesthetic enhancement: role in facial shaping. Plast Reconstr Surg 2003;112:6S–18S.

Fagien S, Cox SE, Finn JC, Werschler WP, Kowalski JW. Patient-reported outcomes with botulinum toxin type A treatment of glabellar rhytids: a double-blind, randomized, placebo-controlled study. Dermatol Surg 2007;33:S2–S9.

Flynn TC. Update on botulinum toxin. Semin Cutan Med Surg 2006;25:115–121.

Flynn TC, Clark RE. Botulinum toxin type B (Myobloc) versus botulinum toxin type A (Botox) frontalis study: rate of onset and radius of diffusion. Dermatol Surg 2003;29:519–522.

Flynn TC, Carruthers JA, Carruthers JA, Clark RE. Botulinum A toxin (Botox) in the lower eyelid: dose-finding study. Dermatol Surg 2003;29: 943–950.

Flynn TC, Carruthers JA, Carruthers JA. Botulinum-A toxin treatment of the lower eyelid improves infraorbital rhytides and widens the eye. Dermatol Surg 2001;27:703–708.

Frankel AS, Kamer FM. Chemical browlift. Arch Otolaryngol Head Neck Surg 1998;124: 321–323.

Gassner HG, Brissett AE, Otley CC, et al. Botulinum toxin to improve facial wound healing: a prospective, blinded, placebo-controlled study. Mayo Clin Proc 2006;81:1023–1028.

Hantash BM, Gladstone HB. A pilot study on the effect of epinephrine on botulinum toxin treatment for periorbital rhytides. Dermatol Surg 2007;33:461–468.

Hexsel D, Mazzuco R, Zechmeister M, et al. Complications and adverse effects: diagnosis and treatment. In: Hexsel D, Trinidade de Almeida A, eds. Cosmetic Use of Botulinum Toxin. Porto Alegre: AGE Editorial, 2002:233–239.

Hexsel DM, De Almeida AT, Rutowitsch M, et al. Multicenter, double-blind study of the efficacy of injections with botulinum toxin type A reconstituted up to six consecutive weeks before application. Dermatol Surg 2003;29:523–529.

Hsu TS, Dover JS, Arndt KA. Effect of volume and concentration on the diffusion of botulinum exotoxin A. Arch Dermatol 2004;140: 1351–1354.

Hsu TS, Dover JS, Kaminer MS, Arndt KA, Tan MH. Why make patients exercise facial muscles for 4 hours after botulinum toxin treatment? Arch Dermatol 2003;139:948.

Huang W, Foster JA, Rogachefsky AS. Pharmacology of botulinum toxin. J Am Acad Dermatol 2000;43:249–259.

Huang W, Rogachefsky AS, Foster JA. Browlift with botulinum toxin. Dermatol Surg 2000;26:55–60.

Humeau Y, Doussau F, Grant NJ, Poulain B. How botulinum and tetanus neurotoxins block neurotransmitter release. Biochimie 2000;82:427–446.

Ipsen. Summary of product characteristics. Dysport: Clostridium botulinum Type A Toxin–Haemagglutinin Complex. Slough: Ipsen, 2004.

Kane MA. Nonsurgical treatment of platysmal bands with injection of botulinum toxin A. Plast Reconstr Surg 1999;103:656–663.

Kane MA. Classification of crow's feet patterns among Caucasian women: the key to individualizing treatment. Plast Reconstr Surg 2003;112: 33S–39S.

Keller JE, Cai F, Neale EA. Uptake of botulinum neurotoxin into cultured neurons. Biochemistry 2004;43:526–532.

Klein AW. Cosmetic therapy with botulinum toxin: anecdotal memoirs. Dermatol Surg 1996;22: 757–759.

Klein AW. Dilution and storage of botulinum toxin. Dermatol Surg 1998;24:1179–1180.

Klein AW. Complications, adverse reactions, and insights with the use of botulinum toxin. Dermatol Surg 2003;29:549–556.

Klein AW, Wexler P, Carruthers A, Carruthers J. Treatment of facial furrows and rhytides. Dermatol Clin 1997;15:595–607.

Landau M. Combination of chemical peelings with botulinum toxin injections and dermal fillers. J Cosmet Dermatol 2006;5:121–126.

Lee SK. Antibody-induced failure of botulinum toxin type A therapy in a patient with masseteric hypertrophy. Dermatol Surg 2007;33:S105–S110.

Lowe NJ, Ascher B, Heckmann M, Kumar C, Fraczek S, Eadie N. Double-blind, randomized, placebo-controlled, dose–response study of the safety and efficacy of botulinum toxin type A in subjects with crow's feet. Dermatol Surg 2005;31:257–262.

Lowe NJ, Lask G, Yamauchi P, Moore D. Bilateral, double-blind, randomized comparison of 3 doses of botulinum toxin type A and placebo in patients with crow's feet. J Am Acad Dermatol 2002;47:834–840.

Lowe P, Patnaik R, Lowe N. Comparison of two formulations of botulinum toxin type A for the treatment of glabellar lines: a double-blind, randomized study. J Am Acad Dermatol 2006;55:975–980.

Mahant N, Clouston PD, Lorentz IT. The current use of botulinum toxin. J Clin Neurosci 2000;7: 389–394.

Matarasso SL. Complications of botulinum A exotoxin for hyperfunctional lines. Dermatol Surg 1998;24:1249–1254.

Matarasso SL. Decreased tear expression with an abnormal Schirmer's test following botulinum toxin type A for the treatment of lateral canthal rhytides. Dermatol Surg 2002;28:149–152.

Matarasso SL. Comparison of botulinum toxin types A and B: a bilateral and double-blind randomized evaluation in the treatment of canthal rhytides. Dermatol Surg 2003;29:7–13.

Meunier FA, Schiavo G, Molgo J. Botulinum neurotoxins: from paralysis to recovery of functional neuromuscular transmission. J Physiol (Paris) 2002;96:105–113.

Monheit G, Carruthers A, Brandt F, Rand R. A randomized, double-blind, placebo-controlled study of botulinum toxin type A for the treatment of glabellar lines: determination of optimal dose. Dermatol Surg 2007;33:S51–S59.

Odergren T, Hjaltason H, Kaakkola S, et al. A double blind, randomised, parallel group study to investigate the dose equivalence of Dysport and Botox in the treatment of cervical dystonia. J Neurol Neurosurg Psychiatry 1998;64:6–12.

Ozsoy Z, Genc B, Gozu A. A new technique applying botulinum toxin in narrow and wide foreheads. Aesthetic Plast Surg 2005;29:368–372.

Paloma V, Samper A. A complication with the aesthetic use of Botox: herniation of the orbital fat. Plast Reconstr Surg 2001;107:1315.

Park MY, Ahn KY, Jung DS. Botulinum toxin type A treatment for contouring of the lower face. Dermatol Surg 2003;29:477–483.

Pena MA, Alam M, Yoo SS. Complications with the use of botulinum toxin type A for cosmetic applications and hyperhidrosis. Semin Cutan Med Surg 2007;26:29–33.

Redaelli A, Forte R. How to avoid brow ptosis after forehead treatment with botulinum toxin. J Cosmetic Laser Ther 2003;5:220–222.

Rzany B, Ascher B, Fratila A, Monheit GD, Talarico S, Sterry W. Efficacy and safety of 3- and 5-injection patterns (30 and 50 U) of botulinum toxin A (Dysport) for the treatment of wrinkles in the glabella and the central forehead region. Arch Dermatol 2006;142:320–326.

Rzany B, Dill-Muller D, Grablowitz D, Heckmann M, Caird D. Repeated botulinum toxin A injections for the treatment of lines in the upper face: a retrospective study of 4103 treatments in 945 patients. Dermatol Surg 2007;33:S18–S25.

Sadick NS. Prospective open-label study of botulinum toxin type B (Myobloc) at doses of 2400 and 3000 U for the treatment of glabellar wrinkles. Dermatol Surg 2003;29:501–507.

Sakaba T, Stein A, Jahn R, Neher E. Distinct kinetic changes in neurotransmitter release after SNARE protein cleavage. Science 2005;309:491–494.

Schantz EJ, Johnson EA. Botulinum toxin: the story of its development for the treatment of human disease. Perspect Biol Med 1997;40:317–327.

Scheinfeld N. The use of apraclonidine eyedrops to treat ptosis after the administration of botulinum toxin to the upper face. Dermatol Online J 2005;11:9.

Scott AB, Rosenbaum A, Collins CC. Pharmacologic weakening of extraocular muscles. Invest Ophthalmol 1973;12:924–927.

Semchyshyn N, Sengelmann RD. Botulinum toxin A treatment of perioral rhytides. Dermatol Surg 2003;29:490–495.

Semchyshyn NL, Kilmer SL. Does laser inactivate botulinum toxin? Dermatol Surg 2005;31:399–404.

Silvestre JF, Carnero L, Ramon R, Albares MP, Botella R. Allergic contact dermatitis from apraclonidine in eyedrops. Contact Dermatitis 2001;45:251.

Solstice Neurosciences. Myobloc (Botulinum Toxin Type B) Injectable Solution (package insert). San Francisco: Solstice Neurosciences, 2004.

Spencer JM, Gordon M, Goldberg DJ. Botulinum B treatment of the glabellar and frontalis regions: a dose response analysis. J Cosmet Laser Ther 2002;4:19–23.

Tamura BM, Odo MY, Chang B, Cuce LC, Flynn TC. Treatment of nasal wrinkles with botulinum toxin. Dermatol Surg 2005;31:271–275.

West TB, Alster TS. Effect of botulinum toxin type A on movement-associated rhytides following CO_2 laser resurfacing. Dermatol Surg 1999;25:259–261.

Wieder JM, Moy RL. Understanding botulinum toxin. Surgical anatomy of the frown, forehead, and periocular region. Dermatol Surg 1998;24:1172–1174.

Wilson AM. Use of botulinum toxin type A to prevent widening of facial scars. Plast Reconstr Surg 2006;117:1758–1766.

Wollina U, Konrad H. Managing adverse events associated with botulinum toxin type A: a focus on cosmetic procedures. Am J Clin Dermatol 2005;6:141–150.

Wyndaele JJ, Van Dromme SA. Muscular weakness as side effect of botulinum toxin injection for neurogenic detrusor overactivity. Spinal Cord 2002;40:599–600.

Yamauchi PS, Lask G, Lowe NJ. Botulinum toxin type A gives adjunctive benefit to periorbital laser resurfacing. J Cosmet Laser Ther 2004;6:145–148.

Fillers

Jamison E. Strahan and Joel L. Cohen

Key Points

- Bovine collagen is the most studied filler and has long been used as a comparison for the development of new fillers.
- Nonsurgical cosmetic procedures now outnumber surgical ones.
- The aim of cosmetic filler usage is to restore a youthful appearance rather than change the patient's natural appearance.

Introduction

The injection of fillers for soft tissue augmentation has become a mainstay procedure in the practice of aesthetic dermatology. The use of injectable hyaluronic acid is second only to the use of botulinum toxin in the number of nonsurgical cosmetic procedures performed. Over the past decade, the increase in nonsurgical cosmetic procedures has greatly exceeded that of surgical ones.

As the baby boomer population begins to experience the effects of aging and solar damage, the interest in minimally invasive procedures will likely expand exponentially. With the increased movement toward nonsurgical facial rejuvenation, fillers have become a staple dermatological tool for the cosmetic patient. Although lasers and chemical peels soften fine lines and superficial wrinkles, they are ineffective in treating deeper rhytides and facial folds. This has led to an explosive innovation in the development of filler substances.

The use of fillers began before the 1900s with autologous fat injection for augmentation. By the 1950s, liquid silicone was making its way into the augmentation arena. Because of the various complications reported with the early, liquid injectable silicon, multiple refinements occurred before its use in North America. However, its use continues to be a polarizing issue among aesthetic physicians, with the central issue being that it has never gained FDA approval for cosmetic use.

Bovine collagen made its debut as a filler in the early 1980s. Today, bovine collagen is still the standard to which all other fillers are compared. Its allergenicity issues, however, precipitated a search for a less immunogenic alternative. By the mid 1990s, hyaluronic acid was making its way into the European marketplace. With mainstream embrace of these collagen and hyaluronic acid products, a race to find an ideal injectable was set into motion, resulting in the investigation and introduction of many additional technologies, including acrylates, hydroxylapatite, and polytetrafluoroethylene, as well as cadaveric tissue transplants.

General principles

Anatomical considerations

A mastery of facial anatomy is critical to optimizing results from soft tissue augmentation procedures. Not only is it important to understand muscular dynamics and age-related anatomic alterations, but it is equally important to be familiar with the vascular network of the face (Fig. 4-1) in order to avoid adverse reactions and complications, which are discussed below. For example, one devastating complication of injecting the glabella is skin necrosis from direct cannulation of the supratrochlear artery or one of its perforating branches. Knowing its position can help guide the appropriate placement of filler to this commonly injected site. In addition, it is important to recognize the vast number of anastomoses between major branches. The arterial tree can be found in a plane deep to the subcutaneous fat and is generally avoided with superficial placement of filler. However, the placement of filler very deep in some areas increases the possibility of arterial puncture. Additionally, high volume filling into a small arteriole may exceed intravascular pressure enough to cause ulceration.

Remember that, although most of the arterial supply to the face is from terminating branches of the external carotid artery, there are several contributions from the internal carotid artery

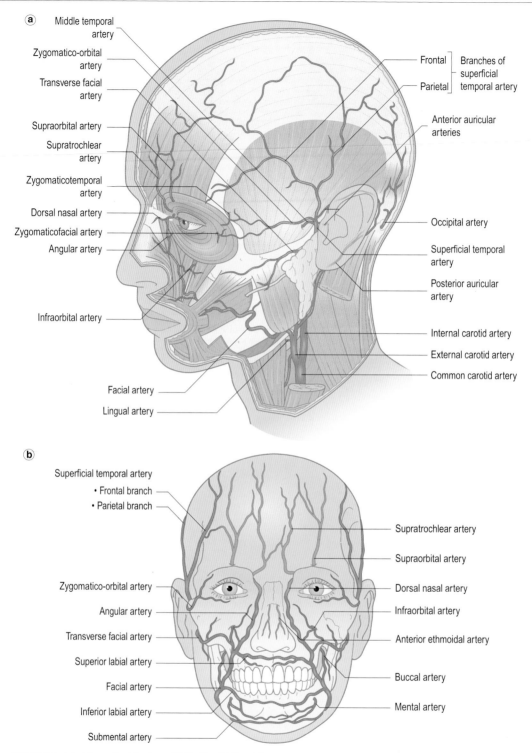

(a)

Middle temporal artery

Zygomatico-orbital artery

Transverse facial artery

Supraorbital artery

Supratrochlear artery

Zygomaticotemporal artery

Dorsal nasal artery

Zygomaticofacial artery

Angular artery

Infraorbital artery

Facial artery

Lingual artery

Frontal   } Branches of superficial temporal artery

Parietal

Anterior auricular arteries

Occipital artery

Superficial temporal artery

Posterior auricular artery

Internal carotid artery

External carotid artery

Common carotid artery

(b)

Superficial temporal artery
• Frontal branch
• Parietal branch

Zygomatico-orbital artery

Angular artery

Transverse facial artery

Superior labial artery

Facial artery

Inferior labial artery

Submental artery

Supratrochlear artery

Supraorbital artery

Dorsal nasal artery

Infraorbital artery

Anterior ethmoidal artery

Buccal artery

Mental artery

Figure 4-1 Arterial supply of the face. (A) Profile. (B) Front view (supraorbital, infraorbital, supratrochlear, infra-trochlear, dorsal nasal arteries). This has relevance to atherosclerotic disease and the changes in flow that accompany stenosis. Occlusion of the common carotid or external carotid artery is less frequent than occlusion of the internal carotid artery. Thus, blood flow through arterial branches of the internal carotid (e.g. medial forehead supply from the supraorbital and supratrochlear) may be less than that through the external carotid in patients with a history of atherosclerosis. Furthermore, a history of internal carotid stenosis may possibly portend a higher risk of skin necrosis from arterial branch cannulation of supratrochlear branches during injection of filler. This is a rare additional risk that should be reviewed with the vasculo-pathic patient prior to proceeding.

The aging face

A commonly taught simplification on aging is that of "triangular reversal" in the shape of the face. Fat distribution continues to change from infancy to late adulthood. As infants, we have large distributions of fat pockets in the lower face and mid-mandible area. With relatively small zygomatic processes at this stage, the appearance is that of an upwardly oriented triangle when looking at the face head on, with its apex at the glabella and the base at the chin and inferior cheek (Fig. 4-2A). As bones continue to develop and fat is redistributed, the chin and zygoma become more prominent and fat infiltrates the medial cheek after adolescence. This gives a reversed appearance of the triangle, with its apex toward the chin and a broad base at the zygoma (Fig. 4-2B). With progression through middle aging, the effects of solar elastosis and muscle atrophy become apparent. There is also a thinning of the subcutaneous layer of the skin of the face. As contours flatten, bony landmarks become more prominent and there is

extensive shadowing of deep folds and facial hollows (Fig. 4-2C).

Replenishment of the subcutaneous fat in some of these areas is an ideal solution to this loss. However, experience with autologous fat grafts remains variable, with publication only of anecdotal reports claiming longevity of weeks to years, depending on technique. Furthermore, there is significant downtime and potential complications associated with the procedure of harvesting and reinjecting fat.

All of these age-related changes cause the epidermal surface to appose more closely the bony skeleton and drop toward the lower face. Thus, the triangular shape again reverses to give the appearance of an aged face. This triangle is further accentuated in patients who are overweight, in whom the appearance of sagging fat can mimic that of infancy.

The goal of facial augmentation is to restore a natural youthful appearance of properly placed volume, rather than creating an effect that differs from the patient's appearance earlier in life. The injector should be wary of the patient who desires a change in anatomic appearance to that of someone other than him or herself, such as a celebrity. It is important to discuss that augmentation for rejuvenation is intended to restore balance, symmetry, and harmony in concordance with an earlier state of life. The astute injector may have the patient bring in photographs from childhood, high school graduation, etc. to help guide the ideal outcome.

Classes of filler

Fillers can be classified according to whether or not they are biodegradable. Biodegradable products are temporary implants that degrade with time. Several modifications can extend their half-life. For example, native hyaluronic acid has a

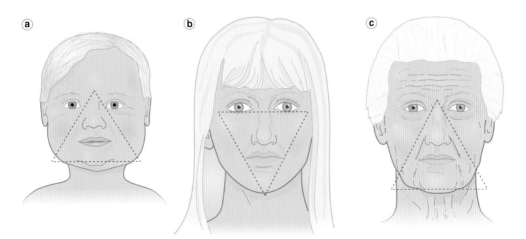

Figure 4-2 Triangle concept to the aging face. (A) Infant. (B) Young adulthood. (C) Older adulthood

half-life of approximately 2–3 days. However, once it is crosslinked, its half-life extends to several months. Biodegradable fillers include collagens, hyaluronic acids (hyalurons), hydroxylapatite, poly-L-lactic acid (PLLA), and cadaveric tissue. Nonbiodegradable fillers are permanent and include polyacrylamide gels, silicone, and synthetic implants. A comparison of filler substances is presented in Table 4-1.

Injection placement

The decision of how deep to place an injectable involves consideration of both the type of product to be used and the type of defect being

Table 4-1 Comparison of different fillers (adapted from Sadick 2007)

Filler	Products	Manufacturer	Approximate duration (months)	FDA approval
Collagen				
Bovine-based	Zyderm® I	Allergan/Inamed, Irvine, CA, USA	3–5	Yes
	Zyderm® II	Allergan/Inamed, Irvine, CA, USA	3–5	Yes
	Zyplast®	Allergan/Inamed, Irvine, CA, USA	3–5	Yes
Human-based	CosmoDerm®	Allergan/Inamed, Irvine, CA, USA	3–5	Yes
	CosmoPlast®	Allergan/Inamed, Irvine, CA, USA	3–5	Yes
	Isolagen®	Isolagen, Exton, PA, USA	12	No
	Fascian™	Fascia Biosystems, Beverly Hills, CA, USA	3–6	Yes
	Cymetra™ (Alloderm™)	LifeCell Corporation, Branchburg, NJ, USA	3–6 (12–24)	Yes
Hyaluronic acid	Hylaform®	Allergan/Inamed, Irvine, CA, USA	3–5	Yes
	Hylaform® Fine Line	Allergan/Inamed, Irvine, CA, USA	3–5	No
	Hylaform® Plus	Allergan/Inamed, Irvine, CA, USA	3–5	Yes
	Restylane®	Medicis, Scottsdale, AZ, USA	6–9	Yes
	Restylane® Touch (previously Fine Line)	Medicis, Scottsdale, AZ, USA	3–6	No
	Perlane®	Medicis, Scottsdale, AZ, USA	6–10	Yes
	Juvéderm™ 18	Allergan/Inamed, Irvine, CA, USA	3–6	Yes
	Juvéderm™ Ultra	Allergan/Inamed, Irvine, CA, USA	6–12	Yes
	Juvéderm™ Ultra Plus	Allergan/Inamed, Irvine, CA, USA	6–12	Yes
	Belotero® Basic	Merz Pharmaceuticals, Greensboro, NC, USA	6–9	No
	Belotero® Soft	Merz Pharmaceuticals, Greensboro, NC, USA	6–9	No
	Elevess™	Anika Therapeutics, Woburn, MA, USA		Yes
	Captique™	Allergan/Inamed, Irvine, CA, USA	3–5	Yes
	Prevelle	Mentor Corp.	3-5	Yes
Calcium hydroxylapatite	Radiesse®	Nioform Medical, San Mateo, CA, USA	9–18	Yes
Poly-L-lactic acid	Sculptra® (New-Fill™ outside USA)	Dermik/Aventis Laboratories, Bridgewater, NJ, USA	24	Yes
Liquid silicone	Silikon® 1000	Alcon Laboratories, Fort Worth, TX, USA	Permanent	Yes[a]
Polyacrylamide gel	Aquamid®	Contura International, Soeborg, Denmark	Permanent	No
Polymethylmethacrylate	ArteFill®	Artes Medical, San Diego, CA, USA	Permanent	Yes

[a]FDA approval only for ophthalmic use

addressed (Fig. 4-3, Table 4-2). Proper choice of filler placement is crucial in reducing the appearance of localized irregularities (Fig. 4-4). In general, the deeper the fold you are trying to correct, the deeper the desired placement of the product. Thus, fine lines should be corrected with placement of product in the papillary dermis, whereas deep folds should be smoothed with subcutaneous deposition of filler. The same is true for product choice. Smaller sized particles work well in the upper dermis, and larger sized particles work better in the subcutaneous fat. Longevity of the product may also be influenced by placement: deposition around the most immunoreactive section of skin for each particular product could potentially enhance its metabolism.

Choosing the right filler

The "ideal filler" has several properties:

- It is safe and offers consistently reproducible results for the restoration of volume without risk of diffusion to surrounding tissue.
- It has low immunogenicity and abuse potential.
- It has no risk of infectious contamination, carcinogenic potential, or teratogenicity.
- It has few preprocedure preparation requirements and is easy to administer.

- It has the potential for multiple applications, from fine lines to deep rhytides.
- It has insignificant breakdown over the desired life of the product.
- It has insignificant postprocedure morbidity and no long-term complications.
- It has Food and Drug Administation (FDA) approval for its safety and target indication.

Although a filler with all of these characteristics is quite unrealistic, several fillers can reliably address some of these traits in certain facial areas.

Many factors must be considered when choosing the appropriate filler (Box 4-1). If the patient has not had previous exposure to fillers, a permanent, nonbiodegradable product may not be appropriate. One advantage of biodegradable fillers is that any unwanted results are temporary. Successive implantation of biodegradable products offers the ability to individualize and perfect the technique to achieve the desired outcome for each patient. Once the desired result has been obtained for a particular patient, consideration may then be given to placement of a more durable or permanent product.

As mentioned above, the depth of defect to be filled will limit the choice of filler. One must identify whether the goal is wrinkle reduction or

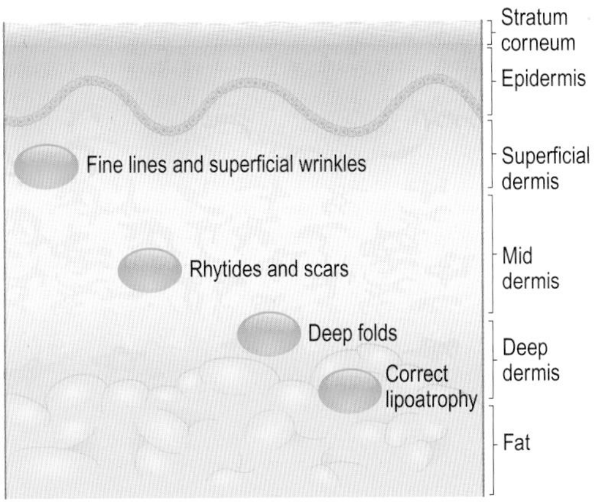

Figure 4-3 Placement of fillers according to indication

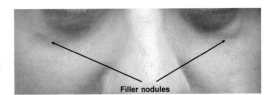

Figure 4-4 Visible nodules resulting from too superficial injection into the periorbital area with Restylane® by a non-physicion

BOX 4-1

Considerations when choosing the appropriate filler

Financial restrictions

Timeliness to important social appearances

- Downtime required
- When effect will be apparent

Previous filler treatments

Allergies

Defect to be corrected (deep versus superficial)

Thickness of skin to be injected

Tolerance to pain

Table 4-2 Ideal locations for each filler	
Ideal location	Appropriate filler
Papillary dermis	Zyderm®, CosmoDerm®, Restylane® Fine Line, Belotero® Soft
Mid-dermis	Zyplast®, CosmoPlast®, Hylaform®, Restylane®, Belotero® Basic
Deep dermis/ subcutis	Zyplast®, CosmoPlast®, Hylaform® Plus, Perlane®, Radiesse®, ArteFill®, Sculptra®

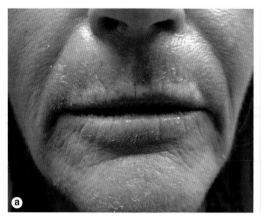 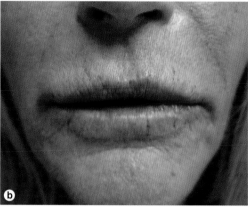

Figure 4-5 Volume was restored to the lips with Restylane® and fine periorbital wrinkles were treated with Cosmoderm®. (A) Before and (B) after treatment

volume restoration. Fine perioral wrinkles may be corrected using injection of the vermillion border with small particulate hyaluron or CosmoDerm® into some etched-in vertical lines on the upper lip (Fig. 4-5). Correction of lipoatrophy below the zygoma, however, requires a denser product such as Radiesse®, Perlane®, or Juvéderm™ Ultra Plus. Some physicians prefer the use of PLLA, with its delayed stimulation of collagen, despite its lack of cosmetic FDA approval.

A study by Lemperle et al. examined 10 common filler products, with biopsies performed at different time intervals to establish product biocompatibility and durability. The authors injected 0.1 mL of each filler into the anterior forearm of a patient and examined the results clinically and histologically (with excisional biopsies) at intervals of 1, 3, 6, and 9 months. The results are summarized in Table 4-3.

Technique

General considerations

In general, most seasoned injectors favor a "zone" approach rather than filling a single rhytid (Fig. 4-6). This addresses the volume depletion in other areas that may accentuate folds for which patients seek treatment. For example, loss of infrazygomatic cheek volume highlights prominent nasolabial folds due to the skin laxity that would fall inferiorly. Thus, by correcting the volume loss in the cheek as well as the nasolabial fold ("zone" filling), the final result can be optimized. In addition, the combination of rejuvenation procedures allows for a more holistic aesthetic restructuring that can maximize satisfaction. This might include chemical peels or lasers for mottled pigmentation, botulinum toxin for dynamic wrinkles, and filler injection for soft tissue volume loss (Fig. 4-7). It is also important to recognize when a filler may not be the best intervention. For example, some thin atrophic periorbital

Table 4-3 Longevity and reaction to 10 different fillers

Filler	Longevity (months)	Reaction
Zyplast®	3–6	NR
Restylane®	6–9	NR
ArteColl®	NR	Encapsulated with collagen and inflammatory cells
Silicone oil (PMS 350®)	NR	Foreign body reaction
NewFill® (Sculptra®)	3–6	Mild inflammatory response
Reviderm®	3–6	NR
Aquamid®	>9	Fine fibrous capsules
Dermalive®	3–6	Lowest cellular response
Evolution®	>9	NR
Radiesse®	>9	NR

NR, not reported

wrinkles may be better managed with a resurfacing procedure rather than a filler.

Injection principles

There is no universal acceptance on the proper implantation technique of fillers. Common techniques include linear threading, serial puncture, fanning, crosshatching, and depot injection (Fig. 4-8). Pain and risk of vessel puncture can be minimized with smaller caliber needles. Retrograde injection may also reduce risk of injection into a vessel.

Linear threading

With a linear threading technique, the area to be filled is punctured with the needle and advanced to the end position for the field to be augmented.

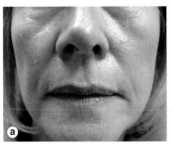
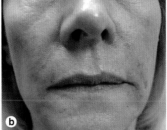
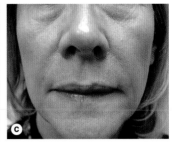

Figure 4-6 Fillers used in both nasolabial folds and oral commissures to rejuvenate the lower face. (A) Before, (B) immediately after treatment, and (C) several weeks later

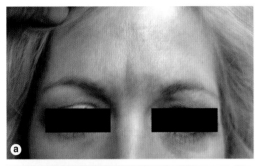
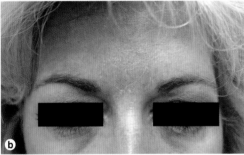
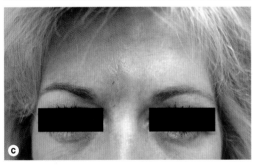

Figure 4-7 Restoration of a youthful appearance to the forehead by combining botulinum toxin A and filler.
(A) Preprocedure, relaxed; (B) after treatment with botulinum toxin; (C) after treatment with botulinum toxin and filler

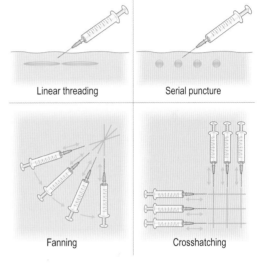

Figure 4-8 Different injection techniques

withdrawn, slow constant pressure is applied to the plunger to deposit filler at an even rate. For deep defects, a layered approach can be adopted, where successive threading is placed at multiple depths. The amount of filler injected depends on the location, depth, and type of filler used.

There are several variations on this technique. One report by Alam and Yoo showed optimal results by varying the depth with a "triangular" approach. This technique was used for correction of the nasolabial fold with calcium hydroxylapatite. With the needle inserted into the mid-nasolabial fold, it was advanced to the alar junction. Successive passes were made at varying depths, 10–20° lower than the initial plane, creating a triangle with an apex at the mid-nasolabial fold and base at the alar junction.

Serial puncture

With this technique, microdroplets (less than 0.03 mL) are deposited with successive injections placed 2–10 mm apart. The skin can be tented up with the needle inserted to ease the deposition of microdroplets. This method has been described to be effective for silicone injection.

For example, for nasolabial fold correction, the midpoint of the fold is punctured, then the needle is advanced to the junction between the ala and nasal side-wall. The needle should be kept parallel to the skin, and filler deposited within the same plane throughout injection. While the needle is

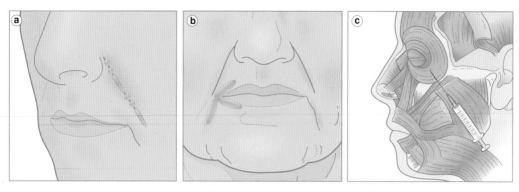

Figure 4-9 Examples of technique modification: (A) combination of serial puncture and linear threading for the nasolabial fold; (B) triangular wedge correction of the marionette line; (C) submuscular injection for tear trough correction

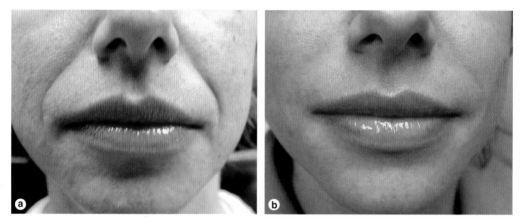

Figure 4-10 Nasolabial fold augmentation with a combination of linear threading and serial puncture. (A) Before and (B) after treatment

Fanning/crosshatching

Techniques such as fanning and crosshatching involve several linear passes of injection next to one another to augment larger areas of tissue. This technique is more commonly used to correct cheek concavity (e.g. lipodystrophy) using agents that require deep dermal or subdermal deposition, such as PLLA or calcium hydroxylapatite. With deeper deposition, the needle can be oriented with the bevel facing up during this technique, in contrast to a downward facing bevel in more superficially placed product. After advancing the needle, the filler is deposited with each withdraw. It may be helpful to outline the area to be injected prior to the procedure for more accurate results. It is key that the distribution of product be uniform. Some injectors describe a finished result as a "fresh dusting of snow." With multiple passes there is an increased risk of bruising. This may be mitigated by using a slower injection rate. Some also argue that anterograde (versus retrograde) injections can hydro-dissect the tissue and push small vessels aside.

Anatomic considerations

There is much variability in injection technique, making soft tissue augmentation an artistic and creative endeavor. Injection technique can be modified, depending on which anatomic rhytides are being corrected.

Nasolabial fold correction

Nasolabial fold correction can be optimized by several retrograde injections into the mid-dermis, followed by serial punctures to bridge these (Figs 4-9A & 4-10). However, a triangular wedge technique might be more suitable for the marionette line. Injection here to the mid and deep dermis, including the commissure, upper lip, modiolus, lower lip vermillion, and marionette groove, can give satisfying results (Fig. 4-9B). This is particularly useful when attempting to correct a "downturned" smile (Fig. 4-11).

Tear trough irregularities

Tear trough irregularities are created by a combination of dermal atrophy in an area of already very thin skin and shifting of the malar fat pad

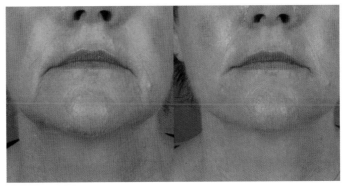

Figure 4-11 Correction of a downturned smile. After initial treatment with botulinum toxin in the depressor anguli oris, a combination of threading and fanning was used to restore the patient's smile. Before (*left*) and after (*right*) treatment. Photograph reprinted from Cohen JL, Hirsch RJ. Skin Aging 2006;14(2):52–53, with permission of the publisher

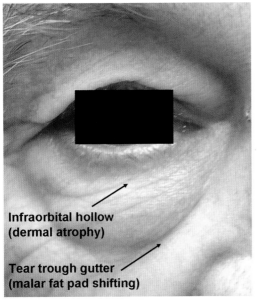

Infraorbital hollow
(dermal atrophy)

Tear trough gutter
(malar fat pad shifting)

Figure 4-12 Example of "double-bubble" appearance of aged infraorbital skin, created by both dermal atrophy and downward shifting of the malar fat pad

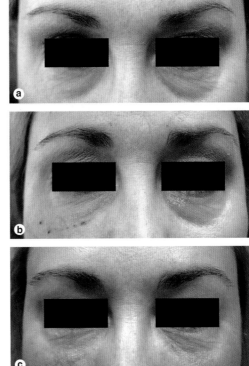

Figure 4-13 Correction of periorbital aging with injection above and beneath the orbicularis oculi muscle. (A) Before, (B) immediately after treating the patient's right side and (C) several weeks after treatment of both side. Photograph reprinted from Cohen JL, Berlin AL. Skin Aging 2007;15(10)28–29, with permission of the publisher

downward. Thus, patients often have both an infraorbital hollow and a tear trough concavity just below this. This results in a protuberance of tissue just below these folds giving a "double-bubble" appearance (Fig. 4-12). For the best aesthetic results, both of these phenomena should be addressed. Because of the high risk of adverse events in this area (nodularity, lumpiness, bleeding, prolonged swelling, etc.), periorbital augmentation should be attempted only by a skilled injector. For the infra-orbital hollow, filler is injected in a subcutaneous fat plane above the orbicularis muscle. For the tear trough itself, filler is best injected deep to the orbicularis muscle at the level of the periosteum (see Figs 4-7C & 4-13).

PEARLS

General principles

Filling in zones, rather than correcting individual lines, can accomplish better cosmetic results.

Biodegradable fillers are ideal initially, and more durable fillers should be considered only for patients who have predictable results after multiple sessions.

Classically, botulinum toxins restore the upper face, whereas fillers help to restore the lower face, but combining these procedures can result in synergy, creating a more complete youthful appearance. Combinations of toxin and fillers in some areas can sometimes optimize results.

Injection technique should be altered for different indications (e.g. linear threading for nasolabial fold correction, and fanning for bulking the zygomatic cheek).

Preoperative evaluation

First consultation

During the initial encounter, it is important to define the patient's expectations. The ideal patient has a realistic view of the potential outcome. An appropriate assessment of the patient's expectations is warranted during this initial visit, as body dysmorphic disorder may be a consideration in some patients. Because this specific subset of patients may have poor satisfaction with cosmetic procedures, caution is advised before proceeding. One should use extreme caution when contemplating to provide augmentation for reasons other than restoring natural anatomic surfaces (Fig. 4-14). As for all procedures, it is best to obtain written informed consent after reviewing the risks, benefits, and alternatives. In particular, patients should be informed of the likelihood of swelling, bruising, and redness, as well as need for massage after the procedure.

It is of paramount importance to document and discuss any preexisting scars, subcutaneous volume differences between facial sides, and any other evidence of asymmetry. This should be discussed thoroughly with the patient prior to the procedure, as patients may not be aware of their naturally occurring asymmetries. It is helpful to point these out with a mirror and take several pictures prior to the procedure. Often, patients pay much more attention to their appearance after injection than they ever did before it. Many patients who return complaining of a lack of efficacy from the injection are convinced that the procedure has worked once you review their before and after photographs with them.

Depending on the type and location of injection, patients may want to defer treatment if they have an important public event within the next 2 weeks. Most patients can be treated the same day as the initial evaluation, provided they meet the preprocedure recommendations, unless they require a product that must be reconstituted

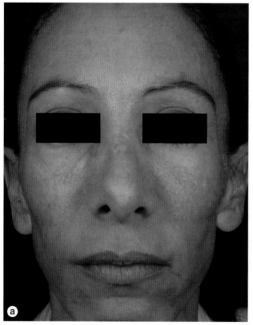
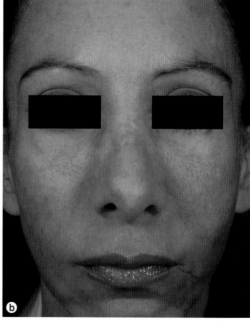

Figure 4-14 Augmentation of the zygomatic region performed by overzealous injection by a non-physician has resulted in an unnatural "chipmunk" appearance. The mid-cheek was later treated by a dermatologic surgeon to help "normalize" contour. (A) Before and (B) after treatment

before use. It is important to underline preprocedure preparation, such as avoidance of elective anticoagulant medications, vitamins, herbs, and supplements (Table 4-4). The decision to discontinue medically indicated anticoagulation, such as warfarin for thromboembolism prophylaxis or aspirin for the prevention of recurrent myocardial infarction, is not recommended as there are more complications due to morbidity for discontinuance versus bleeding from dermatologic procedures, according to a study by Otley in 2003. Although evidence is lacking for herpes simplex virus (HSV) prophylaxis, many practitioners routinely give antiviral prophylaxis for up to 2 days before and after lip augmentation, especially if the patient has a history of multiple recurrent cold sores.

Day of procedure

For many patients, a topical anesthetic may be applied under occlusion for 1 hour prior to injection of many facial sites. Use of ester-based compounds, such as betacaine or tetracaine, should be avoided in patients with a history of para-aminobenzoic acid (PABA) or sulfa allergy. Topical anesthesia is usually all that is needed to minimize discomfort for superficial injections using a small-bore needle; however, procedures around the lip, and fillers that require large-bore needles, may require injection of local anesthetic. Nerve blocks are often ideal in these situations because they preserve the architecture of the target area for injection – unlike field blocks, which sometimes disturb skin contours due to edema from infiltration.

Injection of fillers should be performed only on skin free of make-up and topical agents. This allows a more discriminate examination of the skin surface during the procedure and reduces the very small potential risk of foreign body implantation. Preparation should include the use of an antiseptic such as alcohol, which can be followed by chlorhexidine or chloroxylenol. Because chlorhexidine can cause keratitis and is ototoxic, cautious use around the eyes and ears is advised.

Postprocedure instructions should include application of cold packs intermittently to reduce swelling and bruising, particularly for periocular procedures. Some supplements that potentially decrease bruising, such as arnica and bromelain, have been advocated by some physicians. However, significant supporting data for this are lacking. Massage is an important part of the postoperative management for some fillers, such as Sculptra®. An easy regimen for patients to follow after Sculptra® is the "5-5-5" rule: massage area five times daily for 5 minutes at a time, for a duration of 5 days.

One consideration is to review new patients with filler 2 weeks after injection for assessment of their satisfaction, as well as photographs and potential "touch-up" procedures.

PEARLS

Nerve blocks can safely be performed in the office to achieve pain relief for multiple injection procedures such as lip augmentation.

Discontinuance of anticoagulant therapy should be weighed carefully, as the risk of thromboembolism outweighs the risk of bleeding complications.

Use of arnica, bromelain or vitamin K cream may potentially reduce postprocedure bruising, but data are lacking.

Table 4-4 Agents that increase the risk of bleeding

Medications	Herbs and supplements
Aspirin (and aspirin derivatives)	Arnica (when used with anticoagulants)
NSAIDs	Alcohol
Warfarin (Coumadin®)	Ginger
Clopidogrel (Plavix®)	Ginseng
Dipyrimadole (Aggrenox®)	Garlic
Cilostazole (Pletal®)	Gingko biloba
Ticlopidine (Ticlid®)	Kava kava
	Celery root
	Fish oils
	St John's wort
	Vitamin E
	Feverfew
	Dong quai

Product specifics

Key Points

- Xenographic collagen implantation requires a series of skin testing procedures to assess allergenicity before usage while human-derived collagens can be used the same day without any testing.
- Some injectables (Zyderm®, Zyplast®, Cosmoderm®, Cosmoplast®, ArteColl®) come pre-mixed with lidocaine and thus are contraindicated in patients with a true lidocaine allergy.
- Hylaform is hyaluronic acid that is generated from rooster combs and should not be used in patients with chicken or egg allergies.
- Non-animal hyalurons are derived from bacterial fermentation. Fascian™ may contain trace amounts of antibiotics (polymyxin B, bacitracin, or neomycin) and should not be used in patients with known allergies to these agents.

Collagen

Collagen implantation research began in 1958 by Gross and Kink at Harvard, who showed that a collagen gel could be formed by warming a solution of collagen. However, work toward clinical application did not begin until the 1970s, when elimination of the terminal telopeptides reduced immunogenicity and resulted in successful transplant in animal studies. The first human injection was in 1978, when 28 human subjects were successfully injected with collagen for the treatment of acne scars. Millions of patients have been injected successfully with collagen since it became available in the early 1980s as a treatment for rhytides.

There are three types of collagen fillers: animal-derived, human-derived, and bioengineered autologous collagen. Traditional bovine-derived collagens (Zyplast® and Zyderm®) are potentially immunogenic; skin testing is recommended before use. Thus, they cannot be used on the same day as consultation. Two negative skin tests over a 6-week period are recommended before treatment. For the first skin test, a purified protein derivative (PPD)-like test, is often performed near the antecubital fossa. Most positive results (erythema, induration) occur in the first 72 hours, but may take up to 4 weeks. The second skin test is placed at 4 weeks, often in the skin along the anterior scalp, or sometimes the contralateral arm. Less than 4% of patients will have a positive test, and less than 3% will have a reaction to collagen with a negative skin test. If a patient has gone for more than 1 year without treatment, a repeat skin test is recommended, with evaluation of the test site after 2 weeks. Hypersensitivity reactions usually occur within the first 2 weeks of product placement.

Zyderm® and Zyplast® collagen have been used longer than any other filler and are the standard to which all other injectable fillers are compared. They are bovine dermal-derived collagens that differ in the percentage of total collagen. Zyderm® I, approved in 1981, has 96% type I collagen and 4% type II collagen. The product has 3.5% bovine collagen by weight, suspended in phosphate-buffered saline. Some 2 years after its introduction, Zyderm® II, with a higher 6.5% collagen-containing suspension, was approved. Zyplast®, which contains crosslinked glutaraldehyde that extends its half-life and decreases inflammatory reactions, was introduced shortly afterwards. It has a concentration of 35 mg/mL and was designed for deeper placement.

All of these products are refrigerated and prepackaged in 1- or 2-mL syringes with a 30-gauge needle. Zyderm® is injected into the papillary dermis, with type I being approved for fine lines and wrinkles, and type II for moderate lines and deeper acne scars. Zyplast® is used for deep lines and can be injected from mid-dermis to subcutaneous fat. Because Zyderm® is diluted, overcorrection is needed. Overcorrection of 100% for Zyderm® I and 50% for Zyderm® II will offset absorption of saline. Zyplast® does not require overcorrection. Results with bovine collagen usually last for 3–5 months, with the longer time frame seen more in some areas of repeat use. The products contain 0.3% lidocaine, so are contraindicated in patients who have true lidocaine allergy. Many injectors layer Zyderm® over Zyplast® to address both superficial and deep lines, giving a more uniform result.

CosmoDerm® and CosmoPlast® are human-based allogeneic collagen developed to decrease immunogenicity and provide use without a skin test. They are the only FDA-approved human collagens for facial augmentation. They are generated from a single cell line of human foreskin-derived dermal fibroblasts that undergoes infectious disease testing routinely. The fibroblast cells are seeded onto a three-dimensional nylon mesh that develops into a dermal matrix. As the cells grow, collagen is secreted, and is isolated and then purified for injection.

As they are human derived, these products do not require skin testing. They come in prepackaged syringes that must be refrigerated. Like Zyderm®, CosmoDerm® II is twice the concentration of CosmoDerm® I. CosmoDerm® and CosmoPlast® are packaged in 1-mL syringes and mixed with 0.3% lidocaine. They have the same indications and overcorrection recommendations as Zyderm® and Zyplast®, and may be used simultaneously to correct defects of variable depths (Fig. 4-15). These products also similarly result in correction for 3–5 months. The most commonly reported adverse effect is flu-like symptoms (less than 4% of patients).

There are several cadaveric collagen products on the market as well, including Cymetra™ and Fascian™, although these have not gained widespread use. Cymetra™ is a micronized acellular dermal allograft that comes from approved tissue banks. It is viscous, requiring a large-bore needle. It can be used to treat nasolabial folds and depressed scars, and can sustain augmentation for as long as 9 months. It has the advantage of no skin testing requirement, but is less smooth owing to the large particle size, which involve pain for some patients.

Fascian™ is preserved, particulate, fascia lata. It has a very tight fibrillar collagen weave, making it a dense implant. Its effects last from 3 to 8 months. Because trace amounts of antibiotics (polymyxin B, bacitracin, or neomycin) exist, it should not be used in patients with sensitivity to these antibiotics. A larger bore needle is also required because the filler is so dense.

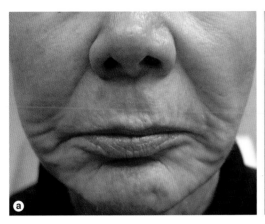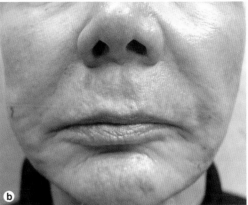

Figure 4-15 Use of Cosmoderm® and Cosmoplast® for lower facial rhytides. Superficial perioral fine lines were corrected with Cosmoderm®, while deeper rhytides were corrected with Cosmoplast®, (A) Before and (B) after treatment

Hyalurons

Hyaluronic acid (hyaluron, HA) is a naturally occurring glycosaminoglycan that is a component of all connective tissues. It does not contain any immunogenic epitopes and its structure does not vary between different tissues or between species. In humans, it is one of the primary constituents of synovial fluid between articular joints and vitreous humor. Its structure contains repeating disaccharide chains of D-glucuronic acid and N-acetyl-D-glucosamine that form long, polyanionic, unbranched polymers. Because of hydrogen binding, it is capable of binding 1000 times its weight in water. Thus, for every gram of HA, approximately 6 liters of water may be bound. The polymers can be broken down rapidly, with a half-life of 2–3 days. Stabilization through crosslinking creates a stiffer product with a long half-life that is suitable for soft tissue augmentation. Crosslinking processes vary between the available products. The higher the degree of crosslinking, the more solidified the product becomes. Thus, highly crosslinked material has a very long lifetime in tissue, but is very viscous.

Normal aging results in reduction of HA. This compromises water-binding capacity and decreases tissue turgor, contributing to the appearance of sagging skin and accentuation of skin folds. Hyaluronidases are tissue enzymes that break down HA, which is then further metabolized by the liver. A recent study by Averbeck et al. showed that ultraviolet B radiation decreases HA content in the dermis and increases the number of degradation products, suggesting that photo-damaged skin may have less dermal production of HA and upregulated hyaluronidase.

It has been suggested that the intense hygroscopic property of HA seen in vivo also exists with injection of HA fillers. Thus, the volume correction should be maintained even as the product is eliminated by the body until a critical HA concentration is reached (isovolemic degradation). This has been heavily disputed and most physicians agree that isovolemic degradation is not observed clinically over the life of the product. Although there is still intense water binding, volume correction does deplete relative to the amount of product remaining.

An additional benefit of HA is the potential to stimulate de novo collagen production. A study by Wang et al. showed synthesis of new collagen production in patients after injection into the forearm of photo-damaged skin. Biopsies and quantitative polymerase chain reaction were performed at 4 and 13 weeks after injection of either saline or cross-linked HA, and new collagen content was compared. At both time intervals, more new collagen was found in the HA-injected skin than in saline-injected samples.

There are several HA products on the market, including Restylane®, Perlane®, Juvéderm™, and Elevess™, along with the fading use of Captique™ and Hylaform® due to less longevity. The major distinction of these products is the source of HA and the polymerized particle size, which varies their clinical applications. The concentration of HA in each product is also different, partially explaining why different products have different residence time in tissue (higher concentration products last longer). However, depth of deposition and injection technique also affect length of time in tissue. Products also differ in the degree of hydration, degree of crosslinkage, percentage of free HA, concentration of HA, types of gel hardener, and homogenization of product.

Hylaform® is derived from rooster combs, and so is contraindicated in anyone with a chicken or egg allergy. It was approved for use in soft tissue augmentation in 2004, and is indicated for moderate to severe facial wrinkles and folds.

The target depth is mid-dermis, with a risk of dyschromia from superficial injection and a risk of lack of success from too deep an injection. Hylaform® is available in a prepackaged syringe with a 30-gauge needle. It lasts for approximately 3–4 months. The particles have a high molecular weight, but the product is formulated in a low concentration of 6 mg/mL. As it is less dense than Restylane®, it has the advantage of less bruising and being more diffusible. Hylaform® Plus is approved for the same indications, but has a larger particle size, making it more ideal for deeper implantation.

All other available HA products are nonanimal-derived products. These are generated through fermentation by streptococci, and are then stabilized by crosslinkage of glycosaminoglycan chains. They have a variety of particles sizes, resulting in indications for fine lines to deep folds, depending on the product. They have higher hydration levels than animal-derived products. For example, Hylaform® and Hylaform® Plus are at equilibrium when injected. Conversely, Restylane® and Juvéderm™ are relatively water deficient, such that the product will swell upon injection, giving longer lasting results.

Restylane®, also referred to as NASHA™ (nonanimal stabilized hyaluronic acid), contains 20 mg/mL of HA, with a particulate size of 100 000 particles per milliliter. Each particle is approximately 400 μm in size. 1,4-Butandiol diglycidyl ether is used to crosslink the HA, resulting in approximately 1% crosslinked. A 30-gauge needle comes prepackaged with the syringe. Restylane® has FDA approval for use in deep wrinkle reduction of the lip, glabellar creases, and nasolabial folds. The manufacturer also makes a similar product with a smaller particle size (200 000 per mL), called Restylane® Fine Line (FDA approval still pending). As it is less dense, this product can be injected with a 30-gauge needle and is more appropriate for superficial wrinkles.

Perlane® is another NASHA™ with a larger particle size of 8000 per mL that must be injected with a 27-gauge needle. Its main use is intended to correct deep rhytides and to enhance lip volume. These three NASHA™ products last for approximately 9 months. The most common side-effects are injection site reaction as well as local swelling and redness, which usually last for a few weeks; however, these side-effects can be more persistent in less than 0.05% of patients.

Captique™ is another bacterial-derived HA filler. It was approved for use in late 2004. It comes packaged in 1-mL syringes and is usually injected with a 30-gauge needle. It lasts for about 3–6 months. Although no controlled trials have compared it with Restylane®, anecdotal reports suggest that its longevity is shorter than that of Restylane®.

Juvéderm™ is one of the newest FDA-approved nonanimal-derived hyaluronic acid products on the market. It is indicated for injection into the mid–deep dermis for correction of moderate to severe facial wrinkles and folds, such as the nasolabial folds. It has a lifespan of at least 6 months, with a recent FDA extension indicating persistence in some patients of up to 1 year. It has one of the highest concentrations of crosslinked HA at 24 mg/mL. It is available in two formulations: Juvéderm™ Ultra and Juvéderm™ Ultra Plus. The latter has more crosslinkage and is indicated for the correction of deeper defects. Adverse effects are similar to those of other HA fillers. Its safety has been established up to 20 mL per 60 kg per year. Juvéderm™ Ultra comes prepackaged in syringes that are formulated for a single patient with a 30-gauge needle, whereas Juvéderm™ Ultra Plus is more viscous and is injected with a 27-gauge needle. It is stored at room temperature and freezing is contraindicated. Optimal results with either product can be obtained with a linear threading or serial puncture technique. There is no need for overcorrection, but touch-up injections may be useful in some patients. In the FDA study, the typical volume needed for augmentation of each nasolabial fold was found to be 1.6 mL.

Allergan performed a split-face study comparing adverse events and longevity of Juvéderm™ Ultra and Zyplast® in 146 patients for augmentation of nasolabial folds over a 24-week period. They found that both products had similar side-effect profiles, including redness, pain, firmness, swelling, lumpiness, and bruising, which occurred in more than half of the patients studied. At the end of the study period, 88% of patients maintained visible augmentation, compared with only 36% of patients treated with Zyplast®. Some 88% of patients polled preferred Juvéderm™ over Zyplast®.

Calcium hydroxylapatite

Hydroxylapatite is a hard, crystalline mineral composed of calcium, phosphate, and hydroxide ions that is the major constituent of mature bone. As it is an inorganic salt found in normal tissue, it has excellent biocompatibility. Hydroxylapatite has been used for more than 15 years as a reconstructive agent in orthopedic surgery, so has been well studied. It is formulated as microspheres that form a scaffold to which fibroblasts anchor and produce new collagen.

Radiesse® (formerly known as Radiance®) is the only product currently available in the USA that uses hydroxylapatite. It is manufactured as an aqueous gel solution that contains these microsphere fragments of calcium hydroxylapatite. The gel (composed of cellulose, glycerin, and water) provides immediate augmentation effects and must be degraded by macrophages to release the hydroxylapatite. This process usually take

2–3 months, at which time new collagen synthesis begins and attaches to the scaffold, which withstands degradation by macrophages for 1–2 years. Thus, this filler is not permanent, and has both immediate and gradual results.

It is FDA approved for the correction of wrinkles and folds around the nose and mouth, as well as for the treatment of lipoatrophy. The package insert states that the microspheres are between 25 and 45 μm in size. This large size impedes macrophage phagocytosis and lymphatic absorption. This leads to its durability. Once macrophages do degrade the matrix, the byproducts are just ions, thus there is limited inflammatory potential. The product is injected into the junction between dermis and subcuticular tissue, or into the deep dermis with a 27-gauge needle. Thus, it is an ideal agent for deeper placement, such as for mid-face augmentation or deeper scars. On average, it lasts approximately 9–14 months. As no lidocaine is mixed with the product, a nerve block should be considered for sensitive patients.

Much of the product (70%) is the gel vehicle, so fast metabolizers could potentially see a decrease in augmentation in the time before the new collagen is generated. In addition, as calcium is radioopaque, the product can potentially be detected with radiological imaging. However, one study by Tzikas et al. showed no interference of X-rays or computed tomography in the evaluation of facial structures with use of hydroxylapatite for augmentation purposes. The lack of interference is also consistent with a report by Carruthers to the FDA looking at hydroxylapatite recipients and radiographic imaging. Because of the large particle size and larger bore needle, excellent technique is critical to prevent clumping of product. Due to reports of delayed lip nodule formation, likely secondary to the mechanical pumping action of the orbicularis oris pushing the product toward the mucosa, this product is not recommended for use in the lips. Radiesse® comes prepackaged in 1.3- and 0.3-mL syringes.

Combination of collagen plus polymethylmethacrylate

ArteColl® is a unique filler that combines bovine collagen with polymethylmethacrylate (PMMA) microspheres. PMMA has been used since the 1950s in medical implants. It is a nonbiodegradable polymer that stimulates tissue fibroblasts to synthesize a capsule around the microspheres approximately 3 months after injection. The microspheres are approximately 20–40 μm in size and are suspended in 3.5% bovine collagen. Because of the bovine collagen, skin testing is required, with a reading after 4 weeks. The product also comes mixed with 0.3% lidocaine and sterile water, and is packaged in preloaded syringes.

The target depth of injection is a plane between the dermis and subcutaneous fat. A 27-gauge needle is used to inject the product. PMMA is not recommended for placement into the lips or fine rhytides, such as in the periorbital area, because of concern for visible nodularities.

In a summary of FDA trials by Cohen et al., more than 60% of patients maintained nasolabial fold augmentation for over 4 years. Because PMMA is not degraded, this is considered a permanent filler. A randomized controlled trial of 251 patients, which compared ArteColl® and bovine collagen (Zyderm® II/Zyplast®) with patient follow-up to 1 year, showed that success and satisfaction with ArteColl® was superior to that with bovine collagen.

ArteColl® has been used widely in Canada and Europe. It was the first generation of a PMMA/collagen microsphere filler. The major complication is granuloma formation, which is thought to result from some of the microspheres being small enough to be engulfed by macrophages, but insoluble enough not to decompose intracellularly. The product underwent reformulation to reduce size variability in the microspheres, to give a second generation that has a reduced incidence of granuloma formation. However, to be used in the USA, FDA approval requires that there be no more than 1% of particles sized less than 20 μm. Thus, a third-generation product was contrived; ArteFill® meets this mandate, with a particle size between 30 and 50 μm.

ArteFill® received FDA approval in October 2006, as the first and only nonresorbable filler available in the USA for use in nasolabial folds and smile lines. It is anticipated that this third-generation product will minimize the granuloma complications even further. Each ArteFill® kit contains three syringes of 0.8 mL and two of 0.4 mL. The product should be stored at 2–10°C and warmed to room temperature before use. A 26-gauge needle is used to deposit the product just above the dermis–subcutaneous interface with a tunneling technique that layers the filler as the needle is passed back and forth. One month after injection, particles are encapsulated by a thin layer of collagen as well as macrophages and fibroblasts. The bovine collagen is believed to be completely resorbed by 3 months after injection and replaced with newly synthesized collagen. Despite approval in 2006, some expert physician have advocated a need for both longer-term studies and histologic evaluation of the effects of this product after cutaneous implantation prior to widespread cosmetic use.

Poly-L-lactic acid

PLLA fillers are composed of α-hydroxy acid polymers with structure similar to that of absorbable suture (e.g. Vicryl™). Similar to hydroxylapatite,

PLLA causes both immediate and delayed augmentation. The immediate effects are due to edema from the fluid in the filler; however, this quickly resolves in 2–3 days, at which time the defect returns to baseline. Once the carrier substance is absorbed, macrophages begin to phagocytose the PLLA, similar to suture resorption. This launches an inflammatory cascade that promotes synthesis of new collagen fibers. As the PLLA is degraded to carbon dioxide and water over several weeks to months after injection, new type I collagen is deposited. By 6 months, less than half of the PLLA can be detected in tissue.

The only available preparation is Sculptra® (called New-Fill™ in Europe). This product is packaged as a freeze-dried powder that must be reconstituted with 5 mL of sterile water with a minimum hydration time of 4 hours before use, but many experienced injectors now reconstitute it several days before injection and keep it refrigerated so that it is available when needed. In addition, many injectors add lidocaine to the preparation a few hours before use. It is injected between the deep dermis and subcutaneous plane with a 26-gauge needle. It was approved by the FDA in 2004 for human immunodeficiency virus (HIV)-associated lipoatrophy of the cheeks. Off-label uses include non-HIV age related lipoatrophy in the cheeks, nasolabial fold and oral commissure. The risk of visible nodules seems to be most frequent when used in the infraorbital area (Fig. 4-16).

According to a study by Valantin et al., when used in patients with HIV infection to correct partial lipoatrophy, 50% reported some lumpiness, although they were satisfied with the augmentation. Foreign body granulomas have been well documented in these patients, particularly those on highly active antiviral therapy. One report by Murray et al. suggested that HIV therapy could restore immunocompetence enough to allow for these types of hypersensitivity reactions. To minimize the occurrence of nodules, post-injection massage is recommended, following the rule of "fives" (five times daily, 5 minutes at a time, 5 days' duration). Although this has become common practice, no studies have shown less nodularity in these patients compared with those who do not massage. Also, larger dilutions and deeper injections can reduce the risk of nodularity. Augmentation typically lasts for 1–2 years or more.

Silicone

Silicone is one of the most controversial and polarizing filling agents in use today. Liquid silicone has been used as a filling agent for decades. Silicone fluid, or polydimethylsiloxane, comes in two forms which have been approved for use by the FDA specifically for retinal detachment: AdatoSil®

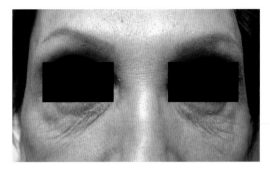

Figure 4-16 Lumpy appearance of infraorbital skin from injection of Sculptra® too superficially by a non-physician

5000 (Bausch & Lomb) and Silikon® 1000 (Alcon Laboratories). The number at the end of the brand name of the product refers to the viscosity in centistokes, with 100 cS defined as the viscosity of water. In facial augmentation, Silikon® 1000 is used by some aesthetic physicians (and sometimes AdatoSil®), although this use is considered off-label.

Silicone fillers have been linked to granuloma formation and nodules for many years. Excessive volumes have also resulted in filler migration. When using silicone, it is recommended to correct a specific area over several sessions using small volumes and microdroplet technique. Disastrous complications from the injection of adulterated, nonmedical grade silicone by inexperienced or unlicenced injectors have been widely publicized. However, when a pure, medical grade silicone is injected by an experienced aesthetic physician familiar with the microdroplet technique, the risk of significant problems is minimized. Potential complications from silicone still include granuloma and nodule formation, ulceration, migration, connective tissue disease, and infection.

On the horizon

Aquamid® is a gel containing 2.5% nonabsorbable crosslinked polyacrylamide that is currently available in Europe, Australia, South America, and the Middle East for the correction of nasolabial folds, mouth corners, perioral wrinkles, glabellar frown-line, and the contouring of chin, cheek, and vermillion borders. It is not FDA approved for use in the USA. It is a permanent filler with a half-life in the human body of more than 20 years. von Buelow et al. detailed a study showed that 93% of 228 patients followed for 12 months post-injection reported satisfactory or very satisfactory results. Unpublished reports of abscess formation in the area of the implant have begun to surface.

Belotero® is a crosslinked HA in a phosphate buffer available in 1-mL prefilled glass syringes.

The manufacturer markets the product as having a monophasic technology with variable density, allowing it to diffuse slightly to give a more smooth appearance post-injection, calling the process cohesive polydensified matrix (CPM) technology. By using a low, even injection pressure, the manufacture asserts that this technology allows for optimal distribution of product without loss of cohesiveness as well as mitigates the pain from implantation. The product is available in two varieties: Belotero® Soft and Belotero® Basic. Belotero® Soft comes in a concentration of 20 mg/mL designed for injection with a 30-gauge needle in the superficial to mid-dermis for the correction of shallow facial depressions, such as fine lines and crow's feet. Belotero® Basic has a higher concentration of 22.5 mg/mL and is more viscous, requiring injection with a 27-gauge needle. It is used to correct deeper wrinkles and for volume restoration of lips and cheeks. It is widely available in Europe but not yet FDA approved for use in the USA.

Evolence™ is an injectable matrix of highly crosslinked, homogeneous, type I porcine collagen. It is currently in phase III clinical trials by the FDA and has been used widely in Canada and Europe for the past few years. Crosslinking extends its life to at least 12 months. During processing, porcine collagen is cleaved with pepsin, then reactive "telopeptides" are removed, dramatically reducing its antigenic potential. With antigenic elements removed, the collagen is linked with ribose sugars into a matrix. Because of low antigenicity, the manufacturer is seeking FDA approval without use of skin testing. It is packaged in a prefilled syringe with a concentration of 35 mg/mL and is injected with a 27-gauge needle. Evolence™ does not require refrigeration. It is used for injection into the nasolabial folds, scars, atrophic areas, and skin graft contour deformities. It has an estimated longevity of 9–12 months. Evolence™ Breeze has a lower concentration of the product and is used with a 30-gauge needle to correct fine lines and medium wrinkles, as well as for lip augmentation.

Complications

Key Points

- Injectors must have a firm grasp of facial anatomy to reduce the risk of complications.
- Acute injection site reactions are the most common filler-associated complication.
- Contour irregularities occur mostly from placement of an improper volume at an inappropriate location or superficial depth.
- Injection of hyaluronidase can sometimes correct hyaluronic acid complications acutely; however, skin testing is required since the enzyme is animal-derived.

BOX 4-2

Potential adverse events associated with dermal fillers

Acute injection site reactions

Superficial or inappropriate placement

Sensitivity

Infection

Necrosis

Filler injections are associated with a wide range of potential complications (Box 4-2). Acute injection site reactions are the most commonly seen adverse event. One randomized-controlled trial by Narins et al. comparing Restylane® with Zyplast® found an event rate of over 90% reported by patients for both products. These reactions typically result in mild to moderate swelling or bruising. They usually last for less than 7 days. Because of the high frequency of bruising and swelling every patient should be informed of this risk regardless of product used. With avoidance of periprocedural nontherapeutic blood-thinning agents (see Table 4-4), this can often be minimized. In the authors' practice, patients taking Coumadin®, Plavix®, or therapeutic aspirin (due to a history of heart attack, stroke, blood clot, etc.) continue these agents as the risk of morbidity from cessation outweighs the benefit of avoiding bruising and swelling.

Inappropriate placement of any product can cause lumpiness, nodularity, or visibility of filler. When HA products are placed too superficially, a nodule with the Tyndall effect can occur, resulting in a visible bluish bump (Fig. 4-17A). Proper injection technique with appropriate depth of placement can minimize the risk of superficial nodules of product. Postprocedure massage (both in the office and at home) can mitigate the appearance of lumpiness.

When surface unevenness occurs with a HA filler, hyaluronidase can be injected to dissolve the HA product (Fig. 4-17B). However, because this is an animal-derived enzyme, skin testing is recommended with an intradermal injection of about 3 units of the enzyme. The patient should be observed for 20 minutes to look for an urticarial-type reaction before administering for corrective treatment. Two commercially available forms of hyaluronidase exist: Amphadase™ (Amphastar Pharmaceuticals, Rancho Cucamonga, CA, USA) and Vitrase® (Ista Pharmaceuticals, Irvine, CA, USA). There have also been reports of successful treatment with hyaluronidase for presumed angular artery impending necrosis after HA placement into the nasolabial folds.

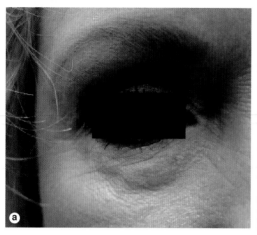
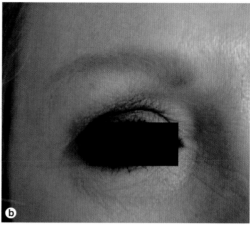

Figure 4-17 (A) Visible product placed too superficially in the nasojugal fold. (B) Correction with injection of hyaluronidase. Photograph reprinted from Hirsch RJ, Cohen JL. Skin Aging 2007;15(1):36–38, with permission of the publisher

Other filler products with which practitioners have also seen issues related to superficial placement include collagen/PMMA, PLLA, and hydroxylapatite. Collagen/PMMA, specifically ArteColl®, has been reported by some injected patients to cause pruritus, erythema, and (less frequently) hypertrophic scar reactions. Topical and intralesional corticosteroids may help itching and redness, while hypertrophic scars may be treated with a combination of intralesional steroids and pulsed dye laser.

Several reports have detailed nodule development after injection of PLLA. This is likely due to poor injection technique rather than being a purely hypersensitivity reaction. Several measures can reduce the risk of nodules. First, the product should be reconstituted with a high volume (mixed with 5 mL or more of sterile water, with 1 mL of lidocaine added prior to injection). Second, reconstitution times should be sufficient for complete dissolution, ideally 8 hours or more before injection. Finally, injections should be made into the high fat, avoiding injection of the precipitate at the end of the syringe.

The management of these nodules and papules due to PLLA depends on the onset. For early-onset nodules, treatment with subcision, sterile water injections, or simple massage may be effective. For later-onset nodules, injection with intralesional triamcinolone or 5-fluorouracil can be helpful, with adjuvant, daily, low-dose tetracycline. Some have also used prednisone to suppress nodularity. When considering intralesional steroid injection, larger concentrations may be required (40 mg/mL) for maximal results. A protocol has recently been published by Stewart et al., identifying treatment options to dissolve clinically apparent nodules of PLLA, especially in the infraorbital area.

Injection of hydroxylapatite too superficially has also resulted in several reports of the development of white nodules; shallow nodules can be treated with a no. 11 blade to nick the skin and express the nodule, or saline can be injected into the nodule to dilute it out. As mentioned, use of hydroxylapatite in the lip may be complicated over time by the migration of nodules due to movement of the orbicularis oris muscle, and thus is not recommended for lip augmentation.

As all fillers contain foreign substances, hypersensitivity reactions may be seen with any of these products. Animal-derived products carry the highest risks of hypersensitivity, given their presentation of xenographic epitopes to recipient immune cells. Bovine collagen injections have been associated with foreign body granulomas, with an incidence of 1.3% in one report from Raulin et al. Skin testing for sensitivity reduces these complications. Delayed granulomas have been seen in the bovine collagen/PMMA product and ArteColl® for up to 24 months after injection. Sensitivity reactions to human collagen have also been reported very rarely. Leonhardt et al. recently reported an angioedema-type reaction has been reported with a NASHA™. There have been a few reports of patients injected with HA who later developed painful, erythematous, inflammatory nodules. Figure 4-18 shows an algorithm for the management of what has been termed "angry red bumps." Some have suggested that inflammatory nodules result from a low-grade infection maintained within a biofilm surrounding the implant.

The potential for hypersensitivity reactions is increased, in theory at least, when patients wear make-up, as these substances can be implanted into the dermis during filler procedures. Thus, it is important for patients to be make-up free

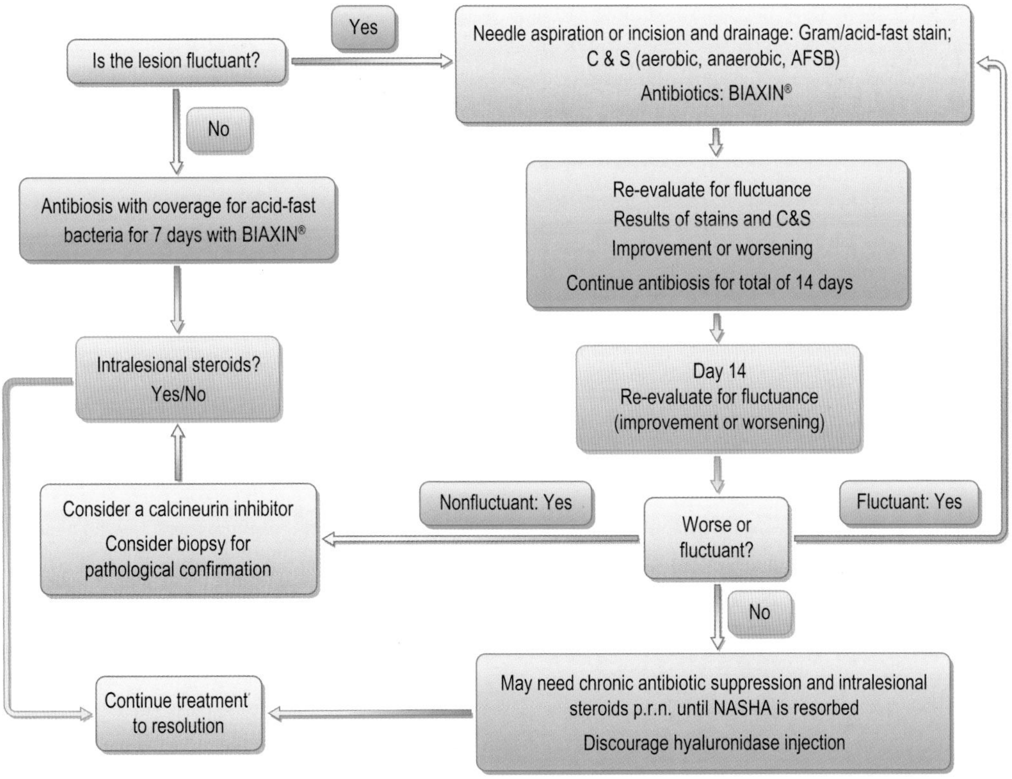

Figure 4-18 Algorithm for the management of angry red bumps. AFSB, aerobic spore-forming bacteria; C&S, culture and sensitivity; NASHA™, nonanimal stabilized hyaluronic acid. Redrawn from Narins RS, Jewell M, Rubin M, Cohen J, Strobos J. Dermatol Surg 2006;32(3):426–434, with permission of the publisher

at the time of injection. Additionally, patients may need to be aware of increased risk of these complications from unrelated proinflammatory medications after the procedure. One recent report by Fischer et al detailed a woman who developed sarcoid-type granulomas and disfiguring facial edema 10 years after injection with ArteColl® when she was treated with interferon and ribavirin for chronic hepatitis C infection. Although allopurinol was used with some success, the patient required several surgical revisions to restore cosmesis. Thus, it is important to counsel patients to include filler injection as part of their medical history when being interviewed by other healthcare practitioners.

Infection is a rare complication, but may be due to reactivation of a latent infection in the recipient or to inoculation with a contaminated product. The most common reactivation infection is herpes labialis (HSV). Contamination is more of a problem with the use of non-FDA-approved imported products. In 2002, there was an outbreak of nontuberculous *Mycobacterium* from injection with an illegal imported filler being used by a non-physician in New York City.

Injection of filler into a vessel or infiltration of tissue with sufficient volume to compress blood flow poses a risk of necrosis. The glabella is the site of necrosis that has been reported with most frequency, owing to compromise of branches from the supratrochlear artery. Precautions to reduce this risk include injecting medially and superficially, using low volumes with treatment spread over multiple sessions, and aspirating before injecting. In the event that vascular compromise is suspected, vasodilatation may be promoted by warm compresses or topical nitroglycerin. For HA fillers, injection of hyaluronidase, as reviewed above, may prevent impending necrosis or mitigate full necrosis. Injection of heparin may promote clot resorption in recalcitrant cases.

Further reading

Alam M, Yoo SS. Technique for calcium hydroxylapatite injection for correction of nasolabial fold depressions. J Am Acad Dermatol 2007;56(2): 285–289.

American Society for Aesthetic Plastic Surgery. Cosmetic Surgery National Data Bank Statistics, 2006. Available: http://www.surgery.org/download/2006stats.pdf (accessed 23 October 2007).

Averbeck M, Gebhardt CA, Voigt S, et al. Differential regulation of hyaluronan metabolism in the epidermal and dermal compartments of human skin by UVB irradiation. J Invest Dermatol 2007;127(3):687–697.

Benedetto AV, Lewis AT. Injecting 1000 centistoke liquid silicone with ease and precision. Dermatol Surg 2003;29(3):211–214.

Berlin A, Cohen JL, Goldberg DJ. Calcium hydroxylapatite for facial rejuvenation. Semin Cutan Med Surg 2006;25(3):132–137.

Carruthers JD, Carruthers A. Facial sculpting and tissue augmentation. Dermatol Surg 2005;31(Pt 2): 1604–1612.

Chang LK, Whitaker DC. The impact of herbal medicines on dermatologic surgery. Dermatol Surg 2001;27(8):759–763.

Christensen L, Breiting V, Janssen M, Vuust J, Hogdall E. Adverse reactions to injectable soft tissue permanent fillers. Aesthetic Plast Surg 2005;29(1):34–48.

Cohen JL, Berlin AL. Challenge: injecting fillers in the infraorbital area. Skin Aging 2007;15(10):28–29.

Cohen JL, Hirsch RJ. Challenge: correcting a downturned smile. Skin Aging 2006;14(2):52–53.

Cohen SR, Berner CF, Busso M, et al. ArteFill: a longlasting injectable wrinkle filler material – summary of the US Food and Drug Administration trials and a progress report on 4- and 5-year outcomes. Plast Reconstr Surg 2006;118(3):64S–76S.

Cohen SR, Holmes RE. ArteColl: a long-lasting injectable wrinkle filler material. Report of a controlled, randomized, multicenter clinical trial of 251 subjects. Plast Reconstr Surg 2004;114(4):964–976.

Cooperman LS, Mackinnon V, Bechler G, Phariss BB. Injectable collagen: a six-year clinical investigation. Aesthetic Plast Surg 1985;9(2):145–151.

Eppley BL, Dadvand B. Injectable soft-tissue fillers: clinical overview. Plast Reconstr Surg 2006;118(4):98e–106e.

Fischer J, Metzler G, Schaller M. Cosmetic permanent filler for soft tissue augmentation: a new contraindication for interferon therapy. Arch Dermatol 2007;143(4):507–510.

Food and Drug Administration Executive Summary, 2006. Radiesse for Soft Tissue Augmentation for the Treatment of HIV-Associated Facial Lipoatrophy: Radiological evaluation of short-term and long-term implantation of Radiesse in the face, protocol numbers 1205191 and 0106198, pp23–28. Available: http://www.fda.gov/ohrms/dockets/AC/06/briefing/2006-4233b1_02.pdf (accessed 30 October 2007).

Friedman PM, Mafong EA, Kauvar AN, Geronemus RG. Safety data of injectable nonanimal stabilized hyaluronic acid gel for soft tissue augmentation. Dermatol Surg 2002;28(6):491–494.

Glaich AS, Cohen JL, Goldberg LH. Injection necrosis of the glabella: protocol for prevention and treatment after use of dermal fillers. Dermatol Surg 2006;32(2):276–281.

Hirsch RJ, Cohen JL. Surgical insights: correcting superficially placed hyaluronic acid. Skin Aging 2007;15(1):36–38.

Hirsch RJ, Cohen JL, Carruthers JD. Successful management of an unusual presentation of impending necrosis following a hyaluronic acid injection embolus and a proposed algorithm for management with hyaluronidase. Dermatol Surg 2007;33(3):357–360.

Hirsch RJ, Lupo M, Cohen JL, Duffy D. Delayed presentation of impending necrosis following soft tissue augmentation with hyaluronic acid and successful management with hyaluronidase. J Drugs Dermatol 2007;6(3):325–328.

Lemperle G, Morhenn V, Charrier U. Human histology and persistence of various injectable filler substances for soft tissue augmentation. Aesthetic Plast Surg 2003;27(2):354–366.

Lemperle G, Romano JJ, Busso M. Soft tissue augmentation with ArteColl: 10-year history, indications, techniques, and complications. Dermatol Surg 2003;29(6):573–587.

Leonhardt JM, Lawrence N, Narins RS. Angioedema acute hypersensitivity reaction to injectable hyaluronic acid. Dermatol Surg 2005;31(5):577–579.

Maloney BP, Murphy BA, Cole HP. Cymetra. Facial Plast Surg 2004;20(2):129–131.

Manna F, Dentini M, Desideri P, DePita O, Mortilla E, Maras B. Comparative chemical evaluation of two commercially available derivatives of hyaluronic acid used for soft tissue augmentation. J Eur Acad Dermatol Venereol 1999;13(3):183–192.

Monheit GD. Hyaluronic acid fillers: Hylaform and Captique. Facial Plast Surg Clin North Am 2007;15(1):77–84.

Murray CA, DeKoven J, Spaner DE. Foreign body granuloma: a new manifestation of immune restoration syndrome. J Cutan Med Surg. 2003 Jan-Feb;7(1):38-42.

Narins RS, Beer K. Liquid injectable silicone: a review of its history, immunology, technical considerations, complications, and potential. Plast Reconstr Surg 2006;118(3S):77S–84S.

Narins RS, Bowman PH. Injectable skin fillers. Clin Plast Surg 2005;32(2):151–162.

Narins RS, Brandt F, Leyden J, Lorenc ZP, Rubin M, Smith S. A randomized, double-blind, multicenter comparison of the efficacy and tolerability of Restylane versus Zyplast for the correction of nasolabial folds. Dermatol Surg 2003;29(6):588–595.

Narins RS, Jewell M, Rubin M, Cohen J, Strobos J. Clinical conference: management of rare events following dermal fillers – focal necrosis and angry red bumps. Dermatol Surg 2006;32(3):426–434.

Oguzkurt L, Kizilkilic O, Tercan F, Turkoz R, Yildirim T. Vertebrocarotid collateral in extracranial carotid artery occlusions: digital subtraction angiography findings. Eur J Radiol 2005;53(2):168–174.

Orentreich DS. Liquid injectable silicone: techniques for soft tissue augmentation. Clin Plast Surg 2000;27(4):595–612.

Otley CC. Continuation of medically necessary aspirin and warfarin during cutaneous surgery. Mayo Clin Proc 2003;78(11):1392–1396.

Raulin C, Greve B, Hartschuh W, Soegding K. Exudative granulomatous reaction to hyaluronic acid (Hylaform). Contact Dermatitis 2000;43(3):178–179.

Sadick N. Soft tissue augmentation: selection, mode of operation, and proper use of injectable agents. J Cosmet Dermatol 2007;20(5):S8–S13.

Schanz S, Schippert W, Ulmer A, Rassner G, Fierlbeck G. Arterial embolization caused by injection of hyaluronic acid (Restylane®). Br J Dermatol 2002;146(5):928–929.

Stewart DB, Morganroth GS, Mooney MA, Cohen J, Levin PS, Gladstone HB. Management of visible granulomas following periorbital injection of poly-l-lactic acid. Ophthal Plast Reconstr Surg 2007;23(4):298–301.

Stolman LP. Human collagen reactions. Dermatol Surg 2005;31(Pt 2):1634.

Toy BR, Frank PJ. Outbreak of *Mycobacterium abscessus* infection after soft tissue augmentation. Dermatol Surg 2003;29(9):971–973.

Tzikas TL. Evaluation of the Radiance FN soft tissue filler for facial soft tissue augmentation. Arch Facial Plast Surg 2004;6(4):234–239.

Valantin MA, Aubron-Olivier C, Ghosn J, et al. Polylactic acid implants (New-Fill) to correct facial lipoatrophy in HIV-infected patients: results of the open-label study VEGA. AIDS 2003;17(17):2471–2477.

Vleggaar D. Facial volumetric correction with injectable poly-l-lactic acid. Dermatol Surg 2005;31(Pt 2):1511–1518.

von Buelow S, von Heimburg D, Pallua N. Efficacy and safety of polyacrylamide hydrogel for facial soft-tissue augmentation. Plast Reconstr Surg 2005;116(4):1137–1146.

Wang F, Garza LA, Kang S, et al. In vivo stimulation of de novo collagen production caused by cross-linked hyaluronic acid dermal filler injections in photodamaged human skin. Arch Dermatol 2007;143(2):155–163.

Chemical peels

Divya Singh-Behl and Rebecca Tung

- Synonyms include chemical resurfacing, chemoexfoliation, chemosurgery.
- Definition: chemical peeling involves the application of a chemical agent that results in exfoliation of skin followed by regrowth of new skin leading to skin rejuvenation.
- Types of peel include very superficial, superficial, medium, and deep.
- Indications include photo-damage, rhytides, dyschromias, epidermal growths, acne scars.
- Recovery time and complications increase with depth of peel.
- Chemical peeling is a technique-dependent procedure; rarely, complications including prolonged erythema, milia, infection scarring, can occur.

Introduction

Skin resurfacing procedures utilizing chemical exfoliation agents have been used for thousands of years. Ancient Egyptians first applied sour milk baths, other fruit acids, and oils for cosmetic skin renewal. However, it was not until 1882 that German dermatologist Unna reported on the unique peeling properties of trichloroacetic acid (TCA), phenol, resorcinol, and salicylic acid. By the middle of the 20th century, physicians had effectively learned to use phenol and TCA peels for facial rejuvenation and the improvement of acne scarring. The much popularized, no downtime, "lunchtime peels" with superficial agents such as α-hydroxy acid (AHA) became widely available by the late 1980s. Even in today's era of lasers, light, and energy sources, the proven safety and efficacy of chemical peels has secured their position in the armamentarium of the cosmetic dermatologist.

Chemical peeling is defined as the application of a topical agent to the skin that results in a variable degree of injury to the epidermis and dermis, depending on type and strength of the chemical. The peel produces a controlled partial-thickness exfoliation followed by second-intention wound healing. The injured epidermis and dermis is regenerated by migration of uninvolved adjacent epithelium and adnexal structures. The end result of this process is an improvement in skin texture, color, superficial wrinkles, and resolution of epidermal growths.

Classification of peels is based on the histologic depth of penetration (Table 5-1)

Preoperative evaluation

- Determination of patient's cosmetic concerns and goals.
- Discussion of downtime and budget.
- Informed consent outlining details of the procedure, common side-effects, recovery time, and wound care.
- Assessment of skin type – Fitzpatrick class.
- Degree of photo-damage – Glogau class.

Consultation

At the initial consultation, it is essential for you and the patient to identify cosmetic concerns, set realistic goals, review downtime issues, and discuss the budget.

Careful analysis of the patient's skin with respect to skin type, amount of pigmentation, and extent of photo-aging is the starting point of the rejuvenation process. The Fitzpatrick classification system standardizes patient assessment by assigning grades from I to VI based on the amount of skin pigmentation and the ability to tan (Table 5-2). This classification can also be used to extrapolate a patient's sensitivity to skin care products, exfoliating agents, and tendency to develop hyperpigmentation after a procedure. Although all skin types require daily broad-spectrum sun protection before and after peeling to reduce the risk of pigmentation abnormalities, patients with skin types I and II have little risk of developing postprocedural dyschromia.

Superficial peels are considered safe for all skin types, but pigmentary complications can be significant with medium to deep peels in patients

Table 5-1 Classification of chemical peels

Type	Target
Superficial	Epidermis to papillary dermis (0.06 mm)
Medium	Papillary to upper reticular dermis (0.45 mm)
Deep	Midreticular dermis (0.6 mm)

Table 5-2 Fitzpatrick skin types

Type	Color	Reaction to sun
I	Very white	Always burns, rarely tans
II	White	Usually burns, rarely tans
III	White–olive	Sometimes burns, average tan
IV	Brown	Rarely burns, usually tans
V	Dark brown	Very rarely burns, usually tans
VI	Black	Never burns, always tans

Table 5-3 Glogau photo-aging classification

Type	Age range (years)	Photo-damage
I – Mild	Usually 28–35	Little or no wrinkling
		No actinic keratosis
		Little or no need for make-up
II – Moderate	Usually 35–50	Early wrinkling
		Early actinic keratosis
		Need for make-up; sallow color
III – Advanced	Usually 50–65	Persistent wrinkles
		Actinic keratosis
		Always uses make-up
		Yellow discoloration and telangiectasias
IV – Severe	Usually 60 to ≥75	Wrinkle at rest
		Actinic damage
		Always uses make-up, but with poor coverage

with darker skin types III–VI. In these predisposed patients, the use of bleaching agents in both the preoperative and postoperative period may prevent postinflammatory hyperpigmentation.

The effectiveness of hydroquinone in the preoperative period is still controversial. When postinflammatory hyperpigmentation develops after resurfacing, studies have confirmed that prompt treatment with bleaching agents such as hydroquinone can speed its resolution.

The sebaceous quality of the patient's skin should also be noted, as increased sebaceous activity can result in diminished effectiveness of exfoliating agents.

The degree of photo-damage is best measured by means of the Glogau classification system (Table 5-3), which stratifies patients into categories I–IV based on the amount of wrinkling, actinic damage, and the need to use concealing make-up:

- Group 1 patients are younger and have minimal photo-aging which is amenable to treatment with superficial peels.
- Group 2 patients have moderate signs of sun damage and are excellent candidates for medium-depth peels.
- Group 3 patients have advanced photo-aging and require at least a medium depth to deep peel for improvement, but may also benefit from targeted ablative laser (carbon dioxide) resurfacing.
- Group 4 patients have severe photo-damage, so a combination approach consisting of surgical lifting (full or partial rhytidectomy) and medium to deep chemical peeling will best address rejuvenation needs.

During the consultation, the physician should clearly delineate what the patient should expect during the procedure and in the postoperative period. Limitations and potential side-effects of the proposed peel should also be discussed. Additionally, patients need to be informed that chemical resurfacing alone may not be able completely to address deeper wrinkles, significant skin laxity, prominent scars, or enlarged pore size. At this point in the conversation, you have a wonderful opportunity to explain how various other minimally invasive procedures (e.g. fillers, botulinum toxin, microdermabrasion, lasers and other devices) may be used in combination with peels for more dramatic rejuvenation. Often, new patients want to start out with a series of light peels regardless of their degree of sun damage in order to become more familiar with your practice, but will graduate to your recommended treatment plan, and even request additional procedures, once they feel comfortable.

The authors find that giving patients a written overview of the proposed peeling procedure, listing indications and frequently asked questions, allows them to plan and prepare with full understanding. Patients also like to see before and after sequential photographs. These images underscore any temporary lifestyle modifications that they may need to make. Detailed written postoperative instructions can maximize cosmetic outcome and avoid any potential side-effects. This regimen includes proper wound care, sun avoidance, and compliance with postoperative medications.

Although superficial peels can be considered pain free, procedural comfort issues during medium and deep peels should also be addressed. Many patients opt to take an oral sedative (e.g. diazepam) before medium-depth peels.

All patients undergoing medium and deep peels should have preoperative and postoperative photographs taken to document the baseline extent of solar damage, scarring, and rhytides, and to demonstrate the degree of improvement.

A signed informed consent form should outline the risks, benefits, alternatives, and limitations associated with chemical peeling. Expected responses to peels include burning and stinging sensations, redness, and peeling. Less common effects following medium and deep peels include prolonged erythema, abnormal pigmentation. Rarely, infection, delayed healing, or scarring may result. Alternative resurfacing procedures such as microdermabrasion, dermabrasion, nonablative and ablative resurfacing lasers should also be mentioned.

Patient evaluation

Key Points

- Take a complete medical, surgical, and psychosocial history along with a skin examination, current and previous medications.
- Photography: consent for before and after photos.

During the evaluation, discussion of relevant history and a careful physical examination are critical to assess the patient's skin problems and to identify any factors that may result in suboptimal results and complications (Box 5-1). The authors suggest having the patient fill out a short questionnaire prior to the consultation regarding their past medical and surgical history, and medications. Pertinent historical details include therapy with oral isotretinoin in the past year or invasive facial surgery within the last 6 months. A time interval of 12 months after isotretinoin therapy is recommended prior to medium-depth peeling. Similarly, resurfacing should be delayed by at least 6 months in patients who have undergone major surgery. Isotretinoin produces atrophy of the pilosebaceous units and can result in delayed

---

BOX 5-1

Patient evaluation

Medication: isotretinoin, minocycline

Active infection

History of radiation to head and neck

History of infections: herpes simplex virus and others

History of keloid formation

History of immunosuppression

Recent facial surgery

---

wound healing and abnormal scarring. Similarly, significant undermining of the underlying soft tissues, as is commonly performed during flap reconstruction and invasive cosmetic facial surgery (i.e. rhytidectomy), can temporarily compromise the blood supply and lead to impaired wound healing.

Patients should also be questioned about active or previous herpes simplex virus (HSV), bacterial, and fungal infections. Current infection is an absolute contraindication to all types of peeling. Medium to deep peels can reactivate HSV during the healing period, creating slow healing and unwanted scarring. For this reason, all patients, regardless of herpetic history, undergoing medium to deep peels should be given prophylaxis with an antiviral medication.

A history of human immunodeficiency virus infection, hepatitis, or immunosuppression due to systemic disease or medications should also be identified as there is a greater risk of infection and its untoward effects in these patients.

Past exposure to radiation in the head or neck is also relevant. Therapeutic irradiation diminishes the number of pilosebaceous units in treated areas and places these patients at increased risk for the development of postoperative scarring. Adnexal structure integrity can be assessed by observing the presence of vellus hairs or by punch biopsy to ensure appropriate re-epithelialization.

Similarly, any history of abnormal scar formation, keloids, warrants extra caution. Patients with ongoing skin disorders such as rosacea, atopic or seborrheic dermatitis should be counseled regarding possible disease exacerbation, prolonged erythema, and hypersensitivity dermatitis following chemical peeling. Test spots treating a small area may be useful to see how the skin responds. Patients taking oral contraceptives, hormone supplementation or minocycline should be alerted that these medications can lead to increased sun sensitivity and predispose to the development of postinflammatory hyperpigmentation. The need for sun avoidance in the postpeel period and

BOX 5-2

Absolute contraindications for medium to deep chemical peels

Open wounds, excoriations

Active infections such as herpes simplex virus and others

Isotretinoin therapy in past 6 months

Pregnancy

Unrealistic expectations, emotional instability

Poor physician–patient relationship

BOX 5-3

Relative contraindications for medium to deep chemical peels

Recent facial surgery in past 6 months

History of keloids or any abnormal scar formation

History of postinflammatory hyperpigmentation

History of irradiation of the head and neck

Fitzpatrick type IV–VI

History of active cutaneous skin disorders, rosacea, atopic or contact dermatitis, seborrheic dermatitis

BOX 5-4

Preoperative patient preparation

Prepeel regimen can maximize cosmetic results and minimize complications

Sun avoidance and broad-spectrum sunscreens with sun protection factor (SPF) 30 or more

Retinoids: tretinoin, tazarotene, adapalene, or retinol

α-Hydroxy acids (AHAs)

Hydroquinones – may reduce the incidence of postinflammatory hyperpigmentation

Antiviral prophylaxis – all patients before a medium or deep peel

Sun avoidance and sunscreens

Key Points

- Avoidance of the midday sun: 10am to 4pm.
- Physical sunscreens are ideal for active outdoor patients or those with a sensitive skin.
- Chemical or combination sunscreens are a good option for patients with limited outdoor exposure.
- Sun protective gear – hats, sunglasses, clothing.

The best defense for combating the signs of aging due to ultraviolet light is prevention. Application of sunscreen is an integral part of a proper skin care regimen. Although complete avoidance of sun is unrealistic, patients should be advised to avoid intense midday sun from 10am to 4pm. In the context of chemical peels, the central purpose of the sunscreen is to reduce baseline pigmentation and minimize potential dyschromia in the postoperative period. Sunscreens that block both ultraviolet (UV) B and UVA should be selected. Extra protection in the UVA range is particularly important as these wavelengths cause tanning and hyperpigmentation. Newer chemical ingredients, such as ecamsule (Mexoryl®) and stabilized avobenzone (Helioplex™), and physical agents (titanium dioxide and zinc oxide) provide more complete protection in the UVA range. A broad-spectrum sunscreen, preferably with sun protection factor (SPF) 30 or above, should be used for at least 2–3 months before the peel, and should become a daily part of the skin care regimen after the peel.

Retinoids

Key Points

- Retinoids are classified as superficial peeling agents.
- Pretreatment with tretinoin accelerates healing after peels.
- Nightly application, starting 6 weeks prior to peel.
- Delay peel if there is active retinoid dermatitis.

regular application with broad-spectrum sunscreens should be emphasized.

Active smoking independently contributes to premature skin aging. It also causes vasoconstriction of small blood vessels to the skin, leading to delayed healing and an increased risk of infection. Smoking also impairs the collagen and elastic fibers, presenting clinically as accelerated solar and actinic damage and increased wrinkling. Although chemical peels can be performed in smokers, they should be forewarned that the results may not be so dramatic.

Overall, superficial chemical peels are safe in all skin types, well tolerated, and considered to be low risk. However, if a patient has an open wound or active infection, the peel should be rescheduled. However, there are absolute and relative contraindications to medium and deep chemical peels, as outlined in Boxes 5-2 and Box 5-3.

Preoperative patient preparation

Starting patients on a good skin care regimen is essential prior to chemical peeling. Box 5-4 lists the factors that may play an important role in optimizing the outcome of chemical peels. These are discussed individually below.

Histologic effects of retinoids

Increased epidermal thickness

Thinned stratum corneum

Increased angiogenesis

Restoration and increased synthesis of collagen, and decreased elastosis

Increase in epidermal and dermal mucin

Decrease in epidermal melanin

Types of α-hydroxy acid

Glycolic acid

Lactic acid

Malic acid

Tartaric acid

Citric acid

Mandelic acid

Histologic effects of α-hydroxy acids

Thin the stratum corneum

Increase the thickness of the photo-aged atrophic epidermis

Thickening of dermis associated with increased production of glycosaminoglycans and collagen

Disperse melanin pigmentation

Reverse of basal cell atypia

The American Academy of Dermatology (AAD) has developed guidelines of the care for chemical peeling. They recommend pretreatment of the skin with tretinoin as well as postoperative tretinoin to promote faster wound healing and maintain cosmetic benefits.

The histologic effects of retinoids are shown in Box 5-5. Clinically, these changes can be seen as an improvement in fine lines and wrinkles, texture, overall color, and pigmentation of the skin. Numerous retinoid products are available, both by prescription and over the counter.

Pretreatment with tretinoin has been shown to speed epidermal healing in patients undergoing any resurfacing procedure. By thinning the stratum corneum, it also increases absorption of the peeling agent. Patients should start using a tretinoin or other tolerated retinoid on a nightly based at least 6 weeks before the chemical peel. Patients with more severely damaged skin and nonsensitive skin can be started on stronger agents, such as tretinoin microgel 0.1% or tazarotene 0.1% cream. Renova® 0.02% should be used as the initial agent in patients with dry, sensitive skin, and increased to a stronger agent based on tolerability. Combining serial glycolic acid peels with topical treatments (adapalene and azelaic acid) improves recalcitrant melasma significantly, compared with topical therapy alone.

Retinoids should be stopped at least 48 h before a peel to ensure an intact epidermal surface. In darker skinned patients, tretinoin increases the depth of peeling agents and the possibility of postinflammatory hyperpigmentation. For this reason, tretinoin may be discontinued as early as 2–4 weeks before a series of chemical peels in at-risk patients. If a patient has active retinoid dermatitis, the peel should be delayed until the inflammation subsides. Tretinoin can be restarted in the postoperative period when erythema has subsided and complete re-epithelialization has occurred.

α-Hydroxy acids

Key Points

- AHAs are naturally occurring acids.
- Strength of the acid is determined by pH.
- They are available in a variety of different vehicles.
- Begin an agent in a low concentration (8–15%) at least 2 weeks before the peel.

The benefits of AHAs on photo-damaged skin are well documented. Box 5-6 lists some commonly known AHAs. The main cosmetic outcomes include moisturization (causing skin to hold onto water), normalization of stratum corneum exfoliation (decreased scales at the surface with better light reflectance, flexibility, and texture), thickening of the epidermis and dermis with increased collagen and mucopolysaccharide synthesis (plumping of fine wrinkles and increased perceived firmness), and dispersal of melanin (promotion of even pigmentation) (Box 5-7). AHAs are useful both as peeling agents and in at-home products designed for use before and after peels.

The clinical response depends on a variety of different factors, including the pH of the specific acid, contact time with the skin (wash off versus leave on), body site, skin condition for which the AHA is being used, the vehicle (cream, lotion, gel), and free acid availability to the skin.

Preparations are available in many vehicles, including creams, lotions, gels, cleansers, and solutions. Products dispensed for home use are typically closer to the natural pH of the skin, which is around 4.2–5.6. The formulations are prepared by using a specific concentration of the particular acid dissolved in the corresponding vehicle. However, formulations with the same concentration of a specific acid are sometimes neutralized with ammonium hydroxide or sodium hydroxide to minimize irritation. This buffering leads to an increase in the product's pH and decreased efficacy of the active agent.

Long-term use of mild preparations of glycolic acid (8%) has been shown to result in a significant improvement of dyschromia, overall sun damage, fine rhytides, and sallowness. It is recommended that a low concentration of a glycolic acid product, between 8% and 15%, is used for at least 2 weeks before the glycolic acid peel. The patient should be instructed to start with the lower concentration and increase as tolerated. As with retinoids, patients should be instructed to discontinue at-home AHA products at least 48 h prior to peels. AHAs can also be safely used in combination with retinoids, with no increase in side-effects. Some studies have suggested possible increased photosensitivity with prolonged use of AHAs, but others have demonstrated a photoprotective effect. The authors always advise that patients continue to use a broad-spectrum sunscreen regularly in conjunction with an AHA program.

Bleaching agents

Hydroquinones are the most commonly used bleaching agents; other products include azelaic acid, aloesin, vitamin C, arbutin, licorice extract, glabridin, mequinol (4-hydroxyanisol), melatonin, niacinamide, paper mulberry, soy, vitamin E, kojic acid, α- and β-hydroxy acids, and retinoids and retinoid combination therapy. In practice, many clinicians recommend both pre- and post-treatment with bleaching agents to minimize the risk of postinflammatory hyperpigmentation in at-risk patients. If postinflammatory hyperpigmentation does develop after a peel, prompt treatment with a bleaching cream such as hydroquinone, or a combination product such as Tri-Luma® (hydroquinone 4% plus tretinoin 0.05% fluocinolone acetonide 0.01%) or Glyquin XM® (hydroquinone 4% plus glycolic 10% acid plus sunscreen) is very effective. Alternating usage of hydroquinone in 4-month cycles with one of the natural depigmenting agents can prevent or reduce the possibility of side-effects such as irritation or even exogenous ochronosis.

Antiviral agent prophylaxis

Key Points

- Not usually necessary for superficial peels.
- Strongly recommended for a medium to deep peel.
- Most common regimen: valaciclovir 500 mg, one tablet twice daily, starting 1 day before the procedure and continuing for 10–14 days afterwards.

There is a significant morbidity associated with a herpetic breakout in the postoperative period of patients undergoing resurfacing procedures. Antiviral prophylaxis is effective at reducing reactivation of HSV following resurfacing and is therefore recommended for all patients undergoing medium full-face to deep peels. As superficial peels do not induce significant injury to reactivate HSV, antiviral prophylaxis is not required. An active herpetic outbreak is an absolute contraindication to any type of peeling and mandates rescheduling of the procedure to a later date.

The most common prophylaxis regimen entails valaciclovir (either 500 mg twice daily or 1 g once daily), commencing 1 day before the peel and continuing for 10–14 days afterwards. When this regimen was used in one study, no episodes of active herpes infection or recurrence in patients undergoing laser resurfacing were found. In another study, a similar HSV prophylaxis regimen of famciclovir (250 mg twice daily) starting 1 day before carbon dioxide resurfacing and continuing for 14 days, reported no reactivation of HSV in any patient. The longer course of therapy is needed because the risk of infection is greatest once re-epithelialization begins, and continues to remain high until healing is complete.

Superficial chemical peels

Key Points

- Discuss with patient the expectations and potential limitations.
- Indications for superficial peels include photoaging, early actinic damage, mild acne, rosacea, lentigines, ephelides, melasma, and postinflammatory hyperpigmentation.
- A series of sessions is recommended; periodic maintenance sessions are suggested.
- Superficial peels cause partial- to full-thickness epidermal injury, occasionally extending to the papillary dermis.
- Depth of penetration and subsequent efficacy depends on several factors.

Owing to their easy application, minimal downtime, low complication rate, relatively low cost, and established safety profile in all Fitzpatrick

BOX 5-8

Advantages of superficial peels

Easy application

Minimal downtime

Low complication rate

Inexpensive

Safe to use in all Fitzpatrick skin types

Multiple sessions result in optimal results

BOX 5-10

Superficial peeling agents

α-Hydroxy acids: 20–70% glycolic acid peels

β-Hydroxy acids: salicylic acid peels (20–30%)

Trichloroacetic acid peels (10–25%)

Jessner's solution

Tretinoin

Solid carbon dioxide slush/liquid nitrogen

BOX 5-9

Indications for superficial peels

Photo-aging

Early actinic damage

Mild acne and rosacea

Lentigines and ephelides

Melasma and postinflammatory hyperpigmentation

Dyschromia

BOX 5-11

Factors influencing depth of superficial chemical peel

Agent used

Concentration of agent used

Preoperative treatment of skin with tretinoin

Skin preparation technique

Application technique

Frequency of treatments

Location of treatment

Sebaceous density at treatment site

skin types, superficial peels have gained tremendous popularity (Box 5-8). Although aggressive marketing of "light peels" to the public has created some degree of misconception and unrealistic expectations, the consultation visit allows you to reorient patients to anticipated benefits and potential limitations of superficial peels. Box 5-9 lists the indications for superficial peels.

It should be emphasized to the patient that a series of chemical peels, typically four to five, in conjunction with an ongoing at-home topical regimen is necessary to obtain and preserve the desired cosmetic result. Furthermore, a maintenance peel, once a season, is usually recommended for photo-damage, acne, and melasma. Patients should also understand that, although multiple superficial peels can improve mild sun damage and other superficial conditions, medium-depth peels are better suited to address more advanced photo-aging, deeper rhytides, and acne scarring.

Several different agents can be used for superficial peeling (Box 5-10). To minimize untoward effects, outdoor and indoor tanning should be avoided, and regular use of a broad-spectrum sunscreen is advocated. Conditioning of the skin with a retinoid should begin at least 4–6 weeks before the peel to promote a uniform peel and speed healing. Patients are instructed to stop using the retinoid at least 2–4 days before the peel. "Active" skin regimen products such as retinoids, AHAs, and antioxidant-containing creams can

be resumed 2–4 days after the peel. During the interim period, the authors advise patients to use bland, nonfragranced, cleansers and moisturizers so that peeled skin is not further irritated.

Superficial chemical peels mainly disrupt and exfoliate all or part of the epidermis, but have also been shown to have dermal effects including stimulation of collagen and glycosaminoglycan production. The depth of penetration and subsequent efficacy depend on several factors (Box 5-11). Even in the same patient, these variables should be re-evaluated prior to each session as they may change over the course of the treatment. The patient should also be asked about their postoperative experience, the degree and length of the postpeel erythema, desquamation, and discomfort so that appropriate adjustments can be made to future treatment.

Procedure for superficial peels

Key Points

• Preoperative skin preparation.
• Developing a consistent application technique.
• Guidelines for use in Fitzpatrick skin type IV and above.

The first step is proper skin preparation. Both preoperative conditioning and skin preparation affect peel depth. Prior to application of the peel, cutaneous lipids should first be removed by use of a gentle cleanser followed by application of a degreasing agent such as alcohol and/or acetone. Care should be taken to avoid excessive scrubbing, as excessive defatting may cause increased penetration of peel. Generally speaking, areas with increased sebaceous glands such as the central face can tolerate more vigorous degreasing without adverse effects. However, the remainder of the face and nonfacial areas such as the hands and forearms that have fewer sebaceous glands should be handled in a lighter fashion.

Becoming comfortable with a variety of agents and developing consistent peeling techniques will produce predictable results for patients and minimize the risk of side-effects. The amount of peeling agent used, type of applicator, duration of contact with skin, degree of rubbing, and the number of coats applied all play a role in penetration depth. Individual application techniques are discussed separately below. As you build your aesthetic practice, you will want to start with the lowest risk procedures (superficial peels) and gradually incorporate more advanced rejuvenation approaches (medium to deep peels) over time.

Although the literature indicates that superficial chemical peels, especially Jessner's, glycolic acid, tretinoin peels, and salicylic acid peels, are well tolerated and effective in patients with Fitzpatrick skin type IV and above, it is best to proceed conservatively in these patients. To minimize postinflammatory hyperpigmentation in these patients, initial contact times should be shorter and titrated up, based on reaction.

If postpeel adverse reactions such as excessive desquamation and irritation occur, patients are treated with medium- to high-potency topical steroids two to three times daily for 2 or 3 days. A previous history of postinflammatory hyperpigmentation or any current erythema and inflammation on the skin can increase the risk of postinflammatory hyperpigmentation.

α-Hydroxy acids

Key Points

- Most common superficial peeling agent.
- Clinical response depends on a variety of factors.
- Application technique and guidelines.
- Expected intraoperative and postoperative responses.
- Safe during pregnancy.

Glycolic acid is the most common AHA used for very superficial peeling. Clinical response depends on a variety of factors, including the pH of the acid, free acid availability to the skin, contact time with the skin, body site, volume applied, and skin condition being treated. The depth of penetration

ranges from stratum corneum to intraepidermal injury, depending on the concentration of agent used and contact time with the skin. A variety of over-the-counter preparations are available, either as prepackaged sachets or as unbuffered and unneutralized solutions in concentrations of up to 70%.

The face should be cleansed with a gentle cleanser and patted dry with a soft cloth in order to avoid excessive scrubbing. In patients with more oily complexions, the skin can be further degreased with alcohol and/or acetone to ensure a uniform peel. Next the solution is applied by means of gauze pads, cotton swabs, or a cotton-tipped applicator. Cotton-tipped applicators or swabs are less abrasive and are preferred periorbitally. Care should be taken to prevent tearing, as this can cause premature neutralization and result in a streaked appearance. A starting concentration of 30–40% glycolic acid is applied and left on the skin for 1–5 min, depending on patient comfort and the degree of erythema.

Conditions such as mild acne and rosacea may be treated successfully with a series of lower concentration (20–40%) glycolic acid peels left on for shorter durations (1–3 min) (Fig. 5-1). Studies have shown that combining a series of glycolic acid peels with topical therapy can provide additional positive effects in the treatment of dyschromias such as postinflammatory hyperpigmentation and melasma (Figs 5-2 & 5-3).

Both the concentration of the solution and contact time may be increased during subsequent treatments, with a maximum concentration of 70% and contact time of 7–10 min, depending on body location and condition. Conditions such as keratosis pilaris on the extremities or acne on the back tend to require higher concentrations (60–70%) of glycolic acid, with longer contact times for clearance.

Studies of the combination treatment of diffuse actinic keratosis with topical 5-fluorouracil (5%) and glycolic acid and Jessner's peels demonstrated clearance of actinic keratosis and improved cosmetic appearance. In a modified technique for the treatment of actinic keratosis and photodamage, patients pretreated their face with 5% 5-fluorouracil cream twice daily for 1–2 weeks until the endpoint of mild erythema and inflammation was achieved. At that point, a 70% glycolic acid in-office peel was administered for 2 min or until epidermolysis (i.e. epidermis turning white) occurred. This combination therapy was effective in treating actinic keratosis with improvement of overall skin cosmesis with a shortened downtime (approximately 1 week).

Glycolic acid peels are neutralized by rinsing thoroughly with either plain water or misting with a 5–10% sodium bicarbonate solution. The patient should be advised to expect a stinging/burning sensation, and in some cases slight discomfort

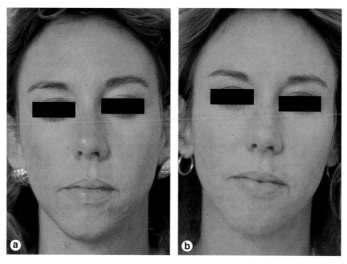

Figure 5-1 (A) Acne rosacea in a pregnant woman. (B) Appearance after a series of 20–50% glycolic acid peels

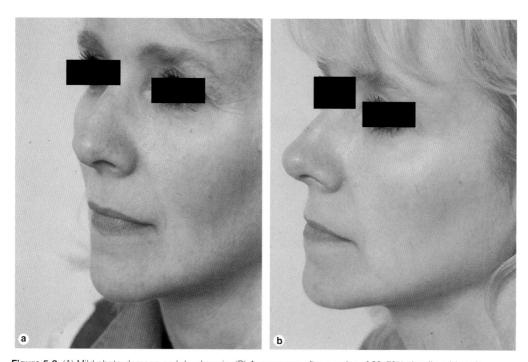

Figure 5-2 (A) Mild photo-damage and dyschromia. (B) Appearance after a series of 20–70% glycolic acid peels

during the procedure. Use of a handheld fan is soothing for many patients. Immediately after the peel, the skin appears mildly erythematous and slightly edematous. In rare instances, vesiculation can occur. To treat these "hot spots," a mild steroid cream is applied immediately and continued twice daily for a 24–48-h period to reduce the severity of the reaction as well as to minimize any potential postinflammatory hyperpigmentation.

A series of four to five peels, spaced 2–4 weeks apart, is required to see maximal cosmetic improvement. A maintenance treatment can be performed every 2–3 months. Topical retinoids and bleaching agents can be resumed in 2–3 days.

Salicylic acid

Key Points

- β-hydroxy acid.
- Application technique.
- Expected intraoperative and postpeel response.
- Ideal as an adjunctive treatment in patients with acne.

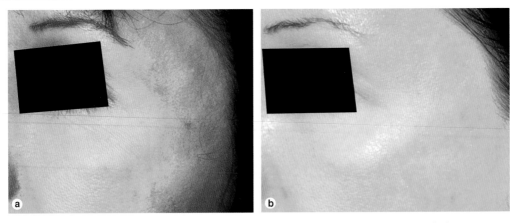

Figure 5-3 (A) Melasma. (B) Appearance after a series of 20–70% glycolic acid peels and at-home topical 4% hydroquinone cream

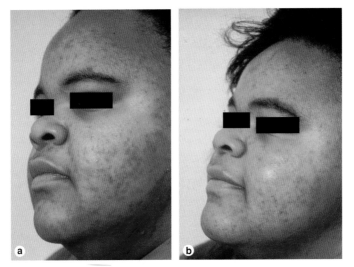

Figure 5-4 (A) Acne vulgaris and postinflammatory hyperpigmentation. (B) Appearance after a series of 20–30% salicylic acid peels

Salicylic acid, a β-hydroxy acid, is a popular ingredient for the treatment of acne and other dermatological conditions (Fig. 5-4). Currently, salicylic acid peels at concentrations of 20–30% are available. Compared with other types of superficial chemical peel, salicylic peels have several advantages (Box 5-12).

An immediate white "frosting," resulting from the precipitation of salicylic acid crystals, is observed at the site of application. No neutralizing agent is required, because once the vehicle has volatilized (within 2–3 min) very little of the active agent continues to penetrate. Salicylic acid has been attributed with anesthetic properties. In some patients, salicylic acid peels can cause significant desquamation, erythema, and edema. Although glycolic acid peels can be performed when a woman is pregnant or breast-feeding, salicylic

> **BOX 5-12**
>
> **Advantages of salicylic acid peels**
>
> Visual cue (frosting) guides uniform application
>
> Self-limited, no neutralizing agent required
>
> Lipophilic – ideal for acne and rosacea
>
> Anesthetic and anti-inflammatory properties

acid peels should not be done in these patients because of the risk of salicylism (presenting as nausea, disorientation, and tinnitus). In addition, salicylic acid peels and products should be avoided by individuals who are allergic to aspirin.

Salicylic acid is lipophilic, which allows it to concentrate in the pilosebaceous unit and exfoliate the pores. As it has both keratolytic and comedolytic properties, salicylic acid peels have been an important adjunctive therapy in patients with acne.

Salicylic acid peels have been proven to be safe and effective for acne, melasma, and photo-aging in all skin types including Fitzpatrick IV and above. One study reported improvement of acne and a whitening effect in Asian patients who underwent bimonthly treatments with 30% salicylic acid over a 3-month period.

Trichloroacetic acid

Key Points

- Recognized as the "gold standard" of medium-depth peels.
- Can be classified as a superficial peel in lower concentrations (10–25%).
- Application technique.
- Expected response during and after the peel.

TCA, when used in low concentrations of 10–25%, is classified as a superficial peeling agent. It creates superficial epidermal exfoliation by precipitation of proteins. If multiple coats of the acid are applied or the skin is aggressively prepared, even a low-concentration TCA peel (10–25%) may lead to intraepidermal, epidermal, or papillary dermis penetration. Using a weight to volume technique of compounding is the preferred method of composing standardized TCA concentrations. For example, a solution of 10% TCA would be made by compounding 10 g (United States Pharmacopoeia [USP] crystals) in 100 mL of distilled water.

Indications for low-concentration TCA peels are similar to those for other superficial chemical peels. A recent study demonstrated that prepeel and postpeel at-home application of topical ascorbic acid significantly improved the results of a 20% TCA peel in the treatment of melasma.

For the application, a saturated but not dripping gauze or a cotton-tipped applicator can be used. Within 1 min of application of a 10–20% concentration, erythema and very light and transient speckled frost is observed. Patients experience a burning/stinging sensation and mild discomfort, which can be relieved with a handheld fan. When using concentrations of 25% and above, a characteristic white frost is seen within a few minutes of application.

Like salicylic acid, TCA peels also do not require neutralization. Cool compresses may be applied immediately afterwards to decrease discomfort. Topical petrolatum-based ointment or Aquaphor is applied at completion of the peel. With lower TCA concentrations (10–20%), the downtime is minimal and the patient may undergo a second treatment within a week or two. However, with applications of 25% or greater healing occurs over 5–7 days. For patients with a darker skin type, starting with lower concentrations

or performing test patches in noncosmetically obvious locations is recommended.

Jessner's solution

Key Points

- This is a combination of 14 g of each of resorcinol, lactic acid, and salicylic acid in 95% ethanol.
- Application technique.
- Expected intrapeel and postpeel response.

Jessner's solution, another type of superficial peel, has been used to treat inflammatory and comedonal acne as well as hyperkeratotic skin disorders since the 1940s. Three keratolytic agents – resorcinol (14 g), salicylic acid (14 g), and lactic acid (14 g) – are compounded in ethanol 95% (up to 100 mL).

Following skin preparation, the Jessner's solution is applied thinly, with one to three coats depending on desired depth of penetration. No neutralizing agent is needed. Instead of a frost, the endpoint is fine white speckles on an erythematous background. Desquamation occurs over the next 2–3 days.

Studies have shown that Jessner's peels are comparably efficacious to 70% glycolic acid peels in the treatment of acne. A series of two to four Jessner's and lactic acid (92%) peels were also found to be similarly effective at treating melasma in patients with skin type IV. Because Jessner's peels can predictably enhance penetration of other peeling agents, they are routinely used in combination with 35% TCA for a reproducible medium-depth peel.

Solid carbon dioxide

Dry ice, or solid carbon dioxide, can be thought of as a physical peeling agent rather than a chemical exfoliant. The cone of dry ice, at −78.5°C, is wrapped in a towel, leaving the tip exposed. It is then dipped in a solution of 3:1 alcohol:acetone, which allows it to be applied to the skin. This carbon dioxide slush is brushed across the surface of the skin, with less than 10 s of contact time at any given location. The amount of pressure and time affect the depth of penetration in the carbon dioxide peel. The immediate expected response is erythema and possibly mild vesiculation. Dry ice can be used alone for a superficial peel or preceding a 35% TCA for a uniform medium-depth peel.

Tretinoin peels

Key Points

- Guidelines for application.
- Efficacy and safety profile.

Topical tretinoin has been used successfully for many years in the treatment of acne, melasma, and postinflammatory hyperpigmentation.

Improvement in melasma, acne, and photo-damaged skin following a series of 1–5% tretinoin peels was reported in one study. Another study further demonstrated the equivalent safety and efficacy of tretinoin 1% peels, compared with 70% glycolic acid peels, in the treatment of melasma in Fitzpatrick skin type III–V; applications of 1% tretinoin peels were performed weekly and left on for 4 h. In a study that examined the effects of 5% retinoic acid peels with and without microdermabrasion, both methods were found to be effective in the treatment of photo-aging.

After the tretinoin peel, the immediate expected response is a slightly yellow coloration of the skin, which is followed by superficial desquamation over the next 2–3 days. Tretinoin peels are very well tolerated, require no neutralization or timing, and are associated with minimal downtime.

Postoperative care and complications

Key Points

- Minimal with a gentle cleanser and a petrolatum ointment.
- Topical low-potency steroid cream for increased erythema and in patients with Fitzpatrick skin type IV and above.
- Resume maintenance regimen once skin has healed.
- Use sun block and sun avoidance.
- Routine prophylactic antiviral and antibiotic drugs are not indicated.
- Complications are limited to transient hyperpigmentation and dyschromia.

Postoperative care for superficial peels is minimal and simple. Immediately after the peel, a thin coat of petrolatum ointment or bland moisturizer is applied. Topical over-the-counter hydrocortisone or a low-potency prescription steroid cream may be substituted if there is an increased degree of erythema or in individuals with darker skin types, both to reduce the recovery time and to minimize the chance of postinflammatory hyperpigmentation. Patients may even apply make-up immediately after the peel if they wish.

At-home care consists of washing the skin twice daily with a gentle cleanser followed by mild emollient cream and application of a steroid cream if needed for the next few days. Topical retinoids or AHA products should be avoided until the skin returns to normal, typically within 2–3 days. Patients may resume to the regular maintenance regimen once the skin has healed. Sun block and sun avoidance should be emphasized as the newly peeled skin is at increased risk of sunburn. Routine prophylactic or postpeel antiviral or antibiotic treatments are usually not required with superficial peels.

Patients can expect mild erythema for a few hours to days, depending on the depth of the peel. Variable amounts of exfoliation also occur over the next few days. Be sure to reassure patients that significant sloughing does not need to occur for results to be seen over the course of time. Although studies have shown that peeled skin returns to its baseline status within 2–6 months without maintenance therapy, good skin care regimens can sustain more long-lasting results. Broad-spectrum sunscreens, retinoids, α- and β-hydroxy acids, other antioxidant cosmeceuticals, and bleaching creams may be recommended singly or in combination as the postpeel skin regimen.

Complications from superficial peels are limited to transient hyperpigmentation or dyschromia, particularly in darker skinned individuals. This is accentuated by sunlight, in a patient who is on an estrogen-containing medication (oral contraceptive or hormone replacement) or other photosensitizing drugs. This hyperpigmentation responds well to bleaching agents such as hydroquinone.

PEARLS

Treatment with superficial peels

Emphasize to patient that a series of peels is required

Manage patient expectations

Address goals of treatment and limitations

Advise that maintenance peels are generally needed

Skin preparation regimen, preferably beginning 6 weeks previously, is preferable

Resume skin care regimen after skin heals

Avoidance of sun exposure before and after peel

Conservative treatment in Fitzpatrick skin type IV and above

Choose the optimal peel based on skin condition

Develop a consistent skin preparation and application technique

Medium-depth peels

Key Points

- Causes injury to the papillary dermis and occasionally upper reticular dermis as a result of keratocoagulation and protein precipitation.
- TCA is the gold standard.
- Several combination medium-depth peels exist.
- Indicated primarily for moderate actinic damage, dyschromia, photo-aging, superficial rhytides, scarring, and epidermal growths.
- Longer downtime than superficial peels: 7–14 days.
- Clinical signs that may represent histologic depth, including Obagi TCA Blue Peel®.

BOX 5-13

Medium-depth peeling agents

Jessner's solution and TCA 35%

Glycolic acid 70% and TCA 35%

Solid carbon dioxide and 35% TCA

TCA 50% (now rarely used)

Phenol 88%

Pyruvic acid

BOX 5-14

Indications for TCA peels

Photo-damage

Epidermal lesions – seborrheic and actinic keratoses

Superficial rhytides

Mild acne scars

Pigmentary changes – melasma, solar lentigos

Blend effects of deeper resurfacing procedures

Medium-depth peeling agents (Box 5-13) cause controlled wounding to the papillary dermis and occasionally to the depth of the upper reticular dermis. This injury leads to epidermal necrosis, papillary dermis edema, and inflammation, and results in an improvement of photo-damage and superficial rhytides.

Indications for medium-depth peels include actinic damage, epidermal growths (seborrheic keratoses, solar lentigines), dyschromias (including melasma), superficial scarring and rhytides, and blending sun-damaged skin with more deeply re-surfaced (either with peels or laser) skin (Box 5-14) (Figs 5-5–5-8).

For many years, TCA at a concentration of 40–50% was the prototypical medium-depth peeling agent. However, over time it was found that TCA peels at strengths of 50% and higher had unpredictable results and carried a substantial risk of associated complications such as scarring and pigment changes. These issues resulted in the development of a variety of combination peeling techniques that aim to produce similar benefits with a lower risk profile and higher predictability. The objective of many different combination peels is the same: initially to cause epidermal injury with a superficial peeling agent followed by application of 35–40% TCA. This two-step process allows for a uniform, controlled, penetration of TCA into the papillary dermis. Combining these two peels prevents the development of "hot spots," which can lead to the undesired

side-effects of scarring and pigmentary alteration. The most common combinations are Jessner's solution with 35% TCA, glycolic acid 70% with 35% TCA, and solid carbon dioxide with 35% TCA. All three combinations are as effective and safer than 50% TCA.

Although most medium-depth resurfacing occurs on the face and neck, a technique to exfoliate nonfacial skin in a controlled manner has been developed. Seventy per cent glycolic acid gel is applied to the skin followed by 40% TCA solution to the same area. The gel vehicle for the glycolic acid is essential because it serves as a partial barrier to TCA penetration. Typically, the endpoint of white speckles appearing on a background of pink skin occurs within 3 min of application. At this point, the treated area is neutralized with sodium bicarbonate 10% solution, and the peel is completed. Reported clinical results included smoother skin texture, decreased wrinkling and striae, and fading of lentigines and other pigmentary abnormalities. Side-effects were limited to temporary postinflammatory hyperpigmentation, which resolved with local hydroquinone treatment.

Another study prospectively compared the effects of 30% TCA peeling, carbon dioxide laser resurfacing, and topical 5% fluorouracil (applied twice daily for 3 weeks) on skin cancer prevention and in the treatment of actinic keratoses. Although all modalities resulted in an 83–92% reduction in actinic keratoses and significantly reduced the incidence of nonmelanoma skin cancer, the TCA peel group showed the greatest reduction in skin cancer incidence.

Serial focal application of high-concentration (95–100%) CTA to atrophic and "ice pick" acne scars has been shown to be effective in improving the appearance and reducing the depth of these types of scar. This procedure, originally termed the CROSS (chemical reconstruction of skin scars) technique, consists of precise application of TCA (65–100%) with sharp wooden applicators every 6 weeks for six sessions. The clinical benefits have been confirmed histologically. TCA, when applied in high concentrations (100%) with the CROSS technique versus simple application of TCA, was more effective at activating fibroblasts in the dermis and increasing the amount of collagen.

Focal TCA application was shown to be a safe and effective treatment for resolving benign pigmented lesions such as seborrheic keratoses and solar lentigines in a study of Asian patients with skin types IV–V using spot application of 65% TCA for seborrheic keratoses and 50–65% TCA for lentigines. Alternately, hyperkeratotic actinic keratoses or seborrheic keratoses can be curetted or frozen after the peel for improved clearance.

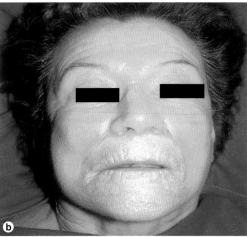

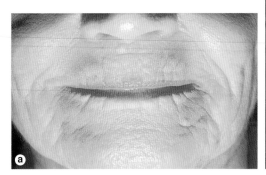

Figure 5-5 (A) Perioral rhytides. (B) Appearance after application of a combination Jessner's solution–35% TCA medium-depth peel

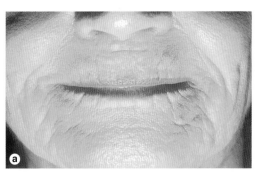

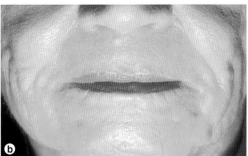

Figure 5-6 (A) Perioral rhytides. (B) Appearance after a combination Jessner's solution–35% TCA medium-depth peel

Many authors have discussed the clinical signs that may indicate the histologic depth of the TCA peels. The degree of whitening or frosting correlates with the depth of TCA penetration. Level I frosting appears as erythema with streaky white frosting. Level II presents as a white enamel color with a background of erythema. Level III signifies penetration to the reticular dermis, and is seen as solid white enamel frosting without background erythema. Most medium-depth peels produce a level II frosting. Only areas of thicker skin and prominent actinic damage should undergo a level III frosting.

The TCA-based Blue Peel® was developed to simplify and standardize the TCA peel by defining depth of penetration of TCA peel with a color guide system. Glycerine and an extract from plant saponin are added to promote uniform application and penetration. Federal Food, Drug, and Cosmetic Act blue number 1 is added as an intraepidermal marker for color guidance. Multiple coats of the peel containing either 15% or 20% TCA are applied to reach the desired endpoints: papillary dermal penetration (light Blue Peel®) or upper reticular dermal penetration (light/medium Blue Peel®).

Procedure for medium-depth peels

Key Points

- Skin preparation.
- Application technique of TCA peel alone and in combination with Jessner's solution.
- Special considerations: treating periorbital and perioral skin, avoiding lines of demarcations.
- Guidelines on achieving an adequate response as judged by frosting.

As for superficial peels, the first step in the procedure is skin preparation. Prior to application of the peel, the cutaneous lipids should be removed first by using a gentle cleanser followed by degreasing agents such as alcohol and acetone until no residual oils can be visualized. The effectiveness of the peel is determined by the depth of penetration and is proportional to the degree of degreasing.

Although a TCA peel can be used singly at a concentration of 40–50%, combining it with a superficial agent leads to more predictable results.

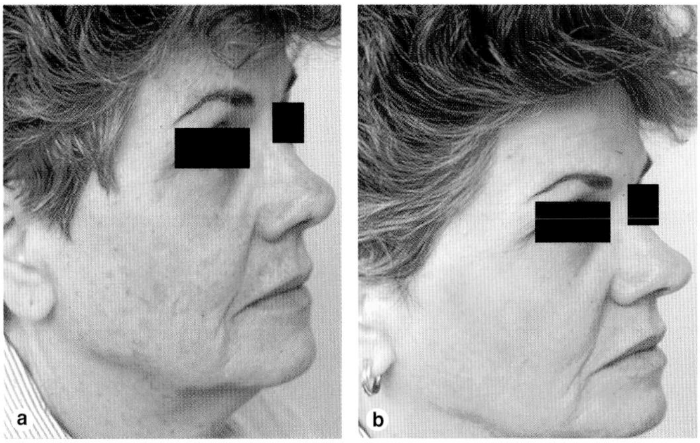

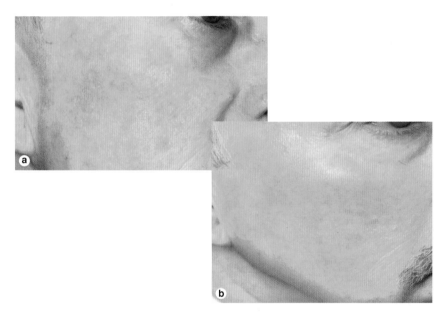

Figure 5-7 (A) Moderate photo-damage and dyschromia. (B) Appearance after a combination Jessner's solution–35% TCA medium-depth peel

Figure 5-8 (A) Diffuse solar damage and actinic keratosis. (B) Appearance after a combination Jessner's solution–35% TCA medium-depth peel

TCA peels at lower concentrations of 25–35% can be used as single-agent peels when a more superficial medium-depth peel is desired, especially in more sensitive skin areas such as the neck or eyelids. Most often, medium-depth peels are performed as a combination technique. The authors use the Jessner's peel with 35% TCA.

Jessner's peel allows for a more uniform, controlled, and deeper penetration of TCA. Using a cotton-tipped applicator, a single coat of Jessner's solution is applied to the face. After it has dried completely, 35% TCA can be applied.

For the treatment of thicker epidermal growths such as thick seborrheic keratosis and actinic keratosis, increased penetration of TCA is required.

This can be achieved either by briskly rubbing the solution into the lesion or by lightly curetting or freezing the lesion before or after the TCA application.

For the application of TCA either 2 × 2-inch gauze or large cotton-tipped applicators can be used. Cotton-tipped applicators have the advantage of increased precision with respect to the volume of solution and degree of pressure applied. When treating the face, 35% TCA should be evenly applied using gauze or cotton applicator, and feathered below the inferior aspect of the mandible. The authors generally start on the forehead and move on to the cheeks, nose, chin, cutaneous upper lip, and finally the upper eyelids.

The perioral and periorbital regions are treated last, owing to the increased sensitivity of these areas.

To facilitate blending, the neck can be treated with 25% TCA. Care should also be taken to feather the peeling agent into the hairline and eyebrows to avoid demarcation between peeled and unpeeled skin. In areas of deeper furrows and rhytides, especially in the perioral region, the skin should be stretched taut to allow for adequate penetration of the peel. The wooden part of the cotton-tipped applicator can be used to treat deeper perioral rhytides. Periorbital skin is thin and delicate, and should also be treated very carefully. The eyelid skin can be peeled within 3 mm of the lid margin. By using a minimally saturated, small cotton-tipped applicator, overapplication of TCA can be avoided. Excess solution should always be removed, so that it does not get in the eyes. If tearing develops, a dry cotton-tipped applicator should be used immediately to dry the area, in order to prevent linear streaking.

Frosting of the treated skin usually begins within 1–2 min of application. If, after 3–4 min, some areas appear to have patchy frosting, they may be lightly retouched with the TCA solution. As the peel is applied, there is an immediate burning sensation, which abates within minutes. Level 2 frosting is appropriate for periorbital skin and most other areas on the face, and level 3 frosting should be reserved for areas with increased sebaceous glands, thicker skin, and areas of heavy actinic damage.

No neutralizing agent is needed for TCA peels. As successive areas are being treated, wrung-out ice water compresses can be applied to peeled areas. These cold compresses are applied over the next 10–15 min until the patient is feeling more comfortable.

The main factors influencing penetration of the peel include degreasing, the amount of peeling agent used, type of applicator, duration of contact with skin, degree of rubbing/pressure of application, the sebaceous nature of the skin being treated, and the number of coats applied.

Postoperative care and complications

Key Points

- Healing time is 7–10 days: erythema and edema in the first few days followed by desquamation.
- Wound care is with acetic acid or normal saline soaks followed by a petrolatum-based ointment.
- Complications include irregular pigmentation, prolonged erythema, infection, delayed wound healing, and scarring.
- HSV prophylaxis is recommended in all patients.

In comparison to superficial peels, postoperative care following a TCA peel is more involved. A petrolatum-based ointment such as Vaseline® or Aquaphor® ointment should be applied. Patients should be advised that the frosting may take 1–2 h to subside completely. Following the peel, erythema is present within the first hour as the frosting completely resolves. Edema also develops in the first 1–2 days and the face starts to appear to have a mild to moderate sunburn. This may be particularly severe in the periorbital region and can raise patient's anxiety. Cool compresses and nonsteroidal anti-inflammatory drugs can be used to reduce the swelling and inflammation. In many patients who are undergoing a full-face procedure, a tapering course of steroids (e.g. a methylprednisolone dose pack) can be prescribed.

A reddish brown appearance occurs at days 2 to 3, followed by complete desquamation by day 4 or 5. Full re-epithelialization is usually complete within a week. Patients should be instructed to avoid the natural urge to pick the peeling skin. The underlying epithelium is initially brightly erythematous and gradually fades to a pinker color. Postoperative care in the first few days after a peel includes cleansing with gauze soaked in either a dilute acetic acid solution (0.25% – 1 pint of water mixed with 1 tablespoon of white vinegar) or saline for 15–20 min four or five times a day. Acetic acid soaks are preferred as the mild acidity has antibacterial effects. This should be followed by liberal application of emollients, such as Vaseline® or Aquaphor® ointment until desquamation is complete.

By postoperative day 7–10, patients can wear make-up to camouflage the erythema. The majority of the erythema resolves within the next 2–4 weeks, and patient can restart their maintenance skin care regimen of retinoids, glycolics, and other products at 6 weeks. Sun avoidance is crucial during the first few weeks after the peel. Sunscreen can be applied as soon as re-epithelialization is complete. The authors see patients in follow-up at 2–4 days and then again at 7–10 days. These follow-up visits serve to note the progress of healing and provide patients with reassurance regarding their course.

The most common complication of chemical peeling is irregular pigmentation. When using lower concentrations of TCA (25–30%) hyperpigmentation is more common, but with a higher concentration of 50% TCA hypopigmentation is more likely. Hyperpigmentation is almost always transient and can be treated effectively with topical hydroquinones. In some cases, a superficial peel (e.g. glycolic acid 30–40%) can also be performed to hasten resolution. Temporary accentuation of lentigines and nevi may also occur because the background sun damage has been cleared.

The expected duration of the erythema depends on the depth of the injury. With medium-depth peels, erythema usually resolves by the second month. If erythema is accompanied by pruritus, burning, or stinging, it may be due to contact with an irritant allergen such as a retinoid or other topical agent, an active infection, or flaring of an underlying skin condition. Persistent erythema needs to be approached aggressively as it may indicate impending scarring. The underlying cause should be determined and possible irritants avoided. Depending on the severity of the erythema, a combination of topical and oral steroids, as well as pulsed-dye lasers, can be used.

Infection, although rare as TCA and phenol are bactericidal, can be seen and may be bacterial, viral, or fungal in origin. The most common cause is poor wound care. Frequent postoperative visits are important to ensure that appropriate at-home wound care is being performed and to minimize the risk of infection. An infection may present as delayed wound healing, folliculitis, or simply as ulceration, superficial erosions, crusting, and drainage. Occlusive dressings should be avoided in the immediate postoperative period because of their propensity to promote both folliculitis and infection with streptococcal and staphylococcal organisms. Infection with other organisms, such as *Pseudomonas* and *Escherichia coli*, has also been documented. If cutaneous candidal infection occurs, it may be related to a recent intake of oral antibiotics or prolonged application of occlusive dressings.

If infection is suspected, the wound should be swabbed for cultures and sensitivity. In some cases, the wound can be lightly debrided and treated, with wound care consisting of acetic acid soaks, a topical antibiotic, and a broad-spectrum oral antibiotic.

Herpes infection can develop after a medium or deep peel and may have serious sequelae, including significant scarring. A negative history of cold sores cannot predict the development of postoperative HSV infection after a procedure. Furthermore, infection may even occur in patients who are on antiviral prophylaxis. All patients undergoing medium-depth peels should be placed on an oral antiviral agent, starting 1 day before the procedure and continued for at least 10–14 days after treatment. Valtrex (500 mg, twice daily) is most often used for prophylaxis. If a herpetic infection develops, it usually presents with intense pain and burning on the skin. If an HSV infection is suspected, the dosage of Valtrex should be increased to 1 g three times daily until the infection resolves.

The risk of scarring increases with higher concentrationsof TCA, especially at 50% or greater. The presentation of early scarring is patchy erythema, which may be indurated. Predisposing

factors include history of smoking, history of isotretinoin use, recent facial surgery that required significant undermining, and recent ablative resurfacing procedures including dermabrasion or laser within 6 months of the procedure, and a past history of other hypertrophic scars or keloids. Treatment should be instituted early, with scar massage, topical, intralesional, or oral steroids, and pulsed-dye laser therapy.

BOX 5-15

Baker–Gordon phenol peel formula

Phenol USP 88%: 3 mL

Distilled water: 2 mL

Septisol liquid soap: 8 drops

Croton oil: 3 drops

PEARLS

Treatment with medium-depth peels

Results are more dramatic following medium-depth than superficial peels.

Combined superficial and TCA peels produce safe, predictable results.

Focal TCA (high concentration) application is useful for treating scars and epidermal growths.

Adjunctive procedures such as botulinum toxin injections can augment results of a medium-depth peel.

TCA peels not only improve the cosmetic appearance of photo-damaged skin but can also reduce the future incidence of nonmelanoma skin cancer.

Meticulous postoperative care is essential.

Deep chemical peeling – phenol peels

Advanced photo-damage requires more extensive resurfacing, with either deep chemical peels or ablative lasers. Although ablative lasers are more commonly used to treat advanced photo-damage in current practice, the Baker–Gordon phenol peel, a deep peeling agent, has a long history of effectively addressing extensive dermal damage (Box 5-15). Candidates for deep peels are ideally patients with skin types I and II, to reduce the risk of potential complications such as hypopigmentation, textural changes ("alabaster skin"), and scarring.

Phenol solution can cause keratolysis and keratocoagulation, depending on the concentration. At full strength, phenol causes immediate coagulation of epidermal keratin proteins and "self blocks" further penetration. However, dilution of the Baker–Gordon formula to 50–55% results in greater penetration, and produces both keratolysis and keratocoagulation. For this reason, if the peeling solution were to enter the eye, it should be flushed with mineral oil instead of water. The Baker–Gordon peel can also be occluded with tape if greater penetration to the midreticular dermis is desired.

As phenol is cardiotoxic, hepatotoxic, and nephrotoxic, it is important to limit systemic levels of phenol due to absorption from the skin. Intravenous hydration with 0.5–1 L of fluid (lactated Ringer's solution) before and during the procedure should be given to avoid renal toxicity. Patients should have cardiac monitoring to detect any electrocardiographic abnormalities (premature ventricular contractions or premature atrial contractions) that would necessitate halting of the procedure. The incidence of cardiac arrhythmias was recently reported as 6.6% in a series of patients undergoing full-face phenol peels. Additionally, full-face procedures should be performed over a 60–90-min period of time. Each cosmetic unit (forehead, cheeks, nose, and perioral and periorbital areas) should be peeled in 15-min increments. Intraoperative oxygen has also been advocated to prevent arrhythmias. Some patients may prefer that the procedure be performed with intravenous sedation and nerve blocks to limit discomfort.

Technique

The face is cleansed and degreased with Septisol followed by acetone. The Baker–Gordon solution is then applied with cotton-tipped applicators. Rapid frosting of the treated areas appears, and coincides with immediate discomfort. This painful sensation initially lasts for only seconds, but returns in 20 min and may last for hours. To minimize lines of demarcation, the peeling solution should be feathered. Periocular peeling should be approached with extra care. After the peel, petrolatum or Aquaphor ointment should be applied. Biosynthetic dressings such as Vigilon can also provide additional patient comfort in the first 24 h.

Scheduled gentle soaks and ointment application, as mentioned above for medium-depth peels, help to keep areas hydrated and prevent crust formation. Re-epithelialization begins after 3 days and is complete at 1–2 weeks. The patient should be advised that the peeled skin may remain erythematous for up to 3 months.

Adjunctive procedures

The combination of peeling procedures with other minimally invasive procedures can synergistically rejuvenate the appearance of the skin by also addressing concomitant cosmetic issues, such as dynamic and static rhytides, volume depletion, and vascular disorders (telangiectasia and poikiloderma). Botulinum toxin injections given 1–2 weeks prior to peeling may allow for more uniform collagen remodeling and healing, because underlying muscles are immobilized and not reinforcing the creation of rhytides. In a study of the effect of preoperative botulinum toxin injections followed by chemabrasion (35% TCA chemical peel application followed by manual dermabrasion with sandpaper) for the treatment of moderate to severe rhytides on the upper lip, botulinum-injected sites showed significantly lower grades on the Facial Wrinkle Severity Scale and enhanced cosmetic outcomes when compared with controls.

Deep furrows and volume loss can be augmented and smoothed with fillers such as the hyaluronans, l-polylactic acid, calcium hydroxylapatite, and others. For many patients, the authors suggest carbon dioxide laser resurfacing for deeper perioral rhytides with a medium-depth peel for the remainder of the face. One study of acne scars evaluated a sequential treatment using a 1450-nm, mid-infrared, nonablative diode laser (four sessions at monthly intervals) followed by two bimonthly 30% TCA peels, and found that patients had a greater improvement with the combination treatment. Vascular conditions, which can actually become more prominent in the early postoperative period, may be treated with vascular lasers or other light devices.

Conclusion

Chemical peels, depending on type, can treat a variety of skin disorders including photo-damage, dyschromias, scarring, and unwanted epidermal growths. By first acquiring a thorough understanding of the limitations and complications associated with all peels, and then developing a consistent technique with the various peeling agents, the most appropriate peeling procedure(s) can be selected to suit the individual needs of patients, and performed safely.

Further reading

Ahn HH, Kim IH. Whitening effect of salicylic acid peels in Asian patients. Dermatol Surg 2006;32. 372–275.

Baumann L. Chemical peels. In: Weisberg E, ed. Cosmetic Dermatology. New York: McGraw-Hill, 2002: 173–186.

Baumann L. Depigmenting agents. In: Day DJ, ed. Understanding Hyperpigmentation. What You Need to Know (Continuing Medical Education Monograph). Aurora, CA: Intellyst Medical Communications; 2004:1–6.

Beeson W. Facial rejuvenation: phenol-based chemexfoliation. In: Coleman W, Lawrence N, eds. Skin Resurfacing. Philadelphia: Williams & Wilkins, 1998:71–86.

Beeson WM, Rachel JD. Valcyclovir prophylaxis for herpes simplex virus infection or infection resuming following laser resurfacing. Dermatol Surg 2002;28:431–436.

Bernstein LJ, Geronemus RG. Keloid formation with the 585-nm pulsed dye laser during isotretinoin treatment. Arch Dermatol 1997;133:111–112.

Bernstein EF. Dermal effects of alpha hydroxyl acids. In: Moy R, Luftman D, Kakita L, eds. Glycolic Acid Peels. New York: Marcel Dekker; 2002: 71–113.

Bisaccia E, Scarborough D. Herpes simplex virus prophylaxis with famciclovir in patients undergoing aesthetic facial CO_2 laser resurfacing. Cutis 2003;72:327–328.

Boyd AS, Stasko T, King LE, et al. Cigarette smoking associated elastotic changes in the skin. J Am Acad Dermatol 1999;41:23–26.

Bridenstine J, Dolezal J. Standardizing chemical peel solution formulations to avoid mishaps. J Dermatol Surg Oncol 1994;20:813–816.

Brody HJ. Variations and comparisons in medium-depth chemical peeling. J Dermatol Surg Oncol 1989;15:953–963.

Brody HJ. Complications of chemical peeling. J Dermatol Surg 1989;15:1010–1024.

Brody HJ. History of chemical peels. In: Brody HJ, ed. Chemical Peeling. St Louis: Mosby Yearbook, 1992:1–5.

Brody HJ. Skin response to chemical peeling. In: Coleman W, Lawrence N, eds. Skin Resurfacing. Philadelphia: William & Wilkins, 1998:37–44.

Brody HJ. Skin resurfacing: chemical peels. In: Freedberg IM, Elsen AZ, Wolff K, Austen KF, eds. Fitzpatrick's Dermatology in General Medicine. New York: McGraw-Hill, 1999:2937–2947.

Brody HJ, Monheit GD, Resnik SS, et al. A history of chemical peeling. Dermatol Surg 2000;226: 405–409.

Burns RL, Prevost-Blank PL, Lawry MA, et al. Glycolic acid peels for postinflammatory hyperpigmentation in black patients. Dermatol Surg 1997;23:171–175.

Butler P, Gonzalez S, Randolph M, et al. Quantitative and qualitative effects of chemical peeling on photoaged skin: an experimental study. Plast Reconstr Surg 2001;107:222–228.

Camacho FM. Medium-depth and deep chemical peels. J Cosmet Dermatol 2005;4:117–128.

Carniol PJ, Vynatheya J, Carniol E. Evaluation of acne scar treatment with a 1450-nm midinfrared laser and 30% trichloroacetic acid peels. Arch Facial Plast Surg 2005;7:251–255.

Cho SB, Park CO, Chung WG, Lee KH, Lee JB, Chung KY. Histometric and histochemical analysis of the effect of trichloroacetic acid concentration in the chemical reconstruction of skin scars method. Dermatol Surg 2006;32:1231–1236.

Chun EY, Lee JB, Lee KH. Focal trichloroacetic acid peel method for benign pigmented lesions in dark skinned patients. Dermatol Surg 2004;30:512–516.

Chung JH, Lee SH, Youn CS, et al. Cutaneous photodamage in Koreans: influence of sex, sun exposure, smoking, and skin color. Arch Dermatol 2001;137:1043–1051.

Coleman W, Lawrence N. The history of skin resurfacing. In: Coleman W, Lawrence N, eds. Skin Resurfacing. Philadelphia: Williams & Wilkins, 1998:3–6.

Cook KK, Cook WR. Chemical peel of nonfacial skin using glycolic acid gel augmented with TCA and neutralized based on visual staging. Dermatol Surg 2000;26:994–999.

Cox SE, Butterwick KJ. Chemical peels. In: Robinson JK, Hanke CW, Sergelmann RD, Siegel DM, eds. Surgery of the Skin: Procedural Dermatology. Philadelphia: Elsevier Mosby, 2005: 463–482.

Cuce L, Bertino M, Scattone L, et al. Tretinoin peeling. Dermatol Surg 2001;27:12–14.

Ditre CM. The treatment of photodamaged skin with 5% 5-fluorouracil peels. Cosmetic Dermatol 2007;20:568–572.

Ditre CM, Griffin TD, Murphy GF, et al. Effects of alpha-hydroxy acids on photoaged skin: a pilot clinical, histologic, and ultrastructural study. J Am Acad Dermatol 1996;34:187–195.

Drake LA, Dinehart SM, Goltz RW, et al. Guidelines/outcomes committee: American Academy of Dermatology. J Am Acad Dermatol 1995;33:497–503.

Dreno B, Nocera T, Verrière F, et al. Topical retinaldehyde with glycolic acid: study of tolerance and acceptability in association with anti-acne treatments in 1709 patients. Dermatology 2005;210:22–29.

Erbil H, Sezer E, Tastan B, et al. Efficacy and safety of serial glycolic acid peels and a topical regimen in the treatment of recalcitrant melasma. J Dermatol 2007;34:25–30.

Falanga V. Occlusive wound dressings. Why, when, which? Arch Dermatol 1988;124:872–877.

Glogau RG, Matarasso SL. Chemical peels. Dermatol Clin 1995;13:263–276.

Goldman MP. The use of hydroquinone with facial laser resurfacing. J Cutan Laser Ther 2000;2:73–77.

Grimes PE. The safety and efficacy of salicylic acid chemical peels in darker racial-ethnic types. Dermatol Surg 1999;25:18–22.

Grimes PE. Glycolic acid peels in blacks. In: Moy RL, Luftman D, Kakita L, eds. Glycolic Acid Peels. New York: Marcel Dekker, 2002:179–186.

Hantash BM, Stewart DB, Cooper ZA, Rehmus WE. Facial resurfacing for nonmelanoma skin cancer prophylaxis. Arch Dermatol 2006;142:976–982.

Helfrich YR, Yu L, Ofori A, et al. Effect of smoking on aging or photoprotected skin. Arch Dermatol 2007;143:397–402.

Hevia O, Nemeth AJ, Taylor JR. Tretinoin accelerates healing after trichloroacetic acid chemical peel. Arch Dermatol 1991;127:678–682.

Hexsel D, Mazzuco R, Dalforno T, Zechmeisler D. Microdermabrasion followed by a 5% retinoic acid chemical peel vs. a 5% retinoic acid chemical peel for the treatment of photoaging – a pilot study. J Cosmet Dermatol 2005;4:111–116.

Kadunc BV, Trindade DE, Almeda AR, et al. Botulinum toxin A adjunctive use in manual chemabrasion: controlled long-term study for treatment of upper perioral vertical wrinkles. Dermatol Surg 2007;33:1066–1072.

Katz BE. The fluoro-hydroxy pulse peel: a pilot evaluation of a new superficial chemical peel. Cosmet Dermatol 1995;8:24–30.

Khunger N, Sarkar R, Jain RK. Tretinoin peels versus glycolic acid peels in the treatment of melasma in dark-skinned patients. Dermatol Surg 2004;30:756–760.

Kligman AM, Leyden JJ. Treatment of photoaged skin with topical tretinoin. Skin Pharmacol 1993;6:78–82.

Kockaert M, Neumann M. Systemic and topical drugs for aging skin. J Drugs Dermatol 2003;2:435–441.

Landau M. Combination of chemical peeling with botulinum toxin injections and dermal fillers. J Cosmet Dermatol 2006;5:121–126.

Landau M. Cardiac complications in deep chemical peels. Dermatol Surg 2007;33:190–193.

Lawrence N, Cox SE, Brody HG. Treatment of melasma with Jessner's solution vs. glycolic acid: a comparison of clinical efficacy and evaluation of the predictive ability of Wood's light examination. J Am Acad Dermatol 1997;35:489–593.

Lee HS, Kim IH. Salicylic acid peels for the treatment of acne vulgaris in Asian patients. Dermatol Surg 2003;29:1196–1199.

Lee JB, Churig WG, Kwahok H, Lee KH. Focal treatment of acne scars with trichloroacetic acid: chemical reconstruction of skin scars method. Dermatol Surg 2002;28:1017–1021.

Maloney BP, Millman B, Monheit G, McCollough EG. The etiology of prolonged erythema after chemical peel. Dermatol Surg 1998;24:337–341.

Marrero GM, Katz BE. The new fluor-hydroxy pulse peel. A combination of 5-fluorouracil and glycolic acid. Dermatol Surg 1998;24:973–978.

Matarasso SL, Glogau RG. Chemical face peels. Dermatol Clin 1991;9:131–149.

Monheit GD. The Jessner's and TCA peel: a medium depth chemical peel. J Dermatol Surg Oncol 1989;15:945–950.

Monheit GD. Chemical peeling for pigmentary dyschromias. Cosmet Dermatol 1995;8:10–15.

Monheit GD. Medium-depth chemical peels. Dermatol Clin 2001;19:413–425.

Monheit GD, Chastain MA. Chemical peels. Facial Plast Surg Clin North Am 2001;9:239–255.

Moy LS, Murad H, Moy RL. Glycolic acid peels for the treatment of wrinkles and photoaging. J Dermatol Surg Oncol 1993;19:243–246.

Nestor MS. Prophylaxis for and treatment of uncomplicated skin and skin structure infections in laser and cosmetic surgery. J Drugs Dermatol 2005;4(Suppl):520–525.

Newman N, Newman A, Moy LS, Babapour R, Harris AG, Moy RL. Clinical improvement of photoaged skin with 50% glycolic acid. A double-blind vehicle-controlled study. Dermatol Surg 1996;22:455–460.

Obagi ZE, Obagi S, Alaiti S, Stevens MB. TCA-based Blue Peel: a standardized procedure with depth control. Dermatol Surg 1999;25:773–780.

Olsen EA, Katz HJ, Levine N, et al. Tretinoin emollient cream: a new therapy for photodamaged skin. J Am Acad Dermatol 1992;26:215–224.

Pathak MA, Nghiem P, Fitzpatrick TB. Acute and chronic effects of the sun. In: Freedberg IM, Elsen AZ, Wolff K, Austen KF, eds. Fitzpatrick's Dermatology in General Medicine. New York: McGraw-Hill, 1999:1598–1607.

Perricone NV, DiNardo JC. Photoprotective and anti-inflammatory effects of topical glycolic acid. Dermatol Surg 1996;22:435–437.

Peters W. The chemical peel. Ann Plast Surg 1991;26:564–571.

Rendon MI, Gaviria JI. Review of skin-lightening agents. Dermatol Surg 2005;31:886–889.

Ridge JM, Siegle RJ, Zuckerman J. Use of alpha-hydroxy acids in the therapy for 'photoaged' skin. J Am Acad Dermatol 1990;23:932.

Roenigk R, Brodland D. A primer of facial chemical peel. Dermatol Clin 1993;11:349–359.

Rubenstein R, Roenigk HH, Stegman SJ, Hanke CW. Atypical keloids after dermabrasion of patients taking isotretinoin. J Am Acad Dermatol 1986;15:280–285.

Rubin M. Manual of Chemical Peels. Philadelphia: Lippincott; 1995.

Sarkar R, Kaur C, Bhalla M, et al. The combination of glycolic acid peels with a topical regimen in the treatment of melasma in dark skinned patients: a comparative study. Dermatol Surg 2002;28:828–832.

Sharquie KE, Al-Tikreety MM, Al-Mashhadani SA. Lactic acid chemical peels as a new therapeutic modality in melasma in comparison to Jessner's solution chemical peels. Dermatol Surg 2006;32:1429–1436.

Soliman MM, Ramadan SA, Bassiouny DA, et al. Combined trichloroacetic acid peel and topical ascorbic acid versus trichloroacetic acid peel alone in the treatment of melasma: a comparative study. J Cosmet Dermatol 2007;6:89–94.

Tse Y, Ostad A, Lee HS, et al. A clinical and histologic evaluation of two medium-depth peels. Glycolic acid versus Jessner's trichloroacetic acid. Dermatol Surg 1996;22:781–786.

US Food and Drug Administration. AHAs and UV Sensitivity: Results of New FDA-Sponsored Studies. Available: http://vm.cfsan.fda.gov/~dms/cosahauv.html (4 February 2008).

Van Scott EJ, Yu RJ. Alpha hydroxy acids: procedures for use in clinical practice. Cutis 1989;43:222–228.

West TB, Alster TS. Effect of pretreatment on the incidence of hyperpigmentation following cutaneous CO_2 laser resurfacing. Dermatol Surg 1999;25:15–17.

Winnington P. Conquer hyperpigmentation after laser resurfacing. Skin Aging 2000;8:43–58.

Yu RJ, Van Scott EJ. Bioavailable alpha hydroxyl acid in topical formulations. In: Moy R, Luftman D, Kakita L, eds. Glycolic Acid Peels. New York: Marcel Dekker, 2002:15–28.

Yug A, Lane JE, Howard MS, Kent DE. Histologic study of depressed acne scars treated with serial high concentration (95%) trichloroacetic acid. Dermatol Surg 2006;32:985–990.

Zachariae H. Delayed wound healing and keloid formation following argon laser treatment or dermabrasion during isotretinoin treatment. Br J Dermatol 1988;118:703–706.

Vascular and pigment lasers

Jillian Havey and Murad Alam

Introduction, definition, and history

Erythema, telangiectasia, leg veins, and cherry angiomas can be treated with vascular lasers and lights (Table 6-1). Similarly, lentigines and tattoos respond to treatment by lasers for pigmented lesions (Table 6-2).

Laser treatment of vascular and pigmented lesions is founded on the theory of selective photothermolysis, as expounded by John Parrish and Rox Anderson in 1983. In layperson's terms, vascular and pigmented lesions are treated by lasers that emit light wavelengths that are selectively and preferentially absorbed by targets, or chromophores, within the blood vessel or pigmented area.

As a general rule, unsightly moles and other melanocytic lesions are seldom treated with laser in the USA. This is based on the solely theoretic risk of energy-mediated malignant transformation within such lesions, as well as the view that worrisome melanocytic lesions should be biopsied to assess their provenance and guide management.

Patient evaluation: examination and history

Preoperative evaluation should assess the nature and anatomic location of the complaint, as well as the patient's skin type. Caucasian patients and those with Fitzpatrick skin types I–III are the best candidates for laser treatment of vessels and pigment. Postinflammatory hyperpigmentation may occur in darker skinned patients. Facial lesions are in general easier to treat than body lesions, as there may be more overlying dermis off the face and healing is also slower on the trunk and extremities owing to reduced blood supply.

Patients undergoing laser treatment for reduction of red and brown areas should have reasonable expectations. Several treatments, usually three to six or more, may be required for significant improvement. Total remission is unlikely. Normal aging and continued sun exposure may also lead to the gradual return of the lesions, which can then be addressed by occasional touch-up treatments.

In general, macular and papular seborrheic keratoses, and other pigmented lesions with texture, are not amenable to laser treatment. If the diagnosis is uncertain because the pigmented lesion appears flat, an initial laser treatment may be attempted and, if unsuccessful, may then militate in favor of a destructive modality, such as low-energy electrodessication.

Melasma (Fig. 6-1) seldom improves with lasers or lights, and may be exacerbated after treatment. Patients with light gray to brown macular confluent pigmentation of the mid-forehead, upper cheeks under the eyes, and upper lip may have undiagnosed melasma. In such patients, a test spot at low settings should be attempted to ensure that lasers or lights do not make the melasma worse.

Erythematous lesions on the face often occupy a malar distribution with superimposed fine telangiectasia around the nose and medial cheeks (Fig. 6-2). Centrofacial redness of this type,

Table 6-1 Lasers and light commonly used for treatment of vascular lesions

Type of laser or light device	Indications	Special considerations
Pulsed-dye laser (585–595 nm)	Superficial vascular lesions	Erythema can be treated without bruising; treatment of telangiectasia may require purpura or stacked pulses
KTP laser (532 nm)	Superficial telangiectasia	Useful for treatment of facial telangiectasia; can be used in combination with other vascular lasers and lights
Intense pulsed-light device	Superficial vascular lesions	Broad emission spectrum permits simultaneous treatment (500–1200 nm) of pigmented lesions; treatment possible without bruising; may require more treatments with more specific lasers
Nd:YAG laser (1064 nm)	Deeper vascular lesions	Long-pulse device can be used in conjunction with other laser and light devices; more painful than other devices

Table 6-2 Lasers and lights commonly used for treatment of pigmented lesions

Type of laser or light device	Indications	Special considerations

Q-switched lasers
  Frequency-doubled Nd:YAG (532 nm)
  Ruby (694 nm)
  Alexandrite (755 nm)
  Nd:YAG (1064 nm)
	Lentigines, tattoos	Darkening and "cayenne pepper"-like stippling may occur for several days after treatment, and then fades; macular seborrheic keratoses and melasma do not respond

Intense pulsed-light device (500–1200 nm)	Lentigines, poikiloderma	Overall treatment of brown–red discoloration achievable; may require more treatments than a Q-switched laser
Fractionated laser and light	Lentigines, poikiloderma	Also, simultaneous treatment of fine lines and wrinkles; resurfacing devices require fewer treatments than light, but some downtime

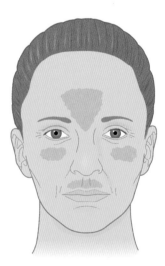

Figure 6-1 Melasma, appearing as confluent gray–tan pigmentation in the mid-forehead, infraorbital skin, and upper cutaneous lip, seldom responds to lasers and lights for treatment of pigmented lesions. In fact, melasma may be temporarily darkened and made more noticeable after laser treatment

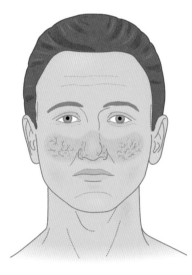

Figure 6-2 Centrofacial redness in a butterfly distribution is common in Caucasian patients. Fine telangiectasia may be superimposed on diffuse redness of the medial cheeks and nose

Table 6-3 Types of cutaneous vascular lesion treatable with laser and light devices

Type of lesion	Type of laser or light commonly used
Diffuse centrofacial erythema	Pulsed-dye, intense pulsed light
Poikiloderma of Civatte	Pulsed-dye, intense pulsed light
Facial telangiectasia	KTP, pulsed-dye, intense pulsed light
Facial reticular veins	Nd:YAG
Venous lakes	Pulsed-dye, Nd:YAG
Cherry angiomas	Pulsed-dye
Leg telangiectatic veins	Pulsed-dye, Nd:YAG, intense pulsed light
Leg reticular veins	Nd:YAG

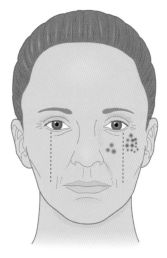

Figure 6-3 Pulsed-dye laser at aggressive settings, such as those required to treat thick telangiectasia, can induce bruising that lasts for days to weeks. Bruising can also be delayed, and may manifest several hours after treatment. Lateral to the midpupillary line, over the malar eminence, bruising may be especially easily elicited, and fluences may need to be decreased when this area is treated. Idiosyncratic bruising occurs when, despite use of consistent settings, one or two areas bruise, but the remainder of the treated area does not

frequently labeled "rosacea" even when other manifestations of that process are not seen, is highly treatable with lasers and lights. Telangiectatic leg veins, as well as deeper reticular leg veins, may respond to vascular lasers and lights (Table 6-3).

Index of devices and device selection

Innumerable laser and light devices are available for treatment of vascular and pigmented lesions. Those used most commonly for vascular lesions can be separated into several categories:

- Pulsed-dye lasers
- Potassium–titanyl–phosphate (KTP) lasers
- neodymium:yttrium–aluminum–garnet (Nd:YAG) lasers
- intense pulsed-light devices.

Pigmented lesions are treated most often with Q-switched lasers and intense pulsed light. Additionally, some minimally ablative fractional resurfacing devices, as well as fully ablative laser and nonlaser devices, can reduce pigmentation.

Pulsed-dye lasers

Key Points

- Pulsed-dye lasers are successful at treating diffuse facial erythema, facial telangiectasia, cherry angiomas, small telangiectatic leg veins, and larger superficial vascular lesions.
- Scarring or textural abnormality following pulsed-dye laser treatment is rare.

Pulsed-dye lasers, which are 585–595-nm devices, are successful at treating a range of superficial vascular lesions. Settings can be optimized for facial diffuse erythema, which can now be treated without bruising by long-pulse pulsed-dye lasers.

Fine facial telangiectasia may also be treated without bruising, but larger telangiectasia and those at resistant sites such as the nasal ala, may require shorter pulse durations that induce mild to moderate ecchymoses, which may be difficult to conceal with make-up and resolve over a week or longer (Fig. 6-3).

Multiple passes can permit the treatment of larger lesions without bruising. Such multiple passes can be separated by some time, or be consecutive at the same site, which may be bombarded with subpurpuric "stacked" pulses until the lesion of interest visibly dissipates. Delayed bruising can manifest several hours after pulsed-dye laser used at near-purpuric settings. Treatment of the lateral cheeks may require less aggressive settings to avoid bruising. The use of special handpieces that compress and blanch superficial vasculature enables the treatment of pigmented lesions with pulsed-dye lasers.

Overall, pulsed-dye lasers have an unsurpassed safety record. Scarring or textural abnormality is extremely rare post-treatment. Postinflammatory hyperpigmentation is a risk in darker skinned patients treated with bruising fluences, but such pigmentation always resolves. Pulsed-dye lasers have been shown to soften scars and induce collagen remodeling; patients receiving such pulsed-dye treatments for vascular lesions may have secondary improvement of skin suppleness and texture.

Pulsed-dye lasers can also be used to treat new-onset venous lakes, including post-traumatic lip lesions which patients may find unsightly. A common application off the face is treatment of cherry angiomas. Many such lesions can be quickly and efficiently treated with settings that bruise only the angioma and not the surrounding skin. Resolution of the angioma is thereby accomplished without the scarring sometimes associated with electric needle ablation. Fine telangiectatic leg veins that are too small to be cannulated by sclerotherapy, as well as telangiectatic mats caused by sclerotherapy, can also be improved with the pulsed-dye laser. Leg vein treatment with the pulsed-dye laser causes bruising, which may resolve slowly. Women, the most frequent recipients of such treatments, may prefer to be lasered in the winter months, when their legs are not exposed.

KTP lasers

Key Points

- KTP lasers are successful at treating fine facial telangiectasia.
- KTP lasers can be combined with other vascular devices to treat more extensive facial vascular lesions.
- If the same site is treated repeatedly, deep indentations can develop as a result of laser-induced focal necrosis.

KTP lasers, usually 532-nm devices, are small lasers with limited but specialized applications. Fine facial telangiectasia can be directly treated by tracing with this device. Disappearance of vessels is immediate, although some may recur. Visualization of fine capillaries may be improved if the operator uses a headset with a polarized light designed to reduce glare. Pattern generators and larger spot sizes are available that allow the KTP laser to treat a wider area more efficiently.

The KTP laser can be combined with pulsed-dye and other vascular devices for the treatment of facial vascular lesions. Grooving, or the formation of deep indentations following laser-induced focal necrosis, may occur if the same site is treated repeatedly; the thick sebaceous skin of the lower nose in men is the most susceptible location.

Nd:YAG lasers

Key Points

- Nd:YAG lasers are successful at treating deeper cutaneous vascular lesions, and are also useful for laser hair removal.
- Although more painful than other vascular devices, the Nd:YAG laser is less likely to cause hyperpigmentation in skin types IV–VI

Long-pulsed Nd:YAG lasers are used for the treatment of deeper cutaneous vascular lesions. Such devices have been used in combination with pulsed-dye lasers, with the former treating the deeper component of a mixed vascular lesion.

Resistant facial vascular lesions may have persistence beyond the depth of penetrance of the pulsed-dye laser and require Nd:YAG treatment (Fig. 6-4). Bluish reticular veins of the face, which may be perioral or periorbital and more visible in patients with fair, near-translucent skin, can also be treated with Nd:YAG. Off the face, reticular leg veins are amenable to Nd:YAG; small intravascular clots may form after treatment, and can be extruded after puncture and compression of

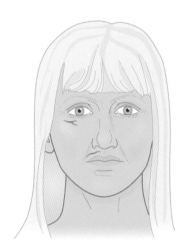

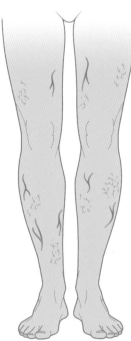

Figure 6-4 Deep blue reticular veins can be seen periorally and periorbitally in patients with fair, translucent skin. These, and similar leg veins, can be treated by long-pulsed Nd:YAG laser. Appropriate cooling is necessary to protect the overlying skin and diminish pain perception. Telangiectatic leg vessels can also be treated by Nd:YAG laser, and pulsed-dye laser may also resolve these smaller, more superficial, vessels

the affected site. Nd:YAG treatment is often eschewed because it is substantially more painful than treatment with other cutaneous vascular devices. However, this laser, which is also used for laser hair removal, is less likely to cause hyperpigmentation in patients with skin types IV–VI.

Q-switched lasers

Key Points

* Q-switched lasers are successful at treating pigmented lesions, lentigines, and tattoos.
* Different wavelengths target specific tattoo colors.
* Incomplete tattoo removal even after numerous Q-switched laser treatments is not uncommon.

Q-switched lasers, including the frequency-doubled Nd:YAG (532 nm), ruby (694 nm), alexandrite (755 nm), and Nd:YAG (1064 nm), have pulse durations in the nanosecond range and are workhorses for the treatment of pigmented lesions. Lentigines and tattoos respond to low and high fluences, respectively. Three to six treatments may be required for reduction of lentigines, and 10 to 20 or more treatments may be necessary for even partial resolution of densely pigmented tattoos. Tan lesions of the face that respond to Q-switched lasers will darken and develop a "cayenne pepper"-like particulate appearance for about a week after treatment; they then become lighter (Fig. 6-5). Lesions that do not exhibit any such darkening and lightening response after treatment may be macular seborrheic keratoses that are amenable only to a destructive modality.

Q-switched lasers are the undisputed first-line treatment for tattoos. Premedication with topical or intralesional anesthetic may increase the tolerability of tattoo treatments. Pinpoint bleeding may be elicited. Different wavelengths target pigment of specific colors, with sky blue, green, yellow, and orange being particularly difficult to remove. Patients undergoing laser treatment for tattoos should be prepared to have uneven removal of pigment at various sites, and some areas may remain minimally improved even after many treatments. Pigment darkening and color change induced by oxidation and other processes can follow attempts at tattoo removal. Often, further tattoo removal treatments will reduce this darkening. Unwanted cosmetic tattoos, such as lip liner and eyebrow tattoos, may be particularly susceptible to color change, and the centrofacial location may make such problems more concerning for patients.

Gold therapy in the distant past can precipitate blue-greenish discoloration, or "chrysiasis," after treatment with the Q-switched laser for lentigines and other complaints.

Intense pulsed-light devices

Key Points

* Intense pulsed-light devices are multi-wavelength lamps that are successful at treating vascular lesions and pigmented lesions.
* When these devices are used by nonmedical personnel, they should be used with great caution to avoid adverse events such as transient hyperpigmentation, permanent hypopigmentation, and scarring.

Intense pulsed-light devices are not lasers but rather lamps that emit at a range of wavelengths. Pioneering devices in this category covered the range from 500 to 1200 nm. Newer devices have

(a)

(b)

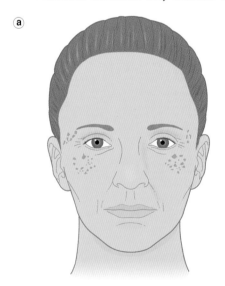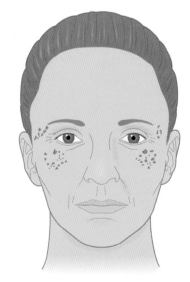

Figure 6-5 After treatment with Q-switched lasers, lentigines darken temporarily. A stippled "cayenne pepper"-like appearance precedes the gradual lightening of these lesions over several days

more specific ranges, which are often augmented by filters that exclude certain wavelengths to focus on a desired subset of wavelengths. Handpieces and filters may be appropriate for vascular lesions, pigmented lesions, or both. Intense pulsed-light devices, by virtue of emitting various wavelengths, offer the promise of simultaneous treatment of vascular and pigmented lesions.

In many US states, intense pulsed devices are regulated more lightly than lasers; this can facilitate delegation of their use to nonphysician and even nonmedical personnel. When used to treat vascular lesions, intense pulsed-light devices may require more iterative treatments than a pulsed-dye laser, but without the risk of bruising. Pigmented lesions treated with intense pulsed light may similarly resolve more slowly than those treated with Q-switched lasers.

Intense pulsed-light devices are versatile and powerful, but, given their many parameter settings and ability to influence multiple chromophores at the same time, should be used carefully by novices. Many adverse events associated with nonphysician laser and light operation have been linked to intense pulsed-light devices, particularly those used for hair removal. Transient configurate hyperpigmentation, permanent hypopigmentation, and scarring are commonly reported (Fig. 6-6).

Method of device or treatment application

Dose setting/selection

There is a dose-related trade-off between comfort and efficacy. Higher fluences and briefer pulse durations are associated with more rapid resolution of pigmented and vascular lesions, but more undesired effects. Pain is increased at higher treatment levels; for cosmetic improvement of skin color, high levels of discomfort may be treatment limiting and impractical. Short-pulse duration treatment with pulsed-dye laser that is effective for larger, resistant, superficial vascular lesions may cause deep blue–black bruising, which can take 3 weeks to resolve completely. Intense pulsed-light devices may require more repeat treatments and yet may be sufficiently gentler so that patients are willing to expend more total time and money. Of course, laser treatments can be similarly decreased in intensity to meet patient preferences. Very intense treatments may be appropriate for patients with a high pain threshold, tolerance for downtime, and a limited budget.

Treatment technique

Once an appropriate device has been selected for a pigmented or vascular lesion, selection of treatment parameters is imperative. Commonly variable parameters include fluence, pulse duration,

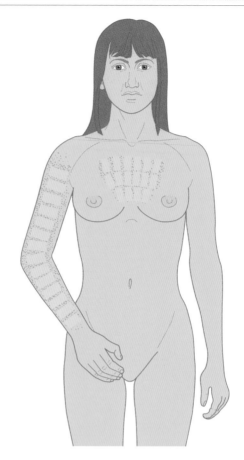

Figure 6-6 Overly aggressive treatment with lasers and lights can result in hypopigmentation at the treated site. Here, treatment of arm and chest lentigines with an intense pulsed-light device has left configurate rectangular hypopigmented areas shaped like the treatment tip

spot size, and cooling settings. Parameters must be appropriate for the lesion characteristics and the patient's skin type. In general, more darkly pigmented patients will benefit from less intense settings, which are less likely to induce undesired pigmentary alteration.

Physical operation of the laser or light device should be done in accordance with manufacturer specifications. Rules of thumb apply. First, eye protection is mandatory for use with medical grade lasers. Patients usually wear opaque goggles, and operators don colored filters. It is imperative to read the inscription on nonopaque eyewear to ensure that it is protective for the wavelength being used. Nd:YAG lasers, if fired into an open pupil, can ablate the retina, causing permanent retinal field defects. Even pulsed-dye lasers, which are extremely safe, have been associated with vitreous floaters if used without adequate eye protection.

Positioning of the handpiece over the patient is important. Some handpieces are meant to be

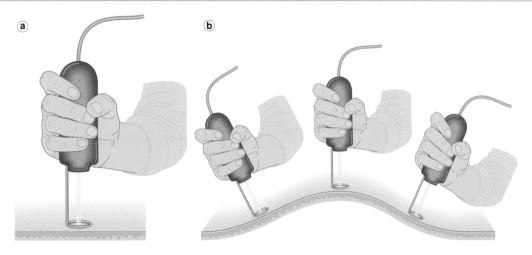

Figure 6-7 The laser or light handpiece should be applied perpendicular to the skin surface. Continual readjustment of the operator's grip is required to maintain this orientation as the handpiece is moved over areas of skin curvature

applied directly to the skin, and some are placed at a fixed distance, which is maintained by a spacer attachment or an aiming beam. The angle of incidence should be perpendicular to the skin (Fig. 6-7). As the handpiece is moved across the face or other curved surface, the angle is continually modified to maintain this flush orientation. Overlap may or may not be desired. For treatment of diffuse vascular and pigmented lesions, such as widespread erythema and lentigines respectively, a modest 10–25% overlap is desirable to avoid lines of demarcation or untreated areas (Fig. 6-8). Intense treatments, such as those with the long-pulse Nd:YAG or treatments of tattoos, may be done with little or no overlap to avoid dermal injury.

During the treatment process, it is important to ensure that the laser or no light source is working properly. Fiberoptic cables that may connect the handpiece to the laser box can be inadvertently broken if bent excessively. Articulated arms that carry handpieces in some devices should not be hit or shocked to avoid misalignment of the mirrors that convey the laser light. Cooling can also fail, and such failures should be noticed immediately. Sapphire windows provided with some Nd:YAG device handpieces need to be pressed against the skin to cool the epidermis; if they are inadvertently lifted off the skin in whole or in part, overtreatment may lead to skin necrosis and scar. Dynamic cooling devices collimated with many pulsed-dye lasers spray a cryogen at the target just before the laser fires; if this spray is interrupted, superficial thermal skin injury can cause scar or hyperpigmentation. Detectors exist to ensure that a blockage in the line carrying coolant is detected automatically, but such detectors can malfunction. It is therefore important to listen for the slight hiss associated with operation of the dynamic cooling device.

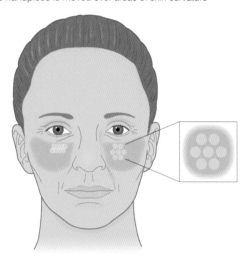

Figure 6-8 "Honeycombing," configurate arrays of residual erythema, can develop if inadequate overlap is used when treating diffuse erythema or poikiloderma. Usually, 15–30% overlap is necessary to ensure that the shape of the treatment tip is not repetitively and recognizably stamped in the field of redness

PEARLS

Treatment of vascular and pigmented lesions

Treatment parameters include fluence, pulse duration, spot size, and cool settings.

More darkly pigmented patients benefit from less intense settings.

Patients and treating medical personnel should wear protective eyeware.

Pay attention to manufacturer specifications for positioning of the laser handpiece and degree of overlap of treatment areas.

Listen for the "hiss" associated with operation of a dynamic cooling device.

Alternative treatment methods

Nonlight treatments can be used to treat vascular and pigmented lesions. Chief among these alternatives are electrodessication and cryotherapy. Facial telangiectasia, angiomas, and venous lakes can be treated with electrocautery, often fitted with fine epilating needle tips. Electrodessication or cryotherapy can be used to treat pigmented lesions. Flat seborrheic keratoses may respond well to light electrocautery, and cryopeeling can remove not only actinic damage but also widespread lentigines or keratoses. Ablative laser resurfacing, medium to deep chemical peels, and dermabrasion can also improve extensive diffuse pigmentation. Fractionated laser and light devices may be successful in treating poikiloderma and mixed pigmented and erythematous lesions on and off the face. Fractionated resurfacing may have a better safety profile and is associated with less downtime than true ablative resurfacing. Several treatments with fractionated devices are usually required to soften skin pigmentation.

Management of adverse events

Adverse events following laser and light treatment of pigmented and vascular lesions tend to be mild and spontaneously resolving. Mild erythema and edema are common after most procedures. Resolution is within a few hours to a day. Purpura, either mild or more evident, and either localized or confluent, can occur after intense treatment with 532-nm Q-switched lasers or pulsed-dye lasers. Ecchymoses will resolve over days to weeks, and can be camouflaged with green-tinged make-up. Pinpoint bleeding and crusting is not uncommon when tattoos are treated aggressively. Emolliation under occlusion or topical steroids can quickly treat such erosions.

More long-lasting adverse events include hyperpigmentation, hypopigmentation, and scar or textural abnormality. Tanned patients should not receive laser or light treatment, as this can increase the risk of hyperpigmentation, even in fair-skinned patients. Darker skinned patients have an increased risk of hyperpigmentation, and this can be mitigated by pretreatment with bleaching agents and the use of less aggressive laser settings. Excessive or insufficient epidermal cooling can both induce hyperpigmentation. Patients with postinflammatory hyperpigmentation can be reassured that this will completely remit; superficial chemical peels, bleaching agents, and sun avoidance may hasten the process slightly.

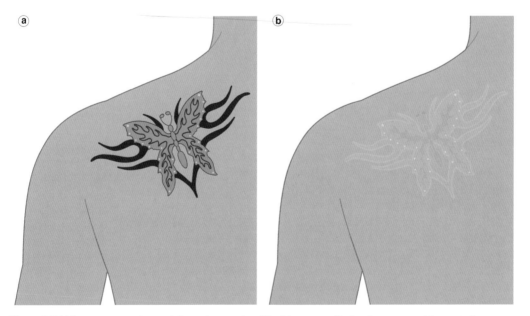

Figure 6-9 Yellow, orange, and green tattoo colors can be difficult to remove. Such colors can persist even as the blue–black framework of the tattoo slowly fades. When Q-switched lasers are used to treat tattoos in patients with darker skin, a halo of hypopigmentation can develop around the edge of the tattoo. Lower fluences and more treatments may help to avoid this

Hypopigmentation is associated with very intense laser treatments. Tattoo laser treatments at high fluence in darker skinned patients may result in hypopigmented halos around the borders of the tattoo pigment (Fig. 6-9). High fluence intense pulsed-light treatments have been associated with rectangular and figurate hypopigmented patches. Laser-induced hypopigmentation can be long lasting to permanent, and is easier to avoid than to treat. Fractional ablation devices are less likely to induce hypopigmentation that traditional ablative lasers.

Scarring is a serious but rare complication. Failure of cooling during the use of long-pulse Nd:YAG lasers for treatment of deeper vascular lesions has been associated with tissue necrosis and development of scar. Scar creation is very rare with the pulsed-dye laser. Erosions, apparent necrosis, and blisters, if they do occur, can be treated with superpotent topical steroids to speed healing and reduce the likelihood of permanent sequelae.

Urticarial-type lesions, which not uncommonly emerge immediately after treatment with Q-switched lasers, usually remit quickly and completely.

PEARLS

Adverse events

Mild adverse events include: erythema, edema, ecchymoses, pinpoint bleeding, and crusting.

Longlasting adverse events include hyperpigmentation, hypopigmentation, and scarring.

Avoid hyperpigmentation in darker skinned patients by pretreatment with bleaching agents, less aggressive laser settings, appropriate cooling, and sun avoidance.

Further reading

Alam M, Dover JS, Arndt KA. Treatment of facial telangiectasia with variable-pulse high-fluence pulsed-dye laser: comparison of efficacy with fluences immediately above and below the purpura threshold. Dermatol Surg 2003;29:681–684.

Alam M, Omura NE, Dover JS, Arndt KA. Clinically significant facial edema after extensive treatment with purpura-free pulsed-dye laser. Dermatol Surg 2003;29:920–924.

Alam M, Dover JS, Arndt KA. Use of cutaneous lasers and light sources: appropriate training and delegation. Skin Therapy Lett 2007;12:5–9.

Alora MB, Arndt KA, Taylor CR. Scarring following Q-switched laser treatment of "double tattoos." Arch Dermatol 2000;136:269–270.

Anderson RR, Parish JA. Selective photothermolysis: precise microsurgery by selective absorption of pulsed radiation. Science 1983;220:524–527.

Bekhor PS. Long-pulsed Nd:YAG laser treatment of venous lakes: report of a series of 34 cases. Dermatol Surg 2006;32:1151–1154.

Goyal S, Arndt KA, Stern RS, O'Hare D, Dover JS. Laser treatment of tattoos: a prospective, paired, comparison study of the Q-switched Nd:YAG (1064 nm), frequency-doubled Q-switched Nd:YAG (532 nm), and Q-switched ruby lasers. J Am Acad Dermatol 1997;36:122–1225.

Holzer AM, Burgin S, Levine VJ. Adverse effects of Q-switched laser treatment of tattoos. Dermatol Surg 2008;34:118–122.

Kauvar AN, Rosen N, Khrom T. A newly modified 595-nm pulsed dye laser with compression handpiece for the treatment of photodamaged skin. Lasers Surg Med 2006;38:808–813.

Mariwalla K, Dover JS. The use of lasers for decorative tattoo removal. Skin Therapy Lett 2006;11:8–11.

Prinz BM, Vavricka SR, Graf P, Burg G, Dummer R. Efficacy of laser treatment of tattoos using lasers emitting wavelengths of 532 nm, 755 nm and 1064 nm. Br J Dermatol 2004;150:245–251.

Ueda S, Isoda M, Imayama S. Response of naevus of Ota to Q-switched ruby laser treatment according to lesion colour. Br J Dermatol 2000;142:77–83.

Varma S, Swanson NA, Lee KK. Tattoo ink darkening of a yellow tattoo after Q-switched laser treatment. Clin Exp Dermatol 2002;27:461–463.

Wang CC, Sue YM, Yang CH, Chen CK. A comparison of Q-switched alexandrite laser and intense pulsed light for the treatment of freckles and lentigines in Asian persons: a randomized, physician-blinded, split-face comparative trial. J Am Acad Dermatol 2006;54:804–810.

Ablative devices

Tina Bhutani and R. Sonia Batra

Introduction

Historically, people in many societies have searched for methods to restore youthful appearance and rejuvenate aging skin. Stories recount the efforts of ancient Chinese emperors and Spanish explorers to seek mythical substances thought to have the ability to reverse the aging process. During the Dark Ages, European alchemists investigated magical methods for prolonging life and restoring youthful beauty. These beliefs have permeated modern society, as people continue to seek assistance for facial skin rejuvenation from healthcare professionals all over the world. In fact, due to the aging population and increasing interest in the field, more options now exist than ever before for reversing cutaneous changes caused by long-term exposure to sunlight. More recently, the spectrum of skin issues for which these methods have been utilized has expanded past the treatment of photo-aging to include many skin problems more common in youth, such as pigmentary disorders and acne scarring.

Laser use on the skin has become one of the most popular methods for achieving a younger and smoother facial appearance. Thousands of physicians are adding cosmetic lasers to their practice. Ongoing laser research and the publication of findings in medical journals have increased

exponentially. The blitz of media attention on the miracles of laser surgeries has caused patients to flood physicians' offices seeking laser firepower to turn back the clocks on their aging faces. Unfortunately, the increasingly widespread availability of cosmetic laser therapy coupled with attendant publicity has created extraordinary, often unrealistic, expectations. Many patients may believe that lasers are magic wands, capable of restoring their skin to the flawless perfection of infancy. Of course, the truth is that cosmetic lasers are not the answer for all dermatologic ills. Although laser surgery is less painful and risky than some of the techniques it has replaced, it is still surgery, with potential complications that may accompany any surgical procedure.

This chapter discusses methods of ablative laser rejuvenation. Although a myriad of techniques are available, the most commonly used lasers, including the carbon dioxide (CO_2) and erbium : yttrium–aluminum–garnet (Er:YAG) systems, are discussed here. In addition, some of the newer modalities, including fractional laser resurfacing and plasma skin regeneration, are described. The goal is to describe the techniques for using these lasers, as well as to enumerate the most common side-effects and the best methods for avoiding these reactions. In addition, information on patient selection and methods to avoid patient dissatisfaction is included.

Clinical examination and patient history

Proper patient selection and assessment of each individual's skin type is crucial prior to determining whether an ablative procedure is indicated. The preoperative consultation is important to identify at-risk patients who are best avoided, or who necessitate an extra-cautious approach, as well as to select patients who are ideal candidates for an ablative procedure. It is imperative to identify the key goals of the patient, such as an improvement in color, texture, or wrinkling, expected timeframe or number of procedures, and patient tolerance for recovery or "downtime" after the procedure. The physician should explore whether a patient may tolerate more downtime or multiple treatments/interventions in order to achieve the primary goal (Box 7-1).

At the time of the initial consultation, the dermatologist must discuss the indications for the procedure; evaluate the patient for relative contraindications; review limitations as well as the potential risks of the procedure; and assess the patient's goals, expectations, and anticipated results. A thorough history should include other medical conditions, past surgeries and complications, including a history of excessive scarring or keloid formation, past resurfacing or laser treatment modalities, if any, and a detailed list of medications. Any history of herpes simplex virus infection should also be elicited. Chronic medical illnesses, prior radiation, chemical or thermal burns, and medications known to delay wound healing may all play a role in scarring and recovery. A history of abnormal scar formation or pigmentary alterations after previous procedures should influence a more conservative therapeutic approach (Box 7-2).

The preprocedure consultation is an opportunity not only to identify and discuss therapeutic options for the patient's chief complaint, but also to understand whether the patient's expectations of the procedure, postoperative period, and results are realistic. It is essential that the patient's goals and expectations are reasonable prior to selecting the patient for a procedure, as this has a strong correlation with postoperative patient satisfaction. The patient must fully understand the potential benefits, limitations, and risks, and an informed consent must be signed before performing the procedure.

Moreover, to achieve a successful procedural outcome, a physician's understanding of cultural differences and preferences among patients from minority ethnic groups is equally as important as the technical proficiency in the procedures to be performed. Cultural preferences can be understood through open discussion with the patient and knowledge of the manner in which cultural variations can affect communication. The doctor should encourage the patient to verbalize concerns and expectations in order to achieve the greatest patient satisfaction ultimately. Care must also be taken to make the patient feel comfortable in the clinical setting and to provide continuous support through the postprocedural period and beyond.

Skin type classification

Owing to the marked variability in skin color across the globe, in 1988 Fitzpatrick developed a standardized method to classify skin types according to color and reaction to sun exposure (Table 7-1). This information can enable the physician better to determine which patients are at higher risk for dyschromias after resurfacing. Patients are classified into a particular skin type by asking them what happens when they are exposed to ultraviolet (UV) radiation. Skin types range from I to VI, with ethnic skin usually classified in the spectrum between types IV and VI.

As melanin is thought to have photoprotective effects, darker skinned individuals are less prone to the direct damage of UV light and are able to maintain a naturally youthful appearance later into life. In fact, studies have shown that about three to four times more UVA light reaches the upper dermis of caucasians when compared to blacks. Consequently, long-term exposure to differing intensities of light produces varied changes between these two groups. While lighter skinned individuals are more likely to present with deep-seated wrinkles, darker patients are usually seen with finer wrinkles, mottled hyperpigmentation, and unique skin lesions such as dermatosis papulosa nigra and actinic lentigines (Fig. 7-1). In addition, patients with Fitzpatrick skin types IV–VI respond to UV injury by producing more melanin. Thus, they are at higher risk for the development of dyschromias after a laser resurfacing procedure. Therefore, it is important to understand the common manifestations of photo-aging in ethnic skin in order to provide the best treatment options. It is critical to determine a patient's skin type before deciding on a procedure, because results and adverse effects will differ accordingly.

Although the Fitzpatrick classification helps to determine the risk of dyschromias after laser resurfacing, it does not assess the degree of damage caused by UV radiation. A classification introduced by Richard Glogau assesses the degree of photo-damage to the skin (Table 7-2). It takes into account the extent of wrinkling, cellular atypia, dyschromias, use of make-up, and degree of acne scarring. Patients with type I damage are typically young with no wrinkling and minimal photo-damage. Those with type IV damage, on the other hand, have significant photo-damage, severe wrinkling, are older, and often have a prior history of skin malignancy.

The Glogau classification system helps the physician determine the depth of damage, and thus offers some indication of what the depth of resurfacing should be. Patients with minimal photo-damage may require ablation of only the upper part of the epidermis. Those with moderate photo-damage may require more extensive resurfacing to the level of the papillary dermis, and so on.

Device or treatment selection

As noted above, the patient's goals and severity of condition will guide the therapeutic plan. All ablative options discussed in this chapter can address photo-aging, pigmentary disturbance, and acne scarring. In general, laser skin resurfacing provides the greatest depth of ablation and is an excellent option for severe acne scarring or photo-aging. However, the potential improvement in texture afforded by this technique must

Table 7-1	Fitzpatrick skin types	
Skin type	Color	Skin characteristics
I	White	Always burns, never tans
II	White	Usually burns, tans less than average
III	White	Sometimes mild burn, tans about average
IV	White	Rarely burns, tans more than average
V	Brown	Rarely burns, tans profusely
VI	Black	Never burns, deeply pigmented

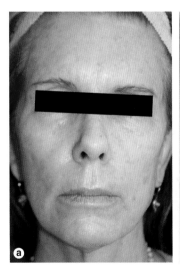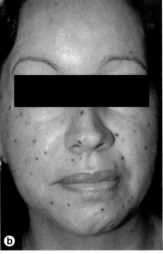

Figure 7-1 Differences in manifestations of photo-aging in light versus ethnic skin. (A) Signs of photo-aging in a lighter skinned individual, including fine lines, fat redistribution and/or volume loss, and loss of skin elasticity. (B) Typical photo-aging changes in darker or ethnic individuals include actinic lentigines; flat, pigmented seborrheic keratoses; and mottled hyperpigmentation. In addition, sun-induced melasma is also more common in this group than in whites (not shown here)

Table 7-2 Glogau classification

Damage	Description	Characteristics
I (mild)	No wrinkles	Early photo-aging: • Mild pigmentary changes • No keratoses • Minimal wrinkles • Patient age: 20s to 30s • Minimal or no make-up • Minimal acne scarring
II (moderate)	Wrinkles in motion	Early to moderate photo-aging: • Early senile lentigines • Keratoses palpable but not visible • Parallel smile lines beginning to appear • Patient age: 30s to 40s • Some foundation make-up worn • Mild acne scarring
III (advanced)	Wrinkles at rest	Advanced photo-aging: • Obvious dyschromias and telangiectasia • Visible keratoses • Static wrinkles present • Patient age: older than 50 years • Heavy foundation usually worn • Acne scarring: make-up cannot cover
IV (severe)	Only wrinkles	Severe photo-aging: • Yellow–gray skin color • Prior skin malignancies • Wrinkles throughout – no normal skin • Patient age: 60s or 70s • Make-up cannot be worn – it cakes and cracks • Severe acne scarring

Adapted from Hoenig & Morrow (1998)

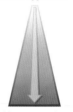

Least aggressive

Microdermabrasion
Superficial chemical peel
Medium-depth chemical peel
Deep chemical peel
Er: YAG lasers
Combination CO_2/Er:YAG lasers
CO_2 lasers

Most aggressive
(greatest depth of ablation)

Figure 7-2 Commonly used ablative modalities for skin resurfacing: spectrum from least to most aggressive

Although not discussed here, an alternate, more conservative, approach is to choose a less aggressive modality, such as chemical peels or nonablative lasers, and for the patient to undergo a series of treatments. This is particularly true for microdermabrasion, which affords the best results with regular therapy sessions. In any ablative modality, strict sun protection must be emphasized to the patient postoperatively to minimize the risk of pigmentary alteration.

Method of device or treatment application

Laser resurfacing

The word laser is an acronym, which stands for *l*ight *a*mplification by the *s*timulated *e*mission of *r*adiation. Laser light has unique properties that allow it to be used therapeutically. Consequently, the popularity of laser procedures has skyrocketed in the past decade as the indications for use and types of lasers available continue to multiply. Laser light is monochromatic (single wavelength), coherent (in phase, both in time and space), and collimated (light waves are parallel). These properties make possible the generation and delivery of high fluence (energy per area), which can interact with the skin. Additionally, the monochromaticity of laser light is essential for selective targeting of structures in the skin that preferentially absorb light of that wavelength. Commonly targeted chromophores in the skin, which each have their own unique absorption spectrum for laser light (Fig. 7-3), include water, hemoglobin, and melanin.

When laser light hits the skin, it may be reflected, transmitted, or absorbed (Fig. 7-4). Absorbed energy is most responsible for the clinical effect because it is converted to thermal energy by absorption of heat by the intended targets. In many cases, complications result from collateral damage created when energy intended for the target chromophore is nonselectively diffused to

be weighed against the greater potential for pigmentary alteration and/or scarring. A greater depth of ablation will usually require increased recovery time, which must also be made clear to the patient. Figure 7-2 depicts the spectrum of ablative modalities in terms of aggressiveness.

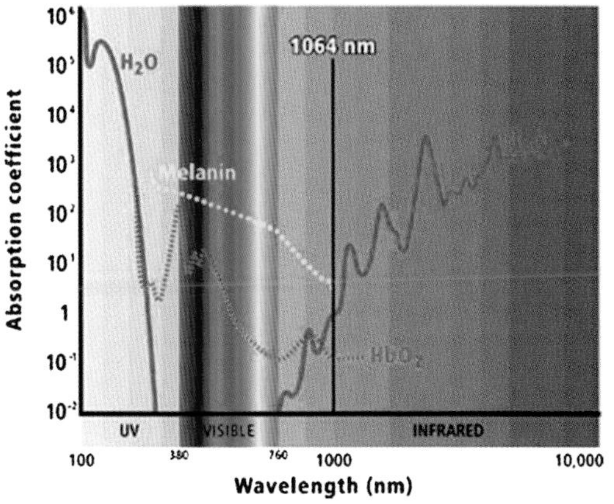

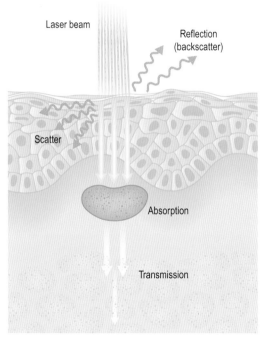

Figure 7-3 Laser chromophore absorption. Adapted from McBurney (1998), p 159

Figure 7-4 Interaction of laser light and tissue. Adapted from McBurney (1998), p 157

Even when wavelengths relatively specific for a particular chromophore were used, their continuous output meant that the amount of tissue exposure to laser light depended on the speed of the surgeon's hand – typically long enough to cause a build-up of thermal energy that diffused to nontargeted adjacent tissue. This led to undesirable rates of adverse effects and complications (notably, scarring), which limited the use of cutaneous lasers.

In the mid 1980s, Anderson and Parrish revolutionized the therapeutic use of lasers with the development of the theory of selective photothermolysis; by using ultrashort pulses of high-energy laser light rather than a continuous beam, collateral thermal damage could be minimized. Pulse duration is considered optimal if it is shorter than the target chromophore's relaxation time, defined as the time required for the targeted site to cool to one half of its peak temperature immediately after laser irradiation. In addition, the majority of cutaneous lasers are now used with systems that cool the epidermis to prevent collateral damage to epidermal structures from laser light intended to target deeper tissues.

Research stemming from these new theories and developments has led to a variety of lasers, electrosurgical, and nonlaser light devices that are currently being used for facial rejuvenation. These devices are divided into those that:

- ablate the epidermis, cause dermal wounding and provide a significant thermal effect (e.g. CO_2 lasers)
- ablate the epidermis, cause dermal wounding, and provide minimal thermal effects (e.g. short-pulsed Er:YAG lasers)
- ablate the epidermis, cause dermal wounding and provide variable thermal effects (e.g. combined CO_2–Er:YAG lasers, variable-pulsed Er:YAG lasers, and ablative radiofrequency devices)
- do not ablate the epidermis, cause dermal wounding, and provide minimal thermal effects (e.g. nonablative lasers and light sources).

and absorbed by surrounding tissue. For example, hyperpigmentation and hypopigmentation noted after CO_2 laser resurfacing are related to damage to melanocytes vaporized along with targeted keratinocytes and fibroblasts in the epidermis and dermis. Similarly, in laser-assisted hair removal, unwanted damage to the epidermis (including melanocytes) may occur despite the fact that follicular melanin is the intended target.

The cutaneous application of laser technology was launched in 1956 with the development of the 694-nm ruby laser by Maiman. The first cutaneous lasers used continuous beams of laser light.

Each of these modalities has specific advantages and disadvantages; however, this chapter focuses on ablative technologies, which fall into the first three categories. Nonablative methods are discussed in Chapter 8.

Carbon dioxide lasers

Key Points

- CO_2 laser resurfacing can be performed in the office or under anesthesia.
- The wavelength 10,600 nm.
- Depth of tissue ablated per pass is approximately 20–30 μm.

- Thermal damage produced is 30–100 μm.
- Time to re-epithelialization is 7–10 days.
- Duration of post-laser erythema is 3–6 months.
- Significant collagen shrinkage and remodeling requires at least two passes.
- A greater number of passes or excess energy densities results in an increased risk of scarring.
- CO_2 systems in pulsed or scanning modes deliver predictable ablation levels and consistent results.
- Advantages include excellent tissue contractions and hemostasis.
- Valuable for treating entire cosmetic subunits, focal lesions, or full-face resurfacing.
- Indications include moderate to severe rhytides and photo-damage, scarring, actinic keratosis, and other superficial lesions.
- In ethnic skin types, more conservative settings and fewer passes can decrease the risk of scarring and pigment alteration.
- Laser "test spots" in inconspicuous areas can be performed in patients at high risk of dyschromia.

Laser skin resurfacing (LSR) with the CO_2 laser remains the "gold standard" for clinical and histologic improvement in severely photo-damaged and scarred facial skin. In fact, the development of high-energy pulsed CO_2 systems in the early 1990s revolutionized aesthetic laser surgery and ushered in a new decade of rapidly evolving laser technology. Producing a wavelength of 10,600 nm, the CO_2 laser penetrates approximately 30 μm into the skin by the absorption and vaporization of water-containing tissues. Energy densities of approximately 5 J/cm^2 must be applied in order to achieve tissue ablation. With each subsequent laser pass, vaporization of very thin (20–30 μm) layers of skin occurs, leaving a small amount of residual thermal necrosis. With each subsequent laser pass, further tissue ablation occurs, but, because the area of residual thermal necrosis increases (effectively reducing the amount of tissue water and hence the targeted chromophore), the amount of ablation with each pass diminishes until a peak of approximately 100 μm is reached. Delivering more than three to four passes, or the use of excessive energy densities, significantly increases the risk of excessive thermal injury and subsequent scarring.

Several CO_2 laser systems are available and can be separated into two distinct groups: pulsed and scanned. The high-energy pulsed CO_2 lasers (e.g. Ultrapulse, Lumenis) produce single, short (1 ms) pulses of very high energy (up to 7 J/cm^2). A computerized pattern generator (CPG) attached to the laser delivery system can rapidly and precisely place 2.25-mm spots in any of several patterns while maintaining appropriate ablation parameters. A large square pattern can be used to treat large areas rapidly. The density of the pattern can be low (nonoverlapping spots)

or high (10–60% overlapping spots). A 3.0-mm collimated handpiece (TrueSpot) is also available for difficult-to-reach areas. The handpiece eliminates the need to focus the laser at a set distance from the target tissue. This provides exact control of spot size and more consistent results. The conventional focusing handpiece can cause irregular ablation and increased thermal damage. Scanned laser systems (e.g. FeatherTouch, Lumenis; Silk-Touch, Lumenis) utilize a computerized scanning device to deliver lower power CO_2 laser energy in the continuous mode rapidly over the skin, thus limiting the tissue dwell time in one area. This system achieves high peak powers by focusing the laser beam to small spot size, and rapidly scans the focused beam over a predetermined geometric pattern, exposing the individual tissue sites for less than 1 ms. A study comparing four different CO_2 lasers found that pulsed systems produced the least amount of thermal necrosis with the greatest subsequent collagen formation (compared with the scanned systems), but equivalent clinical outcomes between all four lasers were observed.

Cutaneous CO_2 laser resurfacing, as currently performed, has been shown to be highly effective in the treatment of photo-damaged skin. In addition to superficial ablation, there is a "tissue tightening" effect following use of these lasers. This effect is thought to be related to heat-induced collagen shrinkage, which occurs maximally at 63°C. Long-term collagen remodeling and neocollagenesis also occur after resurfacing, although the mechanisms behind this are not fully known. It is believed that these effects result from thermal desiccation associated with the concomitant collagen shrinkage. In addition, because there is increased expression of smooth muscle actin after laser treatment, the contracted area may serve as a scaffolding on which new collagen is formed and deposited during wound phase remodeling. These factors are most likely responsible for the long-term clinical improvement seen after resurfacing.

Dose/setting selection

Due to the various parameters involved in the resurfacing technique, settings can vary dramatically according to physician experience and preferences. However, many studies have examined the use of different systems, settings, and ultimate clinical outcomes.

Fitzpatrick and colleagues were among the first to evaluate clinical improvement in mild, moderate, and severe perioral and periorbital wrinkles seen after pulsed laser resurfacing. In their study, multiple passes of confluent singles pulses using the UltraPulse laser (Lumenis) were utilized with a 10% overlap and a 3-mm collimated beam. Pulse energies of 450 mJ were used for the first pass and subsequent passes were treated at 450 mJ (perioral) and 350 mJ (periorbital). Patients were evaluated postprocedure for up to 12 months; an average wrinkle reduction of 45–50% for both treatment areas was found.

Walforf and co-workers, in a retrospective review, performed a similar study to evaluate the clinical results in 47 patients with fine to deep glabellar, perioral, and periorbital rhytides after treatment with the SilkTouch (Lumenis) scanned laser system. One to three passes were provided with a 3-mm spot size (energy 7.5 W, pulse duration 0.2 s) or a 6-mm spot size (18–20 W). In this study, the authors calculated a 60–85% improvement and concluded that the greatest impact was seen in the periorbital area and the least in the glabellar area.

In ethnic patients, more conservative laser settings and fewer passes may decrease the risk of scarring and/or pigmentary change. With an Ultrapulse (Lumenis), the CPG scanner is used primarily and a 3-mm collimated spot for feathering or small areas. Overlap should be 10% or less. The authors prefer a pattern shape of 2 (parallelogram), pattern size 9, density 5, 250 mJ per pulse fluence, 50 W power, and repeat rate 1.5/s. The fluence and power may be decreased at the periphery of treatment to blend with surrounding skin and to minimize the risk of scarring.

Treatment technique

For at least 6 weeks before the procedure, patients may use topical tretinoin in the highest tolerable concentration. If a patient is retinoid intolerant, an α-hydroxy acid may be substituted. Concomitantly, topical lightening agents, such as hydroquinone, soy extract, kojic acid, or azelaic acid, can be used. Patients should be counseled to avoid tanning prior to the procedure and to minimize postoperative sun exposure. Postinflammatory hyperpigmentation (PIH) is a common postoperative side-effect in patients with phototypes IV–VI.

All patients receive prophylactic antibiotics, starting the day before resurfacing and continuing for 1 week. Dicloxacillin 500 mg twice daily or, in penicillin-allergic patients, levofloxacin 500–750 mg daily, are common choices. Prophylactic antiviral therapy with valaciclovir 500 mg twice daily is also begun 2 days preoperatively and continued for 10 days after resurfacing.

Vaporization of epidermal and dermal tissue causes significant pain, and adequate anesthesia must be achieved. This can be accomplished by a combination of topical anesthesia, local infiltration, and regional nerve blocks. Oral sedatives and analgesics may be used adjunctively.

The patient should wash his or her face thoroughly with a gentle cleanser, and thereafter an antiseptic may be used to prepare the skin. Scalp hair may be wrapped with moist towels and Surgilube (Fougera) applied to eyebrows and scalp margins. Corneal shields may be inserted to protect the eyes.

Epidermal ablation can be seen after only one pass with the CO_2 laser; however, collagen shrinkage and remodeling require an additional one to two passes in order to reach the optimal temperature. After the first pass, desiccated proteinaceous debris can be removed by wiping with saline-moistened gauze. Some authors believe that a single pass that leaves the char in place to act as a biologic dressing may minimize the risk of pigmentary change and scarring. Increased passes may be used for areas of deeper wrinkling or scarring. In ethnic or darker skin types, no more than three to four passes should be performed as this greatly increases the risk of scarring.

PEARLS

Preoperative care for CO_2 laser use

Pretreatment regimen: broad-spectrum sunscreens, tretinoin and/or glycolic acid creams, prophylactic oral antibiotics, and antiviral medications

Topical lightening agents: hydroquinone, kojic acid, soy, azelaic acid, and others can also be used to reduce postinflammatory hyperpigmentation.

Anxious patients: oral benzodiazepines such as diazepam (5–10 mg) can be given half an hour before the procedure.

Postoperative care

Following laser skin resurfacing, either open or closed wound care techniques may be employed. Most open wound care regimens consist of frequent soaks with cool compresses of 0.25% acetic acid, normal saline, or cool tap water lasting for 10–20 min every 2–4 h, followed by gentle wiping of the skin. Cold compresses are immediately followed by the application of a bland emollient ointment. Popular ointments include Catrix®-10 (Lescarden) and Aquaphor® Healing Ointment (Beiersdorf). The frequency of soaks and ointment application decreases as re-epithelialization progresses and is tapered off when re-epithelialization is complete.

Studies indicate that closed wound care regimens utilizing occlusive dressings for 48–72 h postoperatively may hasten re-epithelialization and reduce crusting, discomfort, erythema, and swelling. Dressings employed after resurfacing include the composite foam Flexzan® (Dow Hickam Pharmaceuticals), the hydrogel product 2nd Skin® (Bionet), the plastic mesh N-terface® (Winfield Laboratories), and the polymer film Silon-TSR® (Bio Med Sciences). Occlusive dressings are applied for 2–3 days postoperatively.

Longer applications increase the risk of infection with subsequent scarring. The authors employ the Silon-TSR®, a silicone dressing with a polytetrafluoroethylene inner polymer network.

Immediately after resurfacing, the face is blotted dry and the dressing is applied. Openings are cut for the eyelids, nose, and central lips, and a smaller patch of dressing is applied to cover the nasal bridge. Gauze 4×4-inch dressings are applied over the mask to absorb exudates, and held in place by tube gauze. Patients are seen on the first postoperative day and the gauze is removed. The resurfaced area is inspected through the transparent mask, and accumulated exudate or crust is removed from uncovered areas with saline. Patients are instructed to begin iced-water soaks through the mask for 20-min periods at 2–4-h intervals while awake. Patients return again at the third postoperative day and the dressing is removed. They continue soaks at 3–4-h intervals followed by application of Aquaphor® healing ointment.

In both open and closed wound care regimens, by 7–10 days after the procedure soaks are replaced with gentle cleansing, and patients switch to the application of a moisturizer–sunscreen.

PEARLS

Postoperative care for CO$_2$ laser use

Wound care: dilute acetic acid, saline, or tap water soaks every 2–4 h followed by bland emollients are essential for proper healing

Medications: continuation of oral antibiotics and antiviral drugs; short-term pain medications including narcotics should be given if necessary

Follow-up: post-laser follow-up in the office at 2–5 days is valuable to note the quality of the patient's wound care and the progress of wound healing.

Management of adverse events

As noted above, prophylactic antibiotics and antiviral agents should be begun preoperatively, and any sign of infection should be treated aggressively as it may result in scarring. Over 80% of patients note pain in the immediate postoperative period. This can be minimized by intraoperative use of supplemental local anesthesia as well as systemic pain medication. After LSR, ice packs, cold compresses, and acetaminophen help to alleviate pain as well. Approximately 85% of patients require pain medications for the first 3 days postoperatively, and those not relieved by acetaminophen often benefit from acetaminophen with codeine phosphate or acetaminophen with hydrocodone bitartrate.

Pruritus often occurs during re-epithelialization and typically lasts for about 10 days. Pruritus can often be relieved by cool compresses and emollients,

although more than half of patients require oral antihistamines. In more severe cases of severe pruritus, medium-to-high potency topical steroids may be required. Control of pruritus is essential because excoriation may result in scarring. Erythema typically occurs for up to several months after LSR. Erythema can be camouflaged with make-up containing green foundation. As noted above, particularly in ethnic patients, sun protection and avoidance should be encouraged during the entire period of post-LSR erythema to minimize PIH. Edema develops in the first 48 h after LSR. The severity can be controlled with ice packs and head elevation at night. In cases where marked edema develops during or immediately after the procedure, oral corticosteroids may be necessary.

Erbium : yttrium–aluminum–garnet laser

Key Points

- Can be performed in the office or under anesthesia.
- Wavelength 2940 nm.
- Tissue ablated per pass approximately 2–3 μm.
- Thermal damage produced 5–30 μm.
- Time to re-epithelialization 4–5 days.
- Duration of post-laser erythema 3–4 weeks.
- Er:YAG produces less thermal damage than the CO$_2$ laser – multiple passes are needed to ablate to an equivalent level.
- Indications are mild to moderate rhytides and photo-damage, mild to moderate scarring, and superficial lesions.
- Can be a good option in patients with darker skin types.

The short-pulsed Er:YAG laser was developed in the mid 1990s in an attempt to replicate the results of the CO$_2$ laser while minimizing the side-effect profile. The emitted wavelength of 2940 nm has a higher affinity for water and is therefore absorbed 12 to 18 times more efficiently by superficial cutaneous tissues. Approximately 2–5 μm of ablation occurs per pass, with very narrow zones of thermal necrosis. Clinically, this translates into a shorter postoperative healing time with a lower risk of post-treatment erythema and hyperpigmentation than with CO$_2$ lasers.

Several studies have documented the effectiveness of the Er:YAG laser in the treatment of mild to moderate rhytides, photo-damage, and atrophic scars, with the use of multiple passes, high fluences, and/or multiple sessions yielding improved clinical outcomes (Fig. 7-5). The Er:YAG laser has also been shown to be a good option for treatment of patients with darker skin types due to its lower risk of pigmentary alteration, and has been used to treat melasma.

With its higher affinity for water and ultrashort pulses of energy, the skin is removed precisely,

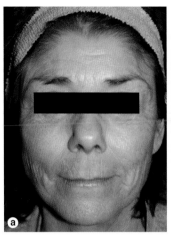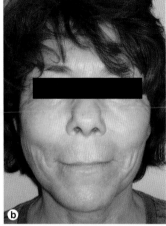

Figure 7-5 Appearance before (A) and after (B) ablative laser resurfacing with the Er:YAG laser

providing safety and reliability. As the Er:YAG laser ablates more efficiently than the CO_2 laser; one might hypothesize that lesser total fluences are required with the Er:YAG in comparison with CO_2. However, this is not the case. Fleming has shown that to achieve equal depth of injury the Er:YAG must ablate deeper than the CO_2 laser because there is minimal laser-induced thermal damage. Hence, multiple passes with the laser are necessary to ablate a similar depth as one pass of the CO_2 laser.

In addition, because the Er:YAG effects are photomechanical rather than photothermal (like the CO_2), intraoperative hemostasis is often difficult to achieve. The thermal damage zone created by this procedure is fixed and very small. In fact, this thermal damage is so shallow that it is insufficient to coagulate dermal capillaries. This explains why Er:YAG-lasered skin bleeds. The lack of thermal damage may also be considered a disadvantage when treating patients with severe wrinkles. Other limitations include the associated noise level and the large amount of plume produced.

Dose/setting selection

With the Er:YAG, approximately 4 μm of tissue is vaporized per J/cm^2 of energy applied. Therefore, a fluence of $5 J/cm^2$ will ablate the epidermis in four passes. Settings can be adjusted, depending on the depth of ablation desired. A repetition rate from 1 to 10 Hz and spot sizes from 3 to 7 mm can be selected with most Er:YAG lasers.

Teikemeier and Goldberg were among the first to evaluate the role of the Er:YAG laser in the treatment of patients with superficial rhytides. Twenty patients with mild periorbital, perioral, or forehead rhytides were treated with a 350-μs pulse duration Er:YAG laser. Pulses of energy varying from 400 to 800 mJ and spot sizes of 2.5 and 5 mm were chosen. The endpoint of treatment was

disappearance of clinical rhytides. Patients were evaluated at 2 days, 1 month, and 2 months for degree of improvement, time of healing, and resolution of erythema. At 2 months, all 20 patients were found to have improvement of wrinkles. This early study demonstrated that the Er:YAG laser was effective in improving superficial rhytides. Quicker re-epithelialization and resolution of erythema was attributed to the minimal thermal damage resulting from Er:YAG laser resurfacing.

Goldberg and colleagues expanded on the previous study by evaluating the Er:YAG laser for the treatment of class III rhytides, defined as generalized deep lines with distinctive textural changes of dermal elastosis. Twenty patients were treated with four 250-μs Er:YAG laser passes at $5 J/cm^2$, a spot size of 7 mm, and a repetition rate of 10 Hz. Three months after the initial treatment, a second treatment with similar parameters was performed. Six months after the initial treatment, a third treatment with identical parameters was performed. Although no improvement was seen after the initial laser session, mild to excellent improvement was noted 6 months after the final treatment. The authors concluded that, with multiple sessions, the Er:YAG laser can successfully treat class III rhytides.

Treatment technique

Patient preparation and anesthesia are performed similarly to those for the CO_2 laser. However, because the Er:YAG laser causes minimal pain, less anesthesia may be necessary for many patients, and topical and local anesthesia will suffice. After the first pass, proteinaceous material may be wiped with moistened gauze; however, after ablation of the epidermis, wiping is not necessary because the amount of debris is minimal. The treated area is covered with moderately overlapping (10–20%) spots. Overlapping of pulses

Table 7-3 Side-effects and complications of ablative laser skin resurfacing

Side-effects	Mild complications	Moderate complications	Severe complications
Transient erythema	Prolonged erythema	Pigmentary change	Hypertrophic scar
Localized edema	Milia	Infections (bacterial, fungal, viral)	Ectropion
Pruritus	Acne		
	Contact dermatitis		

In general, side-effects and complications following Er:YAG laser are similar but less severe and more transient compared with those experienced after CO_2 laser resurfacing

does not create difficulties, as is the case with CO_2 lasers. The surgeon must keep track of the number of passes performed to minimize the risk of scarring and pigmentary alteration.

If using a long-pulsed Er:YAG laser, the effect is similar to that of a CO_2 laser, and initial passes may be performed to induce collagen tightening and coagulation of small dermal vessels. Thereafter, the short-pulse mode may be used for ablation and to remove thermal damage. This technique is similar to that for combination CO_2–Er:YAG resurfacing discussed below, in which the CO_2 laser is used first, followed by one to two passes of an Er:YAG device.

Postoperative care

Wound care is performed similarly to that following CO_2 resurfacing.

Management of adverse effects

Side-effects and complications are varied and greatly influenced by postoperative care, patient selection, and operator skill. In general, the side-effect profile after Er:YAG laser resurfacing is similar but less severe and more transient than that following CO_2 laser resurfacing (Table 7-3). For example, in all CO_2-laser treated patients, postoperative erythema lasting an average of 4.5 months is an expected occurrence and a normal consequence of the wound healing process. Erythema after short-pulsed Er:YAG resurfacing is comparatively transient, lasting for 2–4 weeks. In addition, time to re-epithelialization averages 8.5 days with multipass CO_2 laser resurfacing, compared with 5.5 days after Er:YAG resurfacing.

Hyperpigmentation is a relatively common side-effect, typically seen 3–6 weeks after ablative resurfacing. After CO_2 resurfacing, the reported incidence is 5% in the periorbital area and 17–83% at other facial sites, with an even greater incidence in patients with darker skin tones. Hyperpigmentation also occurs after Er:YAG laser resurfacing. However, when compared with multipass CO_2 laser treatment, hyperpigmentation caused by dual-pass Er:YAG resolves 6 weeks earlier. Hyperpigmentation typically fades spontaneously but dissipates more rapidly with application of any of a variety of glycolic, azelaic, or retinoic acid creams, light glycolic acid peels, and/or hydroquinone

compounds. Hypopigmentation can also be seen after delayed onset (more than 6 months postprocedure), and is more often longstanding and very difficult to treat. Fortunately it is seen far less frequently than is hyperpigmentation.

A potentially more serious complication of laser skin resurfacing is infection – viral, bacterial, or fungal. Even with appropriate antiviral prophylaxis, herpes infection (usually reactivation of latent virus) occurs in 2–7% of patients postoperatively. In addition, patients must be followed closely in the postoperative period and placed on appropriate antibiotics if bacterial or fungal infection is suspected. As noted above, if infections are left undiagnosed or untreated, systemic infections or scarring can result.

Scarring has also been attributed to the use of aggressive laser parameters and/or overlapping or stacking of laser pulses, which leads to excessive residual thermal necrosis of tissue. In addition, resurfacing of the neck and chest has a greater potential for scarring due to the scarcity of pilosebaceous units in these regions and resultant slow re-epithelialization.

PEARLS

Management of adverse events

Hyperpigmentation: continue broad-spectrum sun protection, bleaching creams, and series or superficial peels

Infection: be guided by culture and sensitivity

Scarring: aggressive treatment will lead to resolution. Topical steroid creams with intralesional steroids if hypertrophic scars, series of pulsed dye laser treatments, silicone sheeting, or topical gels. Arrange frequent gratis follow-up visits in your office

Combination CO_2–Er:YAG laser systems and variable-pulsed Er:YAG laser

Key Point

- CO_2–Er:YAG laser systems combine CO_2 energy for coagulation and Er:YAG for finer tissue ablation.

To address the limitations of short-pulsed systems, novel modulated systems have been developed to allow deeper zones of thermal damage and a greater level of hemostasis. Hybrid CO_2–Er:YAG laser systems are capable of delivering both CO_2 energy for coagulation and Er:YAG energy for finer tissue ablation. The dual-mode Er:YAG combines short pulses (for ablation) and longer pulses (for coagulation). The variable-pulsed Er:YAG system has a range of pulse durations from $500\,\mu s$ to $10\,ms$, with the longer pulses effecting coagulation and thermal injury similar to those with the CO_2 laser. As a group, these lasers have been shown to produce deeper tissue vaporization, greater control of hemostasis, and collagen contraction. This translates into greater clinical improvement in skin with mild to moderate acne scars and photo-damage than their short-pulsed predecessors, and thus represent a good compromise between CO_2 and earlier generation Er:YAG lasers.

CO_2 laser studies have demonstrated that this modality ablates approximately $100\,\mu m$ of skin, leaving an additional 50–$300\,\mu m$ of collateral thermal damage. As described above, this thermal damage promotes collagen contraction and remodeling. However, it can also lead to prolonged recovery time and complications. Studies with short-pulsed Er:YAG lasers, with their higher water absorption rate and shorter pulse duration than CO_2 lasers, demonstrate tissue ablation of 20–$40\,\mu m$ with each pass, and collateral thermal damage of 5–$30\,\mu m$. This amount of tissue ablation and thermal damage is typically much less than that seen with CO_2 laser resurfacing.

In theory, combining the deep tissue penetration of a CO_2 laser with the fine depth control of an Er:YAG laser may improve clinical outcome, and decrease both recovery time and associated complications (Fig. 7-6). The use of combinations of CO_2 lasers and Er:YAG lasers prompted the development of alternative laser resurfacing technology. One such system, the Derma-K laser (Lumenis), is a combined CO_2–Er:YAG laser. This system combines simultaneous low-fluence CO_2 laser and short-pulsed Er:YAG laser delivery. Such a laser delivers the combined deep thermal damage and associated collagen remodeling of a CO_2 laser with the more precise ablative capacity of an Er:YAG laser. Another approach to laser resurfacing is found in the CO_3 (Cynosure) and Contour (Sciton) variable-pulsed Er:YAG lasers. The CO_3 laser is a single variable pulse-width Er:YAG laser. The Contour laser is, in fact, two separate Er:YAG lasers that fire almost simultaneously. One of these lasers is a short-pulsed Er:YAG laser; the other emits a longer, variable pulse-width Er:YAG laser pulse. The variability seen with both of these lasers allows the user to choose various levels of tissue ablation and/or thermal effect. These choices can provide a unique degree of control in resurfacing that is not provided by either standard short-pulsed Er:YAG or CO_2 lasers.

Manuskiatti and colleagues performed one of the earliest clinical evaluations of sequential CO_2 and Er:YAG laser treatment. In this study, 30 patients were treated with full-face CO_2 laser resurfacing. Some were then treated with a short-pulsed Er:YAG laser in an attempt to remove a portion of the CO_2 laser-induced residual thermal damage. Postoperative follow-up varied with each patient. According to the authors, all deep rhytides and all deep acne scars responded better to a sequential CO_2/Er:YAG laser treatment compared with CO_2 laser treatment alone. Healing times were on average 2–3 days faster with sequential treatment.

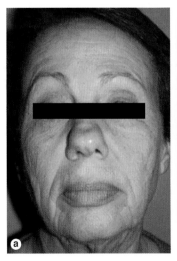 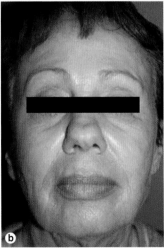

Figure 7-6 Appearance before (A) and after (B) ablative laser resurfacing with a combination CO_2–Er:YAG laser in a caucasian patient with typical signs of photo-aging

Goldman and Marchell were among the first to evaluate the effect of combined CO_2–Er:YAG lasers. In one study, 11 patients were treated with two passes of a combined CO_2–Er:YAG laser. The patients were monitored for 2 weeks postoperatively and then re-evaluated at 3–6 months. Physician evaluation revealed moderate improvement in skin color and a marked improvement in skin texture and wrinkling for all patients. Most patients felt that they had a 75–100% improvement in their skin texture. The overall patient satisfaction rating was 75–100% in 10 of the 11 patients, with one patient giving a rating of 50–74%. No hypopigmentation or scarring was found in this study. Similar results may be seen with the variable-pulsed Er:YAG lasers.

Increasing accumulated data about both the combined CO_2–Er:YAG lasers and variable-pulsed Er:YAG lasers now exist. Their effect and healing response appear to be a good compromise between the more aggressive, yet highly effective, CO_2 lasers and the less aggressive, albeit not as effective, short-pulsed Er:YAG lasers.

Fractional lasers

Key Points

- Fractional laser devices produce rejuvenation and collagen remodeling by creating thousands of microscopic wounds called microscopic treatment zones (MTZs) with sparing of adjacent skin.
- Indications include mild to moderate rhytides and photo-damage, acne scars, melasma and other pigmented lesions, and actinic keratoses.

While ablative skin resurfacing with CO_2 and Er:YAG lasers has proven highly effective in reversing the signs of facial photo-aging and atrophic scars, the associated lifestyle hindrance and potential complications are often unacceptable to patients. In recent years, focus has shifted to nonablative technologies that deliver either laser, light-based, or radiofrequency energies to the skin without alteration of the epidermal surface. Although effective for collagen contraction and popular for a low side-effect profile and minimal recovery period, the use of nonablative lasers for more severe photo-damage has revealed inconsistent results with no epidermal resurfacing effects.

Fractional lasers attempt to bridge this gap between ablative and nonablative laser modalities, and are now being used in many centers to treat the epidermal and dermal effects of skin aging. By targeting water as a chromophore, the 1550-nm erbium fiber laser induces a dense array of microscopic, columnar, thermal zones of tissue injury that do not perforate or impair the function of the epidermis. In addition, for every MTZ (microthermal zone, or microscopic treatment zone) that the laser targets and treats intensively,

it leaves the surrounding tissue unaffected and intact (Fig. 7-7). This "fractional" treatment allows the skin to heal much faster than if the entire area were treated at once, owing to the presence of residual viable epidermal and dermal cells. The skin remodeling that ensues can be used to treat, with less downtime, epidermal pigmentation, melasma, and rhytides, as well as textural abnormalities that include acne-related and surgical scars (Fig. 7-8).

The spatially precise columns of thermal injury produce localized epidermal necrosis and collagen denaturation at 125 or 250 MTZ/cm^2. The depth of penetration of each MTZ is energy dependent and can be tailored to the characteristics of the treatment area (facial versus nonfacial skin). Histologic evaluation of the MTZ demonstrates homogenization of dermal matrix and the formation of microscopic epidermal necrotic debris, which represents the extrusion of damaged epidermal components by viable keratinocytes at the lateral margins of the MTZ. The stratum corneum remains intact during the process, thereby maintaining epidermal barrier function.

The fractional laser contains an intelligent optical tracking system that utilizes OptiGuide Blue™ tint, a water-soluble Federal Food, Drug, and Cosmetic Act (FD&C) dye. The optical mouse in the laser handpiece recognizes subtle differences in the density of blue dye on the skin's dermatogliphs. The mouse communicates with the laser to lay down an even MTZ spot pattern independent of handpiece velocity. This system allows for a more even placement of MTZs, which is important in fractional tissue treatment where the optimal spacing between lesions allows for rapid re-epithelialization and prevents negative sequelae associated with fully ablative treatment at depths of 300–800 μm.

Fractional ablative CO_2 systems (10,600 nm) have been shown to produce similar results to traditional bulk CO_2 lasers with significantly less downtime and a reduced risk of adverse events. These lasers deliver focused CO_2 energy as opposed to confluent zones of tissue ablation. Clinical indications include photo-damage, rhytides, textural irregularities, dyschromia, and scars.

Dose/setting selection

Using the 15-mm handpiece on the 1550-nm erbium-doped fiber laser (Fraxel, Reliant Technologies), it is recommended that facial skin receive eight passes at a fluence of 8 mJ/cm^2 and a density of 250 MTZ/cm^2 to an endpoint of approximately 2000 MTZ/cm^2, or approximately 3 kJ. Treatment may be used consecutively every 3–4 weeks until desired results are achieved. Clinical improvement is greatest 3 months after a series of fractional photothermolysis treatments,

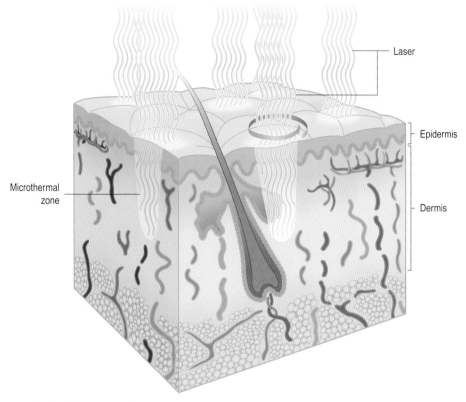

Laser

Epidermis

Microthermal
zone

Dermis

Figure 7-7 Fractional laser resurfacing

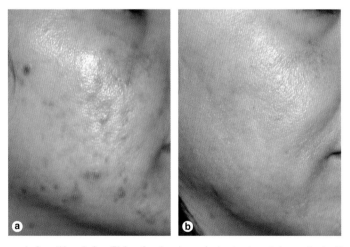

Figure 7-8 Appearance before (A) and after (B) four fractional resurfacing treatments in a patient with acne scarring. The patient was treated concomitantly for active acne vulgaris

a finding that stands in contrast to results seen after purely nonablative, mid-infrared lasers where optimal efficiency was obtained 6 months after treatment.

Treatment technique

Pain management is one of the most significant hurdles of the procedure. Discomfort from the laser treatment is managed by use of a topical anesthetic prior to the procedure. Oral anxiolytics and analgesics may be required in a small minority of patients who cannot tolerate the procedure with topical anesthetic alone.

Forced air cooling (Zimmer), which is often used concurrently with fractional laser treatment, increases patient comfort significantly. Histologic analysis reveals a slight reduction in thermal damage zone width, but no statistically significant change in lesion depth. Forced cooled air should be used at the lowest possible setting to minimize alteration in the MTZs. When treating for superficial indications such as pigmentation and melasma, the Zimmer setting should be 1–2. When treating deeper indications such as deeper rhytides or scars, higher forced air settings, in combination with higher laser settings, may be used.

Adverse effects and postoperative care

Postoperatively, patients can apply sunscreen and/or make-up. There is no oozing because there is no disruption in the stratum corneum, but some patients may experience excessive desquamation and some crusting following an aggressive treatment. The majority of patients experience some degree of erythema, which resolves within 2–3 days after gentle to modestly aggressive treatment. Erythema may persist for up to 1 week after more aggressive treatments. This often resembles a sunburn.

Post-treatment edema is very patient dependent. Some have little swelling. The average patient experiences edema for 1–3 days, more than 5% of patients for up to 1 week. The risk of edema also increases with higher-level treatments. This can be alleviated by applying ice at 10-min intervals for the first 24 h after treatment, and by sleeping with the head elevated on extra pillows. Although some physicians advocate the use of topical or short-course systemic steroids following treatment, the inflammatory cascade that leads to subsequent upregulation of collagen production may be best left unaltered.

There is always a risk of postinflammatory pigmentary alteration following any type of inflammatory process in the skin, and fractional laser treatments are no exception. One review of this technique indicated an approximately 10–12% incidence of hyperpigmentation after fractional treatments. This is most common in patients with a history of PIH or melasma. PIH is more common in patients with darker skin types; hence, a precautionary 6-week pretreatment with hydroquinone and a strict sun protection regimen are advisable for these individuals.

Lastly, bulk heating can result from treating too large a fraction of the skin at one time, or from inadequate cooling between laser passes. To reduce the risk, the density of MTZs per pass should be halved to $125\,MTZ/cm^2$ when using energies above 15 mJ. Treating a small area without allowing the skin to cool between passes can lead to bulk heating, even at lower energies. Treatment of more than 35–40% of the skin in a single session may lead to adverse sequelae. Maintaining sufficient normal tissue between the deep zones of coagulate epidermis and dermis is essential for rapid healing following fractional treatments.

Plasma skin regeneration

Key Points

- Plasma skin rejuvenation delivers plasma energy into the dermis while leaving the skin surface intact, leading to neo-epithelialization and collagen synthesis.
- Indications include fine to moderate rhytides and photo-damage, dyschromias, scars, and superficial lesions.

A newer modality uses energy delivered from plasma rather than light or radiofrequency. Plasma is a unique state of matter in which electrons are stripped from atoms to form an ionized gas. The plasma is emitted in a millisecond pulse to deliver energy to target tissue upon contact without reliance on skin chromophores. The Portrait® plasma skin regeneration (PSR) device (Rhytec) is approved by the US Food and Drug Administration for multiple, single-pass, low-energy treatments and for single-treatment, one-pass, high-energy treatment of facial rhytides and superficial skin lesions. In a pilot study evaluating the use of a single full-facial treatment at high energy (3–4 J), a mean improvement in overall facial rejuvenation of 50% was found by 1 month.

The Portrait® PSR device consists of an ultra-high-frequency radiofrequency generator that excites a tuned resonator and imparts energy to a flow of inert nitrogen gas within the handpiece. The activated ionized gas is termed plasma and has an optical emission spectrum with peaks in the visible range (mainly indigo and violet) and near-infrared range. Nitrogen is used for the gaseous source because it is able to purge oxygen from the surface of the skin, minimizing the risk of unpredictable hot spots, charring, and scar formation. On formation, the plasma is directed through a quartz nozzle out of the tip of the handpiece in a 6-mm diameter spot. As the plasma hits the skin, energy is rapidly transferred to the skin surface, causing instantaneous heating in a controlled uniform manner, without an explosive effect on tissue or epidermal removal.

Dose/setting selection

The depth of thermal effect is determined by the energy setting. The energy can be adjusted from 1 to 4 J per pulse. There is a self-calibration feature within the generator that verifies that the energy delivered matches the preset level. By using different energy settings, the technology can be used to affect different depths of the skin, from superficial epidermal effects similar to microdermabrasion to deeper dermal heating similar to CO_2 resurfacing. Preliminary studies examining a single pass of 1–4 J over postauricular skin showed that at 1–2 J thermal energy was limited to the epidermis and dermoepidermal junction. At 3–4 J, thermal energy reached the papillary dermis. The frequency of pulses can be varied from 1 to 4 Hz as well.

There are three recommended treatment guidelines: PSR1, PSR2, and PSR3. The PSR1 protocol uses a series of low-energy treatments spaced 3 weeks apart. The first treatment is performed at 1.0–1.2 J, and fluences are increased as tolerated at subsequent visits. Recovery time is 3–4 days. The PSR2 protocol uses one high-energy pass (3.0–4.0 J) with a recovery time of 5–7 days, and the PSR3 protocol uses two high-energy passes with a recovery time of 6–10 days. A series of treatments in the mid-energy group (1.5–3.0 J) produced good results in improving skin texture and discoloration, but involved only slightly less recovery time than a single high-energy treatment, and less skin tightening. Thus, most practitioners prefer to use the suggested PSR1, 2, or 3 protocols.

Preoperative considerations and treatment technique

The first step is to assess the patient and determine the goals of treatment. Low-energy PSR1 treatments can normally be performed under local anesthesia with a topical agent. For mid to high energies, patients require adjunctive oral anesthesia such as meperidine or a codeine derivative, in addition to a topical agent. Patients should arrive early so that the topical anesthetic cream can be applied and left on for approximately 1 h. Oral anesthesia should be administered 30–45 min before the procedure begins. To avoid unexpected downtime, it is important for the physician to develop a standard protocol for removal of topical anesthesia and delay time before starting the procedure. Hydration of the epidermis influences the amount of energy that is absorbed and the depth of thermal insult achieved, with drier tissue absorbing more energy.

Generally, it is a good idea to work in aesthetic segments of the face, removing the anesthetic cream for each area immediately before treating that area, rather than removing the cream for the entire face all at once. This helps to standardize the delay time between anesthetic removal and treatment. Anesthetic should be gently wiped off with dry gauze. Again, it is not necessary to use water or alcohol-soaked gauze as this will change the hydration properties of the skin.

Once a facial segment is ready for treatment, the tip of the handpiece should be held approximately 5 mm from the skin surface. The pulses are delivered in a paintbrush fashion in one direction across the treatment area. The pulses should be delivered in rows of one direction (either all right to left, or all left to right) because a zig-zag pattern has been found to cause heat build-up at the corners where direction is changed to start the next row. Pulses should not be overlapped

by more than about 10%. To avoid lines of demarcation in the high-energy protocol, the borders of the treatment area should be feathered by increasing the distance of the nozzle from the surface of the skin to about 1 cm. Feathering can be achieved by holding the handpiece nozzle at an angle with respect to the skin surface, or by reducing the power setting. There is no need for feathering in the low-energy PSR1 protocol.

Postoperative care

Patients should be instructed to avoid sun exposure and to apply a bland ointment to the face at frequent intervals after the procedure while the skin is healing. Low-energy PSR1 treatments may cause only erythema, for 2–3 days. High-energy treatments will cause erythema and a "dirty" look to the skin, which will resolve in 5–10 days as re-epithelialization occurs and the photo-damaged epidermis is sloughed off. It is important for patients not to excoriate peeling skin, in order to avoid prolonged erythema or scarring.

Major side-effects are likely to be rare with this modality. As for all procedures utilizing heat energy, side-effects that could occur include erythema, edema, epidermal de-epithelialization, scarring, and hyperpigmentation. At the time of writing, there have been no reported instances of hypopigmentation. Erythema and edema are common postprocedure, and usually resolve within several days. Edema can be decreased by the application of ice after the procedure. Epidermal de-epithelialization is possible at higher energies, and should be treated with appropriate wound care and liberal application of bland ointment, as for ablative laser skin resurfacing.

Considerations in ethnic skin

The most common complication in dark-skinned patients after laser surgery is PIH, as mentioned above. Although this is transient in nature, it can last for several months and so is poorly tolerated by most patients. Recent advances in skin cooling, longer laser wavelengths, and shorter pulse durations have improved treatment outcomes, but PIH still remains an important issue.

Due to the higher risk of postoperative complications and less deep wrinkling in dark-skinned patients, nonablative technologies are currently the first-line therapy. However, when ablation is required for deep-seated damage, a combination approach, in which three passes of CO_2 laser are followed immediately by one pass of Er:YAG laser, can be employed. This combination has been associated with reduced erythema and hyperpigmentation. More recently, long-pulsed Er:YAG lasers have been used with the aim of achieving better hemostasis and some degree of collagen contraction. Jeong and Kye studied the use of such a system in 28 patients with skin types III and IV with pitted acne scars. They found an excellent response in 26 (93%) of these patients, but erythema lasting more than 3 months was seen in 54%. Patients should be warned that several treatments may be necessary to achieve a significant degree of improvement, but there will be less downtime and lower risk of hyperpigmentation. Single-pass CO_2 laser resurfacing has also recently been shown to be effective in the treatment of acne scar and wrinkle reduction in dark-skinned patients. with a reduction in the severity and duration of laser-associated complications.

In addition, just as in all other patients, sun avoidance and sun protection prior to surgery are encouraged in order to reduce the risk of PIH. It is not uncommon for patients to misunderstand the meaning of sun avoidance, and avoid only sunbathing. Therefore, it is important to emphasize to all patients that they should apply a broad-spectrum sunblock (preferentially containing physical blockers such as titanium dioxide or zinc oxide) for 2 weeks daily before and for 6 weeks after laser surgery, whether or not they engage in outdoor activities. UV light-protected clothing and a broad-rimmed hat are also useful.

Recent studies have also shown that application of a moderate potency topical steroid immediately after laser surgery may reduce the risk of hyperpigmentation. The use of topical bleaching agents before and after surgery, such as combinations of tretinoin, hydroquinone, topical steroid, α-hydroxy acid, kojic acid, and azelaic acid, has been advocated. A sample regimen is a combination of 0.025% tretinoin cream mixed with 4% hydroquinone and a moderate potency steroid twice daily preoperatively and then postoperatively for a further 4 weeks. If PIH develops despite the use of such agents, the addition of 5% glycolic acid in the morning may further reduce pigmentation. Depending on the degree of irritation, other bleaching agents may be added, including vitamin C, vitamin E, and kojic acid. If hyperpigmentaion persists, a mild glycolic acid peel may be performed about 6–8 weeks after surgery. The use of microdermabrasion may also be effective as an adjunctive means to improve superficial pigmentation.

Although newer technologies such as fractional lasers and plasma skin resurfacing have shown promising results in many large-scale studies, none thus far has focused on the effects in patients with a darker skin complexion. Early data have shown that PIH is less common with these modalities. Consequently, further large-scale studies examining their use in the treatment of photoaging in darker skinned patients are necessary. In the meantime, caution must be taken with these modalities in patients with Fitzpatrick skin types IV–VI so as to avoid possible side-effects.

PEARLS

Considerations in ethnic skin

Nonablative technologies are considered first-line because of a lower risk of postoperative complications.

However, ablative therapies (combination treatment with CO_2 and erbium lasers, single-pass CO_2 laser, or long-pulsed Er:YAG systems) can be used in a conservative fashion to treat advanced damage and scarring.

Pre- and post-procedural sun protection and bleaching creams can minimize the risk of postinflammatory hyperpigmentation.

In the post-laser period, short-term use of a medium potency steroid cream may also reduce the hyperpigmentation risk.

If postinflammatory hyperpigmentation develops, glycolic acid peels and microdermabrasion can hasten resolution.

Conclusion

Multiple ablative modalities can be used to address cosmetic concerns in many patients. Common goals include improvement of photo-damage and rhytides, pigmentary dyschromia including PIH and melasma, and acne scarring. Traditional ablative lasers, such as CO_2 or Er:YAG, may be combined to achieve optimal results. Newer ablative modalities, such as fractional lasers or plasma devices, may decrease patient recovery time and pose a lower risk of adverse events. With any ablative modality, treatment must be pursued cautiously and with specific precautions against scarring and pigmentary alteration. Further research and development of new ablative and nonablative devices and techniques may bring physicians and patients ever closer to achieving the age-old quest for the "fountain of youth."

Acknowledgments

The authors thank Ava T. Shamban, MD for sharing clinical photos, and Isabella Toma for helping with figure preparation.

Further reading

Alster TS. Preface. In: Manual of Cutaneous Laser Techniques. Philadelphia: Lippincott-Raven, 1997.

Alster TS. Preoperative preparations for CO_2 laser resurfacing. In: Coleman WP, Lawrence N, eds. Skin Resurfacing. Baltimore: Williams & Wilkins, 1998:171–180.

Alster TS. Cutaneous resurfacing with CO_2 and erbium:YAG lasers: preoperative, intraoperative, and postoperative considerations. Plast Reconstr Surg 1999;103:619–632.

Alster TS. Clinical and histologic evaluation of six erbium:YAG lasers for cutaneous resurfacing. Lasers Surg Med 1999;24:87–92.

Alster TS, Doshi S. Laser skin resurfacing. In: Burgess CM, ed. Cosmetic Dermatology. Berlin: Springer, 2005:111–126.

Alster TS, Garg S. Treatment of facial rhytides with a high energy pulsed carbon dioxide laser. Plast Reconstr Surg 1996;98:791–794.

Alster TS, Lupton JR. Erbium:YAG laser for cutaneous laser resurfacing. Dermatol Clin 2001;19:453–466.

Alster TS, Lupton JR. Prevention and treatment of side effects and complications of cutaneous laser resurfacing. Plast Reconstr Surg 2002;109:308–316.

Alster TS, Nann CA. Famciclovir prophylaxis of herpes simplex virus reactivations after laser skin resurfacing. Dermatol Surg 1999;25(3):242–246.

Alster TS, Kauvar ANB, Geronemus RG. Histology of high-energy pulsed CO_2 laser resurfacing. Semin Cutan Med Surg 1996;15:189–193.

Alster TS, Nanni CA, Williams CM. Comparison of four carbon dioxide resurfacing lasers: a clinical and histopathologic evaluation. Dermatol Surg 1999;25:153–159.

Anderson RR, Parrish JA. Selective photothermolysis: precise microsurgery by selective absorption of pulsed radiation. Science 1983;220:524–527.

Batra RS. Ablative laser resurfacing – postoperative care. Skin Therapy Lett 2004;9:6–9.

Batra RS, Ort RJ, Jacob C, Hobbs L, Arndt KA, Dover JS. Evaluation of silicone occlusive dressing after laser skin resurfacing. Arch Dermatol 2001;137:1317–1321.

Batra RS, Dover JS, Hobbs L, Phillips TJ. Evaluation of the role of exogenous estrogen in postoperative progress after laser skin resurfacing. Dermatol Surg 2003;29(1):43–48.

Batra RS, Jacob CI, Hobbs L, Arndt KA, Dover JS. A prospective survey of patient experiences after laser skin resurfacing: results from 2½ years of follow-up. Arch Dermatol 2003;139:1295–1299.

Bogle MA. Plasma skin regeneration technology. Skin Ther Lett 2006;11(7):7–9.

Bogle MA, Arndt KA, Dover JS. Evaluation of plasma skin regeneration technology in low-energy full facial rejuvenation. Arch Dermatol 2007;143:168–174.

Carniol PJ. Laser resurfacing technique: Feather-Touch, SilkTouch, and SureTouch resurfacing lasers. In: Carniol PJ, ed. Laser Skin Rejuvenation. Philadelphia: Lippincott-Raven, 1998:115–122.

Chan HL, Kono T. Laser treatment in ethnic skin. In: Goldberg D, ed. Procedures in Cosmetic Dermatology Series: Lasers and Lights – Volume II. Philadelphia: WB Saunders, 2005:89–101.

Fitzpatrick RE, Goldman MP, Satur NM, et al. Pulsed carbon dioxide laser resurfacing of photoaged facial skin. Arch Dermatol 1996;132:395–402.

Fitzpatrick RE, Smith SR, Sriprachya-anunt S. Depth of vaporization and the effect of pulse stacking with a high energy, pulsed carbon dioxide laser. J Am Acad Dermatol 1999;40:615–622.

Fitzpatrick TB. The validity and practicality of sun-reactive skin types I through VI. Arch Dermatol 1998;124(6):869–871.

Fleming D. Controversies in skin resurfacing: the role of the erbium:YAG laser. J Cutan Laser Ther 1999;1:15–21.

Goldberg DJ. Lasers for facial rejuvenation. Am J Clin Dermatol 2003;4(4):225–234.

Goldberg DJ, Cutter KB. The use of the erbium:YAG laser for the treatment of class III rhytides. Dermatol Surg 1999;25:713–715.

Goldman MP, Marchell NL. Laser resurfacing of the neck with combined CO_2/Er:YAG laser. Dermatol Surg 1999;25:923–925.

Goldman MP, Marchell N, Fitzpatrick RE. Laser skin resurfacing of the face with combined CO_2/Er:YAG laser. Dermatol Surg 2000;26:102–104.

Hanke CW. The coherent UltraPulse. In: Carniol PJ, ed. Laser Skin Rejuvenation. Philadelphia: Lippincott-Raven, 1998:103–114.

Hoenig JA, Morrow DM. Patient evaluation. In: Carniol PJ, ed. Laser Skin Rejuvenation. Philadelphia: Lippincott-Raven, 1998:65–86.

Hruza GJ, Fitzpatrick RE, Arndt KA, Dover JS. Lasers in skin resurfacing. In: Kaminer MK, Dover JS, Arndt KA, eds. Atlas of Cosmetic Surgery. Philadelphia: WB Saunders, 2002:328–350.

Jackson BA. Cosmetic considerations and non-laser cosmetic procedures in ethnic skin. Dermatol Clin 2003;21:703–712.

Jeong JT, Kye YC. Resurfacing of pitted facial acne scars with a long pulsed Er:YAG laser. Dermatol Surg 2001;27(2):107–110.

Kaufman R, Hibst R. Pulsed erbium:YAG laser ablation in cutaneous surgery. Lasers Surg Med 1996;19:324–330.

Kauvar ANB, Grossman MC, Bernstein LJ, et al. Erbium:YAG laser resurfacing: a clinical histopathologic evaluation. Lasers Surg Med 1998;Suppl 10:33.

Kilmer S, Fitzpatrick R, Bernstein E, Brown D. Long-term follow-up on the use of plasma skin regeneration (PSR) in full facial rejuvenation procedures. Lasers Surg Med 2005;36(Suppl 17):22.

Lanzafame RJ, Naim JO, Rogers DW, et al. Comparisons of continuous-wave, chop-wave, and super pulsed laser wounds. Laser Surg Med 1988;8:119–124.

Lowe NJ, Lask G, Griffin ME. Laser skin resurfacing: pre and post treatment guidelines. Dermatol Surg 1995;21:1017–1019.

Manaloto RMP, Alster TS. Erbium:YAG laser resurfacing for refractory melasma. Dermatol Surg 1999;25:121–123.

Manuskiatti W, Fitzpatrick RE, Goldman MP. Treatment of facial skin using combinations of CO_2, Q-switched alexandrite, flashlamp-pumped pulsed dye, and Er:YAG lasers in the same treatment session. Dermatol Surg 2000;26:114–120.

McBurney EI. Physics of resurfacing lasers. In: Coleman WP, Lawrence N, eds. Skin Resurfacing. Baltimore: Williams & Wilkins, 1998:155–160.

McCurdy JA. Facial surgery in Asian patients. In: Matory WE, ed. Ethnic Considerations in Facial Aesthetic Surgery. Philadelphia: Lippincott-Raven, 1998:263–284.

Munavalli GS, Weiss RA, Halder RM. Photoaging and nonablative photorejuvenation in ethnic skin. Dermatol Surg 2005;31:1250–1261.

Pathak MA. The role of natural photoprotective agents in human skin. In: Fitzpatrick TB, Pathak MA, eds. Sunlight and Man. Tokyo: University of Tokyo Press, 1974:725–750.

Polnikorn N, Goldberg DT, Suwachinda A, et al. Erbium:YAG laser resurfacing in Asians. Dermatol Surg 1998;24:1303–1307.

Pozner IN, Roberts TL. Variable pulse width Er:YAG laser resurfacing. Clin Plast Surg 2000;27:263–271.

Rahman Z, Rocha CK, Test Y, Lee S, Fitzpatrick R. The treatment of photodamage and facial rhytides with fractional thermolysis. Lasers Surg Med 2005;36(Suppl 17):32.

Rahman Z, Alam M, Dover JS. Fractional laser treatment of pigmentation and texture improvement. Skin Therapy Lett 2006;11(9):7–11.

Rubenstein R, Roenik HH, Stegman SJ, Hanke CW. Atypical keloids after dermabrasion of patients taking isoretinoin. J Am Acad Dermatol 1986;15:280–285.

Ruiz-Esparza J, Barba Gomez JM. Long-term effects of one general pass laser resurfacing: a look at dermal tightening and skin quality. Dermatol Surg 1999;25:169–173.

Sapijaszki MJA, Zachary CB. Er:YAG laser skin resurfacing. Dermatol Clin 2002;20:87–96.

Stuzin JM, Baker TJ, Baker TM, et al. Histologic effects of the high-energy pulsed CO_2 laser on photoaged facial skin. Plast Reconstr Surg 1997;99:2036–2050.

Tanzi EL, Lupton JR, Alster TS. Review of lasers in dermatology: four decades of progress. J Am Acad Dermatol 2003;4:1–32.

Teikemeier G, Goldberg DJ. Skin resurfacing with the erbium:YAG laser. Dermatol Surg 1997;23:685–687.

Tremblay J, Moy R. Treatment of post-auricular skin using a novel plasma resurfacing system: an in-vivo and histologic study. Annual Meeting of the American Society for Laser Medicine and Surgery, April 3, 2006; Dallas, TX.

Waldorf HA, Kauvar ANB, Geronemus RG. Skin resurfacing of fine to deep rhytides using a char-free carbon dioxide laser in 47 patients. Dermatol Surg 1995;21:940–946.

Walia S, Alster TS. Prolonged clinical and histologic effects from CO_2 laser resurfacing of atrophic acne scars. Dermatol Surg 1999;25:926–930.

Walsh JT Jr., Deutsch TF. Er:YAG laser ablation of tissue measurement of ablation rates. Lasers Surg Med 1989;24:81–86.

Wanner M, Tanzi EI, Alster TS. Fractional photothermolysis: treatment of facial and nonfacial cutaneous photodamage with a 1550-nm erbium-doped fiber laser. Dermatol Surg 2007;33:22–28.

Weinstein C, Scheflan M. Simultaneously combined Er:YAG and carbon dioxide laser (Derma K) for skin resurfacing. Clin Plast Surg 2000;27:273–285.

Nonablative laser and light sources

8

Joy H. Kunishige and Paul M. Friedman

Key Points

- Synonyms include nonablative remodeling.
- Nonablative lasers heat the papillary and reticular dermis, without damaging the epidermis, to stimulate collagen synthesis.
- Applications include photo-aging, acne, and acne scars.
- Compared with ablative procedures, nonablative resurfacing provides more modest improvements, but with essentially no downtime and an excellent safety profile.

Introduction

Ablative carbon dioxide (CO_2) and erbium: yttrium–aluminum–garnet (Er:YAG) lasers remove sheets of epidermis and dermis. These are associated with many side-effects, risks, and prolonged downtime. After Anderson and Parrish published their principles of "selective photothermolysis" in 1983, the pulsed-dye laser (PDL) was designed to treat port-wine stains and other vascular structures, without destroying overlying tissue. Other lasers have since been developed to meet growing patient interest in less invasive treatment options.

Nonablative lasers refer to those that heat the papillary and reticular dermis without damaging the epidermis. This leads to fibroblast activation and synthesis of new collagen, resulting in dermal thickening and skin rejuvenation. This technology has been demonstrated to benefit photo-aging, acne, acne scars, and other conditions (Box 8-1).

Initially, available lasers were used to achieve nonablative resurfacing, such as the PDL and various neodymium:yttrium–aluminum–garnet (Nd:YAG) lasers. Devices were then modified and some were specifically engineered for nonablative rejuvenation. Longer wavelengths, improved epidermal cooling devices, and fractional technology have expanded the armamentarium of devices available. Compared with ablative procedures, nonablative resurfacing provides more modest improvements, but with essentially no downtime and an excellent safety profile.

This chapter is organized into three parts. First, possible mechanisms of action and efficacy of this new technology is explored. Second, various devices are outlined with published evidence for their use. Finally, practical considerations before, during, and after treatment are reviewed.

Mechanism of action

Photo-damaged skin contains increased levels of metalloproteinases, which degrade and disorganize collagen fibrils. Ultraviolet (UV) radiation induces free radicals, which further damage collagen. Damaged collagen is replaced by increased glycosaminoglycans and thickened elastic fibers (solar elastosis). Most of these changes occur between 100 and 500 μm below the skin surface.

The "gold standard" for laser rejuvenation remains ablative CO_2 and Er:YAG lasers. Histologic studies of CO_2 laser resurfacing show thermal alteration of collagen fibrils at depths of up to 300 μm. During the first 3 days of laser resurfacing, collagen is denatured and shrinks acutely, stimulating a wound healing reaction (Fig. 8-1). Injured papillary dermal fibroblasts proliferate and migrate into the wound, where they synthesize type I procollagen and other matrix molecules. Thirty days after treatment, denser collagen fibers, oriented parallel to the skin surface, are visible. By 90 days after treatment, the collagen and elastic fibers in the upper dermis are more organized. It is believed that this long-term wound healing process is responsible for rhytid reduction.

Nonablative lasers attempt similarly to heat and stimulate the wound healing process in the dermis, but without removing epidermis. This is often referred to as dermal remodeling, subsurface resurfacing, or laser toning. In theory, dermal heating should be aimed at tissue 100–500 μm below the skin surface. More superficial injury may be ineffective and result in epidermal injury, whereas

Reported indications for nonablative lasers

Photodamage

Rhytides

Pigmentary dyschromia

Lentigenes

Melasma

Telangiectasia

Erythema

Acne

Acne scarring

Atrophic scars

Hypertrophic scars

Surgical scars

Hair removal

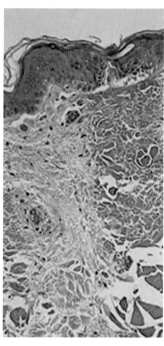

Figure 8-1 Histopathology of untreated and treated skin. Left side: untreated; right side: immediately after treatment with a 1500-nm ER:glass fractionated laser

deeper injury may result in scarring. Too much dermal injury, even within this zone, may result in irreversible damage to the microvasculature and dermis, resulting in necrotic tissue that cannot be regenerated. Each type of laser is associated with a different depth of penetration (Fig. 8-2), which is reciprocal to the absorption coefficient of water (μ_{water}) (Table 8-1). Based on this table, the 1.45-µm diode laser should be the optimal light source.

However, depth is also influenced by scatter, fluence, pulse duration, number of pulses, repetition rate, and, sometimes, epidermal cooling. In addition, lasers associated with deeper injury have been used safely.

The effect of the major chromophores in the skin – water, hemoglobin, and melanin – should be considered (Fig. 8-3). Water is the main target for most of the nonablative lasers, including fractionated lasers. Targeting water results in bulk heating, and the heating of epidermal water is limited by epidermal cooling methods. Bulk heating is not spatially selective, and can result in damage to adjacent tissues, scarring, and more pain than that associated with spatially selective heating.

Spatially selective heating can be obtained by utilizing the chromophores hemoglobin or melanin. Hemoglobin absorbs light between 577 and 595 nm; the PDL or a low-fluence potassium–titanyl–phosphate (KTP) laser can be used to heat dermal blood vessels and adjacent perivascular collagen. Damage to the endothelium may lead to cytokine-mediated induction of collagen remodeling. Melanin is concentrated in the basal layer, located 50–100 µm below the skin surface. Heating melanin may result in subjacent dermal collagen heating and contribute to desired histologic changes. However, excessive melanin absorption can result in epidermal injury and dyspigmentation, and also reduces the amount of heat that reaches the dermis. Regardless of chromophore, the overarching concept is that gentle dermal heating will stimulate new collagen deposition.

Acne vulgaris

For the treatment of inflammatory acne vulgaris, the mechanism of action may be different. It was first postulated that carotenoids in sebum were the chromophore, with an absorption range of 425–550 nm. The most current theories are that light targets *Propionibacterium acnes*, the sebaceous gland, or the infrainfundibulum of the follicle. Light converts *P. acnes*-produced porphyrins into free radicals that destroy the bacterium. However, *P. acnes* regenerates rapidly, so this is unlikely to be the main mechanism by which laser achieves its long-lasting reduction of inflammatory acne.

Histologic examination following irradiation with the 1450-nm diode reveals sebaceous gland necrosis, which correlates with reports that sebum excretion is reduced. However, other studies have reported no changes in the sebaceous gland or sebum excretion. An alternative mechanism of action may be that light increases the activity of transforming growth factor (TGF)-β. TGF-β both suppresses inflammation and stimulates neocollagenesis, perhaps explaining how nonablative lasers can be used to treat both acne and acne scarring. PDLs may cause selective photothermolysis of the dilated vessels associated with inflammation.

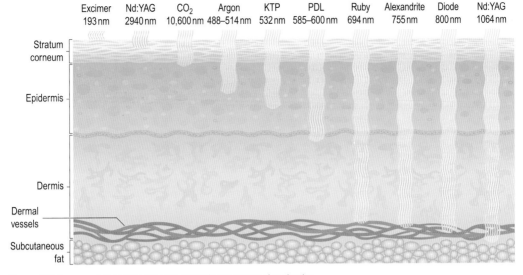

Figure 8-2 Laser and light sources with approximate penetration depths

Table 8-1 Depth of penetration as a function of radiation wavelength (Nelson et al 2002)

Laser	Wavelength (nm)	μ_{water} (per mm)	Depth of penetration (μm)
Diode	980	0.0448	32 000
Nd:YAG	1064	0.0177	81 100
Nd:YAG	1320	0.204	7000
Diode	1450	3.04	470
Er:glass	1540	1.18	1200
Er:YAG	2940	1220	1.2
CO_2	10 600	84.4	17

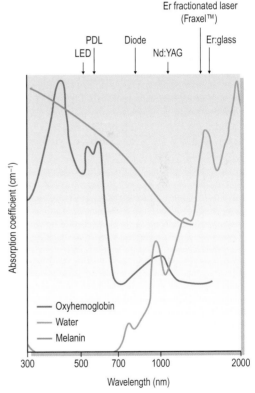

Figure 8-3 Absorption spectra

Most of the literature regarding laser treatment of acne involves the use of 585- or 595-nm PDL, 1450-nm diode, and 1320-nm Nd:YAG, reviewed in more detail below.

Studies on efficacy

Several studies have demonstrated the histologic and clinical efficacy of nonablative technology. After 1540-nm Er:glass laser treatment, biopsies showed keratinocyte damage, homogenization of the dermis, and fibroblast proliferation. Spreading the energy over a train of pulses enabled fibroplasia without keratinocyte damage. Another study of the 1540-nm Er:glass laser found new collagen and decreased elastotic material, also without epidermal effects. Eleven studies using the PDL, 980-nm diode, 1320-nm Nd:YAG, Q-switched 1064-nm Nd:YAG, intense pulsed light (IPL), and Er:glass lasers all demonstrated increased epidermal thickness and increased collagen density.

From these studies, it appears that many different devices lead to similar histologic responses. Further, the amount of new collagen formation correlates with the number of treatments received.

This wound healing effect may be directed by alterations in various molecules. After a single laser treatment, there are significant increases in type I procollagen messenger RNA, and type I procollagen protein. Variable increases in type III procollagen, various matrix metalloproteinases, interleukin (IL)-1β and TNF-α also occur. Matrix metalloproteinases remove collagen fragments and restore collagen biosynthesis. Nonablative laser therapy might result in fundamentally similar, but quantitatively more modest, biochemical changes to those seen with CO_2 laser resurfacing. Variable molecular responses may explain the spectrum of efficacy seen clinically.

Variable response to treatment is a major concern regarding nonablative treatments. Some patients report remarkable improvements, whereas others achieve changes detectable only by sophisticated measuring instruments. The literature regarding the consistency of efficacy is also muddled. Clinical improvement may not correlate with histologic assessments. Patients may perceive more improvement than physicians.

Part of the problem is the lack of objective measures of efficacy. Most studies report clinical efficacy via patient surveys, physician evaluations, and photographic comparisons. More objective measures of efficacy have been sought, including noninvasive attempts to measure texture via profilometry, ultrasonography, silicone replicas, and three-dimensional in vivo skin imaging systems. Silicone replicas yield results that correlate with histologic findings, ultrasonographic imaging, and clinical observations. Three-dimensional imaging systems that show real-time skin topography have also been used to demonstrate reductions in roughness that concur with clinical assessments.

The development and validation of objective tools or grading systems, and the refinement of technology and treatment protocols, may improve the validity and consistency of results. Future studies should explore various patient characteristics that may predict efficacy, such as age, severity of photo-damage, sex, race, skin type, and number of previous treatments.

Epidermal cooling

Minimizing epidermal injury is an integral part of nonablative rejuvenation. Less scatter and deeper penetration are generally associated with longer wavelengths, up to about 1200 nm, after which water is greatly absorbed and epidermal injury becomes more of a concern (see Fig. 8-3). Uncontrolled epidermal heating manifests as blistering, loss of epidermal barrier, dyspigmentation, and scarring. Epidermal cooling selectively cools the superficial layers of the skin before, during, and after laser irradiation, protecting it from damage. The epidermis should never reach temperatures above 60–65°C, the temperature at which denaturation occurs. Ideally, the epidermis should reach 40–48°C, which correlates with a dermal

BOX 8-2
Epidermal cooling devices
Ice
Aluminum roller
Cooled gels
Cooled pads
Sapphire plate
Precooled air
Cryogen spray

temperature of 55–65°C, required for collagen contraction and simulation of neocollagenesis.

Several different methods for cooling are available (Box 8-2). Contact cooling involves the conduction of heat from the skin to an applied solid, such as a transparent plate cooled by an external cooling system. Highly conductive materials, such as sapphire, are used to make the cooling plate. Air, bubbles in applied gel, hair, and other substances can block the contact between the cooling plate and the skin surface, decreasing the ability to extract heat from the skin. In practice, if a patient feels pain during laser irradiation, the impulse to remove the handpiece should be ignored, as continued application of the cooling plate will help alleviate damage.

Transparent fluid gel, such as that used during ultrasonography, can be refrigerated and applied to the skin before treatment. As the gel is heated, it can become opaque and impair the visibility of underlying structures. The gel can also collect debris, which may stick to the laser head, and usually needs to be reapplied throughout the procedure; this is time consuming and messy. Recently, cooling hydrogel pads have been designed for application to the skin before and during treatment. The pad adapts to the contours of the treatment area, and the laser head glides smoothly over the material. The pad can be recooled throughout the procedure, and the patient can take the pad home for relief and reuse later.

Precooled air as low as −30°C (probably about −10°C at the exit nozzle) can be blown onto the skin surface (Fig. 8-4). Air cooling is the least efficient method, as heat transfer for forced convection in gas is very low, so long cooling times (up to several seconds) are required. The hose emitting cooled air is held over the general area throughout the treatment, resulting in nonspecific "bulk" cooling of adjacent and deeper tissue. Still, precooled air is easy to use and can also mediate pain.

The most rapid and spatially selective cooling is achieved with cryogen spray cooling. The only cryogen currently approved by the Food

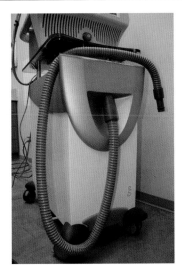

Figure 8-4 Precooled air delivery system. The nozzle emitting precooled air is held approximately 6 cm from the treatment area, moving in concert with the laser handpiece. The nozzle should not be directed at the same area for a prolonged period of time. One advantage is that this cooling device can be used with multiple different laser systems

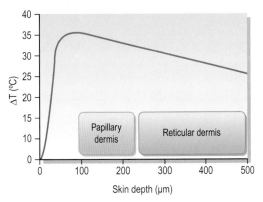

Figure 8-5 Computed temperature increase as a function of depth after 1320-nm Nd:YAG laser treatment with cryogen spray cooling. Although the most superficial depths of the skin are cooled, the targeted depth (100–500 μm) retains heat. Adapted from Nelson et al (2002)

and Drug Administration (FDA) for use in dermatologic surgery is the chlorofluorocarbon substitute tetrafluoroethane (TFE), a nonflammable, nontoxic, freon substitute that does not deplete atmospheric ozone. TFE is dispersed as a fine liquid spray that evaporates during flight, creating temperatures between –40°C and –60°C at the skin surface. Patients usually feel a burst of cool air, but may instead feel a pricking sensation. This provides spatially selective cooling, which is necessary to avoid cooling the nearby target (the upper dermis) (Fig. 8-5). There are some disadvantages: surrounding humidity may cause the vapor to form a layer of ice on the epidermis that

concentrates the fluence or impairs heat transfer. Cryogen spurt durations longer than 40 ms can result in dyspigmentation in patients with darker skin. Also, TFE inhalation can cause nervous system depression and should be used in well ventilated areas. Cryogen spray cooling has been incorporated into multiple systems by Candela Corporation.

Index of devices available

Key Points

- Pulsed-dye lasers (PDLs) were the first modality to be used for nonablative remodeling and shown to improve acne vulgaris.
- Neodymium : yttrium–aluminum–garnet (Nd:YAG) lasers benefit rhytides and acne scarring.
- 1450-nm diode is effective for rhytides, acne, and acne scarring, but is associated with some pain.
- 1540-nm erbium:glass may be used for rhytides or acne.
- Fractionated erbium lasers are nonablative with a growing list of applications.
- Intense pulsed light (IPL) (500–1200 nm) is not a laser, but instead emits multiple wavelengths of light, so is useful for both color and textural changes.

The first two lasers discussed here target either hemoglobin or melanin, whereas the others target water. IPL is not a laser, but a device that delivers several different wavelengths of light, and therefore targets multiple chromophores. Light-emitting diodes also emit a range of wavelengths, but at low intensity. All of these modalities result in similar histologic changes and the overall appearance of more even skin.

585- and 595-nm pulsed dye lasers

In 1999, Zelickson demonstrated that the PDL induced a Grenz zone of new, healthy appearing, collagen in the papillary dermis and set the stage for nonablative laser rejuvenation.

PDL was also one of the first lasers to be used for the treatment of acne, albeit with variable results. In one study, 41 patients were assigned randomly to treatment with the 585-nm PDL or placebo. Acne severity was graded using the Leeds acne grading system, which compares patients' skin with standardized photographs. The Leeds score in the PDL arm (1.5 or 3 J/cm², 5-mm spot, pulse duration 350 μs) was lowered by 1.9, and that in the placebo group by 0.1. Another study using similar parameters (3 J/cm², 7-mm spot, pulse duration 350 μs) found no changes in Leeds score. Both studies administered only one treatment session and followed patients for 12 weeks.

The new long-pulsed 595-nm PDL has already been reported to be successful in treating acne. When combined with topical 5-aminolevulinic acid (ALA), all 14 patients with recalcitrant acne achieved complete clearance after one to six treatments. In this study, ALA was applied for 45 min, followed by one minimally overlapping pass (7–7.5 J/cm², 10-mm spot size, pulse duration 10 ms, dynamic cooling spray of 30 ms with a 30-ms delay).

In addition to acne, PDL treatment also benefits acne scarring. A 48% reduction in the depth of acne scars was achieved in ten patients following a single treatment (585 nm, 5-mm spot size, pulse duration 350 μs, average fluence 2.33 J/cm²). PDL in combination with 1450-nm diode benefits both acne and scars. Previously, the treatment options for acne scarring were dermabrasion, deep chemical peels, punch excision, punch grafting, subcision, and ablative resurfacing. The use of PDL, and now multiple other lasers, is a welcome option for patients with acne scars, which are traditionally difficult to treat.

Neodymium : yttrium–aluminum–garnet lasers

Nd:YAG lasers are currently available in 1320-nm long-pulsed, 1064-nm long-pulsed, 1064-nm short-pulsed, and 1064-nm Q-switched versions. This category of laser has been used to benefit photo-damage (Fig. 8-6), mild rhytides, and acne scarring, and is historically safe in darker skin types.

Ten patients with periocular and periorbital rhytides underwent treatment with a long-pulsed 1064-nm Nd:YAG laser (Altus Vantage; Cutera, San Francisco, CA) every 2 weeks for a total of three treatments (spot size 5 mm, fluence 13 J/cm², pulse duration 300 ms, repetition rate 7 Hz). Patients had skin types II–IV. At 6 months, patients' subjective improvement was 40%, physician-assessed improvement was 40%, and imaging program improvement was 50%. Still, 30% of the participants were not satisfied with the result. Peak results were reached at 2 months, suggesting that additional treatments may have been needed.

Combination therapy using both the 532-nm KTP and long-pulsed 1064-nm Nd:YAG laser may better address the multiple aspects of photo-damage, and have a synergistic effect on collagen stimulation. In one study, 150 patients were treated with KTP laser alone, Nd:YAG laser alone, or KTP followed immediately by Nd:YAG laser. Variable parameters were used. Patients underwent three to six monthly treatments. All patients exhibited at least mild to moderate improvement in rhytides, skin tone and texture, and redness and pigmentation. For all of these efficacy points, combination therapy achieved higher scores than KTP monotherapy, which was better than Nd:YAG monotherapy. The combination group also achieved a thicker zone of new collagen, as measured from histologic samples.

Technology that increases collagen formation and improves rhytides should also benefit atrophic acne scars. A study comparing the 1064-nm (Lyra; Laserscope, San Jose, CA) with the 1320-nm Nd:YAG (CoolTouch II; ICN Pharmaceuticals, Cost Mesa, CA) showed comparable and good results for both systems (22–28% overall improvement by independent observers). Patient surveys and prolifometric studies demonstrated comparable improvement. Other studies have confirmed the efficacy of the 1320-nm Nd:YAG laser for acne scars; even better results may be achieved with concomitant subcision – the use of a tri-beveled hypodermic needle to undermine and untether the scar.

All patients improved after treatment with a novel, short-pulsed 1064-nm Nd:YAG laser (5-mm spot size, 14 J/cm², 0.3-ms duration, 7-Hz repetition rate, 2000 pulses per side of face). Patients underwent eight treatments, 2 weeks apart. Some 89% of patients noted a greater than 10% improvement in acne scarring; the mean improvement was 29%. The advantage of this short-pulsed system is

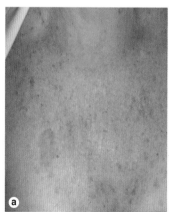 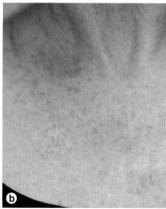

Figure 8-6 Photo-damage before (A) and after (B) Nd:YAG treatment

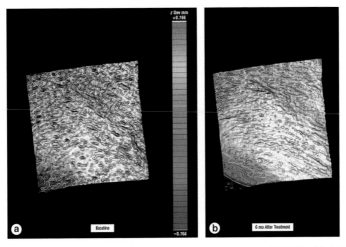

Figure 8-7 Skin roughness, as determined by a three-dimensional imaging device (PRIMOS). (A) At baseline and (B) 6 months after final treatment. Mean improvement at 6 months was 39.2%. Reprinted from Friedman et al (2004), with permission

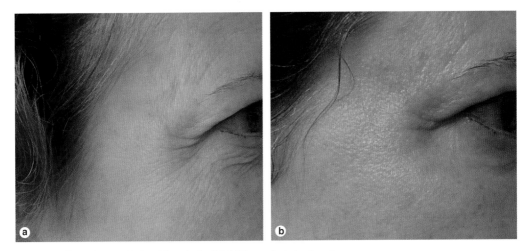

Figure 8-8 Photo-damage before (A) and after (B) 1450-nm diode treatment

that the target was not water, but gradual heating of the small dermal vessels, so contact cooling was not needed.

The efficacy of the Q-switched laser was shown in a study of 11 patients with mild to moderate atrophic acne scarring who underwent five treatments with a 1064-nm Q-switched Nd:YAG laser (Medlite IV; Continuum, Santa Clara, CA) (6-mm spot size, average fluence 3.4 J/cm^2, 4–6-nm pulse duration, repetition rate 10 Hz). Skin roughness, as determined by a three-dimensional imaging device (PRIMOS; GFM, Teltow, Germany), improved increasingly at 1, 3, and 6 months after the fifth treatment, indicating ongoing collagen remodeling (Fig. 8-7). Mean improvement at 6 months, after the fifth treatment, was 39%.

In a patient satisfaction study after treatment with the 1320-nm Nd:YAG laser, patients rated overall improvement of acne scarring as 5.2 on a scale from 1 to 10, and 62% were satisfied with the treatment.

1450-nm diode

The most popular long-pulsed diode laser is a 1450-nm system with an integrated dynamic cooling device (DCD) that uses TFE (Smoothbeam; Candela, Wayland, MA). This laser has been used for the treatment of photo-damage (Fig. 8-8), rhytides, acne vulgaris (Fig. 8-9), acne scars, and other atrophic scars.

In one study, 25 patients with mild to moderate facial rhytides were treated with four monthly Smoothbeam laser treatments (4-mm spot size, fluence 15–20 J/cm^2, 210-ms pulse duration). Peak histologic and clinical improvements were noted at 6 months, and maintained at the end of the 12-month follow-up period. Periocular improvement was especially significant, possibly

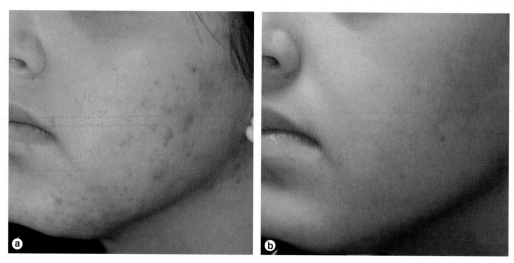

Figure 8-9 Acne before (A) and after (B) 1450-nm diode treatment

secondary to thin skin allowing either more thermal injury or enhanced perception of neocollagenesis.

The same authors also applied the 1450-nm laser to transverse neck rhytides, which are inherently difficult to treat. Twenty patients received three monthly treatments (fluence 10–13 J/cm², other parameters not published), and underwent in vivo three-dimensional skin surface microtopography measurements. Mild to moderate improvement was achieved in all patients. Scores from patient surveys and physician assessments paralleled topographic measurements The only side-effects were transient erythema and edema lasting for up to 48 h.

This laser is the most widely published for the treatment of acne and acne scarring. Sebaceous glands reside 200–1000 μm below the skin surface, and the diode laser penetrates to 435 μm. Histologic examination demonstrates that the 1450-nm diode causes thermal damage at 50–800 μm below the stratum corneum, particularly around adnexae.

Confirming that more is not always better, a split-face comparison of two different fluences reported slightly better results with 14 J/cm² than with a prototype laser emitting 16 J/cm² (Candela, Wayland, MA). After one treatment, 43% (14 J/cm²) and 34% (16 J/cm²) reductions in acne count were achieved, and after three monthly treatments the reductions were 75% and 71% respectively. Notably, lesion counts were maintained at 12 months. Improvements in acne scarring and sebum production were also noted. Overall, there was no significant difference in efficacy or adverse events between the two fluences. All 20 patients tolerated these higher fluences with premedication with topical lidocaine 5% cream (Ela-Max; Ferndale Laboratories, Ferndale,

MI) under occlusion for 1 h before each treatment. Pain was rated as moderate for both fluences, and improved with subsequent treatments.

A study designed to determine optimal parameters found that low-energy, double-pass treatment yielded similar results to high-energy, single-pass treatments. This supports the above findings and suggests that lower energies can be used to reduce discomfort.

A split-face comparison of the 1320-nm Nd:YAG laser with the 1450-nm diode laser showed greater clinical improvement in acne scars with the diode. For both lasers, maximal improvement was attained at 6 months, which corresponded to increased dermal collagen on histologic examination. There was slightly longer lasting erythema and more hyperpigmentation (7% versus 3%) with the diode, but all hyperpigmentation resolved with hydroquinone within 6 weeks. Patients also reported more pain, but greater satisfaction, with the diode laser. The use of trichloroacetic acid peels after 1450-nm diode treatment may further improve results.

A study of 57 Asian patients treated with the 1450-nm diode (6-mm spot size, fluence 11–12 J/cm², pulse duration 250 ms, DCD duration 50 ms, repetition rate 1 Hz) confirmed efficacy and safety for the treatment of acne scars in skin types IV and V. Although 22 patients (39%) developed hyperpigmentation, this was rated as mild in 17 patients and moderate in 5. The authors attributed the high incidence of hyperpigmentation to the long DCD spray duration and high fluence. After completing this study, they found that decreasing the DCD spray duration from 50 to 40 ms resulted in less hyperpigmentation. No hypopigmentation or blistering occurred.

In summary, the diode laser targets water and is associated with moderate but tolerable pain.

Side-effects are usually limited to mild erythema and edema, lasting for less than 24 h. Hyperpigmentation, especially in darker skin, may be reduced with shorter cryogen spurt times. The long-term remission achievable with laser treatment along with the uniform clinical efficacy and minimal adverse effects make the 1450-nm diode laser a suitable first-line, second-line, or adjuvant treatment modality for moderate to severe acne. This laser also offers the added benefit of improving atrophic scars. Results may be maintained for as long as 12 months, which is significant when compared to that associated with antibiotics or topical treatment.

1540-nm erbium:glass laser

The 1540-nm erbium-doped phosphate glass laser is another mid-infrared range laser that targets intracellular water. This wavelength has the least amount of melanin absorption compared with the 1320- and 1450-nm laser systems – an advantage when approaching darker skin types.

An early histologic study suggested that the damage induced by this laser might be too deep, but recent studies have reported significant increases in dermal thickness and improvements in appearance of rhytides. One study demonstrated clinical and histologic improvement in fine periorbital and perioral rhytides after three monthly treatments (4-mm spot size, 10 J/cm^2 fluence, 3.5-ms pulse duration, 2-Hz repetition rate). It was reported that these changes may peak at 14 months and persist for 35 months.

Significant improvements in pustular and nodular acne have been reported. After four bimonthly treatment sessions (1540-nm Aramis; Quantel Medical, Clermont-Ferrand, France) (4-mm spot, 3.3-ms pulse duration, 500 ms between pulses, contact cooling +5°C), patients reported a 68% improvement and physicians a 78% improvement, maintained at 9 months. There were no objective changes in sebum measurements (Sebumeter SM-815; Courage-Khazaka, Cologne, Germany).

Fractionated lasers

Key Points

- Synonym: fractional photothermolysis.
- Fractionated lasers deliver energy to vertical columns of skin to create microscopic treatment zones (MTZs).
- Inter-MTZ skin remains untreated and serves as a reservoir of healthy skin to speed healing.
- Multiple passes and treatment sessions are needed to treat a given area completely.
- Results are probably somewhere between that of nonablative and ablative laser therapy, although efficacy differs widely from patient to patient.

Fractional photothermolysis is the delivery of energy to vertical columns of skin, instead of parallel sheets of skin. The basic concept was introduced in 2003. Initially, a 1500-nm laser was focused to produce arrays of microscopic columns of thermal injury. There are now three commercially available fractional devices: Fraxel re:store™ (Reliant Technologies, Palo Alto, CA), Lux-IR Fractional™ (Palomar Medical, Burlington, MA), and Affirm (Cynosure, Westford, MA). Fractional delivery may be superior to traditional uniform delivery of heat for three reasons:

- Higher irradiation within the columns results in more damage and increased wound healing response. This can be achieved without increasing the power of the optical source.
- Faster healing response due to increased surface-to-volume ratio of the microwounds. The interface between injured and normal skin, where most neocollagen formation occurs, is maximized.
- Larger safety margin as fractional resurfacing is less likely to result in infections and scarring.

The Fraxel re:store™ laser is an Er:glass laser that emits 1500-nm light to create tiny vertical columns of injury, called microscopic treatment zones (MTZs) (Fig. 8-10). The density of MTZs and amount of space between them can be varied. The original handpiece looked at blue dye applied to the skin to track handpiece velocity, which determines the laser repetition rate needed to achieve the prechosen MTZ density. MTZ densities of 400, 1600, and 6400 MTZ/cm^2 correspond to inter-MTZ distances of 500, 250, and 125 µm respectively. The total density in a treatment session is calculated by multiplying the density setting by the number of passes. Current handpieces work with a rollerball tip, which reads the reflection from a clear gel applied to the skin. In the currently marketed SR system, the user chooses a treatment level that corresponds to the percentage coverage, and, depending on energy level and number of passes, to total MTZ density (Fig. 8-11). Energy levels from 4 to 70 mJ correspond to depths of penetration from 382 to 1379 µm. A kilojoule (kJ) counter is used to monitor total treatment output.

After treatment with the Fraxel re:store™ laser, histologic studies show damage to columns that are approximately 100 µm wide and at least 300 µm deep. Columns may be wider and deeper (up to 1400 µm) at higher fluence settings. The stratum corneum always remains intact, but the lower epidermis may separate from the dermis. By 24 h, the lower epidermis and basal cell layer are restored, and microscopic epidermal necrotic debris (MEND) has formed. MEND represents damaged keratinocytes and melanin that migrate upward through viable keratinocytes at the margin of the MTZ, and is extruded by day 7 (Fig. 8-12). MEND formation is associated with a mild bronze color clinically, which can persist for several weeks. Collagen III staining gradually increases from the first to the seventh day, and is more prominent in the dermis that surrounds the MTZ, especially below the MTZ (Fig. 8-12). Dermal alteration and inflammation resolves by 3 months.

The main use of this technology is for nonablative rejuvenation for improvement of photoaging. Mild to moderate improvements in solar lentigines, skin texture, dilated pores, and fine rhytides can be expected, whereas deeper lines are less amenable to treatment, as with other nonablative modalities.

The Fraxel re:store™ laser is also used for the treatment of atrophic scars, including acne scars (Fig. 8-13), and surgical scars (Fig. 8-14). All types of acne scarring – rolling, boxcar, and ice-pick – are amenable to treatment with the Fraxel re:store™ laser. How the same technology can improve both atrophic acne scars and hypertrophic scars is not yet known. It has been postulated that thermal injury can be made strong enough to destroy individual blood vessels irreversibly in hypertrophic scars.

Two other exciting indications for the Fraxel re:store™ laser are the ability to treat nonfacial areas and modest success with melasma. Even the neck and chest, which are difficult to treat and often associated with dyspigmentation and scarring, can be treated. Large areas on the trunk and extremities can be treated quickly with the rolling handpiece. Melasma treatment results are promising, but not always permanent. Marked reduction in pigmentation has been reported, even in patients with previously refractory melasma, and in those who are not typically candidates for laser therapy because of darker skin type. Multiple other indications for the Fraxel re:store™ laser are being reported (Box 8-3).

Side-effects reported with Fraxel re:store™ include erythema, edema, xerosis, flaking, superficial scratches, pruritus, bronzing, dyspigmentation (short term), herpes simplex virus (HSV) activation, increased sensitivity, and acneiform eruption.

The two other commercially available fractional devices use the traditional stamping method.

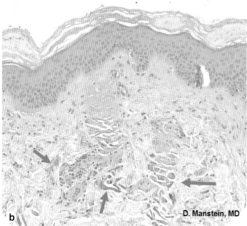

D. Manstein, MD

Figure 8-10 Microscopic treatment zones (MTZs) are treated vertical columns of tissue surrounded by untreated tissue. (A) Clinical photograph. (B) Procollagen III stain is most prominent at the interface between the MTZ and uninjured tissue (arrows)

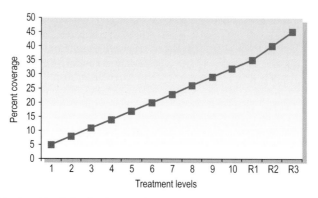

Figure 8-11 Fraxel SR treatment levels for all pulse energies

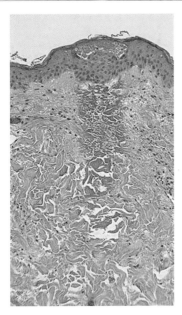

Figure 8-12 Microscopic epidermal necrotic debris (MEND) represent damaged keratinocytes and melanin, and migrate upward to be extruded by day 7

The Lux-IR Fractional™ emits light from 850 to 1350 nm through a 12 × 28-mm handpiece and patterned optical window with 3-mm wide apertures. No dye, and often no anesthetic premedication, is required. The device is marketed for the treatment of photo-damage, mild rhytides, and acne scars. The Affirm™ uses a microlens array to divide a 1440-nm Nd:YAG beam into microspots.

Intense pulsed light (500–1200 nm)

IPL is not a laser emitting a single coherent wavelength, but rather a device that emits multiple different wavelengths of light at the same time. Most systems emit wavelengths of 500–1200 nm, and cut-off filters can be used to block out lower wavelengths. The multiple different wavelengths of light can target simultaneously all aspects of photoaging – vascular, pigmentary, and textural (Fig. 8-15). It is generally safer, quicker because large spot sizes are available, and less painful than other devices, but overall may yield less impressive results.

When IPL is used for general photorejuvenation, a low cut-off filter is used that allows most of the different wavelengths of light to pass through. Theoretically IPL is best suited for the various aspects of poikiloderma. In a study of 135 patients with poikiloderma of Civatte who received one to five treatments on the neck or upper chest, 75% of hyperpigmentation and telangiectasias cleared; improved skin texture was also noted. The authors used an 8 × 35-mm spot size and concluded that, in general, the best parameters were: 3 ms, 515-nm filter, and 25–28 J/cm². In a separate study, the same authors reported 50–75% improvement of telangiectasia.

IPL may be combined with various nonablative lasers and trichloroacetic acid peels to improve outcome.

Light-emitting diodes

The science of light-emitting diodes (LEDs), which emit low-intensity noncoherent light of multiple wavelengths, is new. The light excites atoms and molecules, resulting in chemical reactions that are postulated to influence fibroblast proliferation. Gentlewaves (Light BioScience, Virginia Beach, VA) is the first LED to be approved by the FDA for the treatment of periorbital rhytides (Fig. 8-16). This technology is being explored for prevention of radiation dermatitis and as a light source for photodynamic therapy.

Pretreatment considerations and safety precautions

Nonablative technology is not a replacement for ablative laser resurfacing or surgery. Patient selection is key. Patients should understand that the overall appearance of their skin will be improved because lines, textural differences, and pigmentary changes will be softened, but not eradicated. Skin changes are usually subtle and gradual. Nonablative procedures require a number of treatments over a period of months before the full benefits can be appreciated. A total of three to six treatments is usually required, at 3–4-week intervals. Patients seeking improvement of a particular feature, such as a specific wrinkle or lentigo, are better treated with a laser specific for that indication.

Some physicians recommend that patients stop topical retinoids, α-hydroxy acids, and vitamin C derivatives 48 h before and after each treatment. Relative contraindications are a previous history of skin cancer, Kaposi's sarcoma, lupus erythematosus, or other photosensitivity. Patients should wait 6 months after completing isotretinoin therapy before undergoing laser treatment. Individuals with a suntan or history of keloid scarring should not be treated. Although there is no scientific evidence regarding this, patients who are pregnant should not undergo laser treatment.

Although antibiotic prophylaxis is required for all patients undergoing ablative laser resurfacing, it is not necessary in patients having nonablative laser therapy. Antiviral prophylaxis may be appropriate for some patients. Patients with a history of HSV infection should be started on antiviral prophylaxis 1 day before treatment. An example prophylactic regimen is valacilovir 500 mg by mouth twice daily for 3 days, starting 1 day before treatment.

Not all types of nonablative laser necessitate premedication with topical anesthetics. Topical anesthetics are recommended prior to treatment

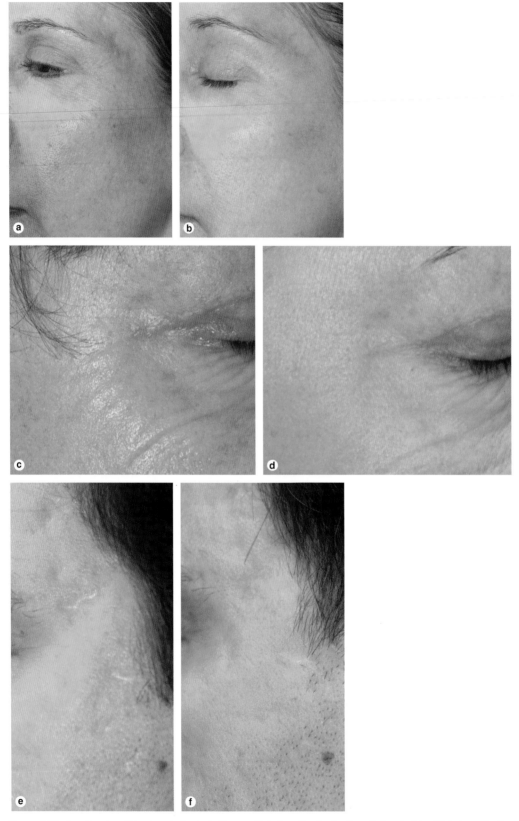

Figure 8-13 Fraxel re:store™ treatment of solar lentigenes (A, before; B, after treatment), fine rhytides (C, before; D, after treatment), and acne scarring (E, before; F, after treatment). Parts E & F reprinted from Glaich, Rahman, Goldberg, et al (2007), with permission

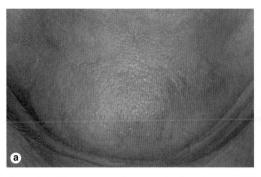
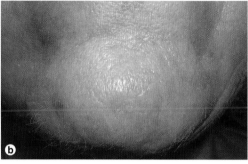

Figure 8-14 Surgical scars improve after Fraxel re:store™ therapy. (A) Baseline photo taken 4 weeks after Mohs excision of basal cell carcinoma. (B) Post-treatment photo taken 2 weeks after a single treatment. Reprinted from Behroozan DS, Goldberg LH, Dai T, et al (2006), with permission

---

Reported indications for Fraxel re:store™

Photodamage

Poikiloderma of Civatte

Rhytides

Hyperpigmentation

Lentigenes

Becker's nevus

Melasma

Telangiectasia

Erythema

Acne

Acne scarring

Atrophic scars

Hypertrophic scars

Hypopigmented scars

Surgical scars

Striae distensae

Actinic keratosis

Disseminated superficial actinic porokeratosis

---

with the 1450-nm diode and the Fraxel re:store™ laser. Lidocaine 5% cream (Ela-max) is applied 1 h before treatment, and is removed immediately before the laser is started. Anesthesia lasts for 1–2 h after removal. Beware of allergic reactions and, if lidocaine is applied for longer periods of time or to large surface areas, toxic reactions. Lidocaine allergy manifests as pruritus, urticaria, angioedema, laryngeal edema, pulmonary edema, and diarrhea. Lidocaine toxicity begins with tinnitus, circumoral pallor, metallic taste, lightheadedness, and talkativeness. As blood

levels increase, patients can demonstrate slurred speech, nystagmus, muscle twitching or tremors, bradycardia, hypotension, seizures, and ultimately coma.

Topical anesthetics may superhydrate the dermis (increase tissue water from 65% to 80%), so that heating with devices targeting water is more superficial than usual. Anesthetics such as EMLA (EMLA; Astra Zeneca, Wilmington, DE), or those containing epinephrine, may blanch the skin, cooling the epidermis and superficial dermis. This may protect the epidermis, but may also decrease the peak dermal temperature reached and the efficacy of treatment. It is important not to blunt the patient's pain response, as this is a good gauge of optimal treatment fluence.

Local infiltration, tumescent, intravenous, or general anesthesia is not recommended. Oral analgesics and short-acting anxiolytics can be taken an hour before the procedure.

Eye protection is very important and should always be used by both the patient and any providers present in the room during laser use. Lasers targeting pigment can cause retinal damage, whereas lasers targeting water can damage the cornea. Protective eyewear is color coded, and the wavelengths that the lenses protect against are typically printed on the glasses themselves. When planning to treat inside the orbital rim, adhesive eyepads or eyeshields should be used; after lidocaine solution is dropped onto the conjunctiva, eyeshields are inserted like contact lenses for the duration of treatment.

When using long wavelengths, such as the diode or Nd:YAG systems, gauze should be placed inside the mouth to protect teeth and fillings.

Pretreatment photos are especially important for this type of therapy, where improvements may be subtle and undetected by the patient. Preoperative and postoperative pictures should match in lighting and position. A pretreatment checklist is provided in Box 8-4.

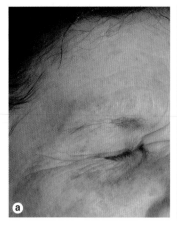
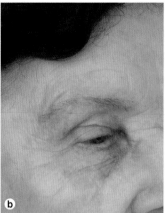

Figure 8-15 Intense pulsed light improves solar lentigenes. (A) Before treatment; (B) after treatment. Photo courtesy of Ramsey Marcus MD

BOX 8-4

Pretreatment checklist

Number of treatments that will be required

Amount of improvement to expect – show realistic before and after pictures

Avoid certain medications for 1 week before and after certain laser procedures:

- aspirin
- ibuprofen
- vitamin E
- anti-inflammatory medications
- photosensitizing medications
- alcohol

Stop topical medications for 2 days before and after:

- tretinoin topical
- α-hydroxy acids
- vitamin C derivatives

Confirm no contraindications for laser treatment:

- pregnancy
- history of keloids
- current suntan
- isotretinoin therapy within 6 months
- lupus erythematosus or other photosensitivity

If history of herpes simplex virus, prescribe valaciclovir 500 mg by mouth twice daily for 3 days. Start 1 day before procedure

If pretreatment anesthesia needed, prescribe topical anesthetic such as EMLA cream to treatment area 1 h before treatment under plastic wrap occlusion

Pretreatment photos in a reproducible position and lighting

Eye protection for patient and physician

Teeth protection for patient

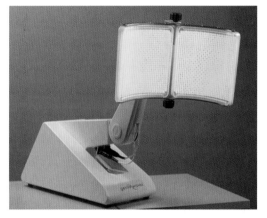

Figure 8-16 Light-emitting diode panel. Photo courtesy of GentleWaves, Virginia Beach, VA

PEARLS

Counseling the patient for nonablative laser treatment

Discuss realistic expectations and show before and after photographs.

Multiple monthly treatments will be needed to achieve full benefit.

General improvement in skin texture, fine rhytides, or acne can be expected; deep wrinkles and lentigines are better treated with a laser for that indication.

Confirm there are no contraindications to laser therapy, such as isotretinoin use in past 6 months.

Topical retinoids, α-hydroxy acids, and vitamin C should be discontinued 48 h before treatment.

Optional aspirin, ibuprofen, vitamin E, and alcohol should be avoided for 1 week prior to treatment.

Consider pre- and post-treatment with hydroquinone in darker skin types.

Advise patients not to present for laser treatment with a tan.

Query patient for history of herpes simplex and give prophylaxis accordingly.

Discuss anesthesia options.

Sign consents and take baseline photographs.

Device selection

In general, rhytides and acne scars are best treated with mid-infrared lasers such as the 1320-nm Nd:YAG, 1450-nm diode, 1540-nm Er:glass, or nonablative fractional devices (Fig. 8-17). Textural changes also respond to nonablative fractional devices. Photo-damage with prominent vascular lesions responds well to the PDL, IPL, long-pulsed Nd:YAG, and even the vascular specific 532-nm KTP laser. Photo-damage with prominent hyperpigmentation is best treated with the Q-switched lasers, IPL, and nonablative fractional devices. Textural and pigmentary improvements usually accompany each other, regardless of device selection, although IPL is touted as being particularly effective in treating both simultaneously.

A combination of lasers can also be used to address multiple concerns in the aging or acne-ridden face. With time, improved and tailored combination treatment protocols will likely be determined.

Dark-skinned patients should undergo treatment with a longer wavelength, infrared-emitting device. KTP lasers are associated with hyperpigmentation and hypopigmentation and should be avoided in this population.

Practical considerations during treatment

General considerations

A test spot in a nonauspicious area, such as the preauricular cheek, should be performed, and parameters adjusted to achieve mild erythema. Suggested starting parameters for fair-skinned individuals are listed in Table 8-2. The handpiece should be held exactly perpendicular to the skin. If there is a contact cooling device, the cooling window should be in complete contact with the skin, and should remain in contact even after light delivery. The cooling window is cleaned to remove debris that may heat the window and attenuate the beam. If there is a cryogen spray cooling system, the handpiece must be perpendicular to ensure alignment of the cryogen spray and laser pulse (Fig. 8-18). Second passes are often used to provide subsequent and gentle heating. However, after the first pass, inflammation ensues. This results in increased perfusion and temperature, so a second pass over this mileu may result in higher temperatures and more damage.

The neck, chest, and hands are more hazardous. These areas have decreased sebaceous glands and follicular units, so fewer stem cells are available for re-epithelialization and wound healing.

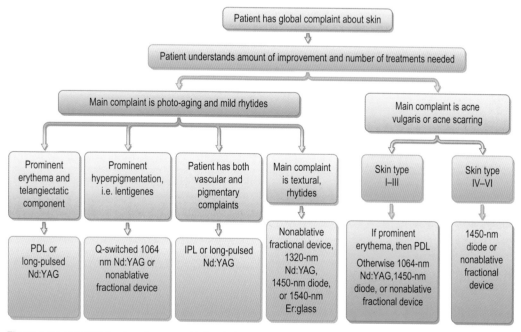

Figure 8-17 Algorithm for choosing a nonablative device

Table 8-2 Selected nonablative light sources and suggested parameters

Laser	Wavelength (nm)	Indications	Parameters
Long-pulsed PDL (V-beam, Candela, Wayland, MA)	595	Photo-damage; acne vulgaris	7–8.5 J, 6–20 ms, 10-mm spot
Nd:YAG (Gentle YAG; Candela, Wayland, MA)	1064	Photo-damage	3.5 J/cm^2, 6-mm spot (28-ns pulse duration is standard)
Q-switched Nd:YAG (Medlite IV; Continuum, Santa Clara, CA)	1064	Acne scars	3–4 J/cm^2, 4–6-ns pulse duration, repetition rate 10 Hz, 6-mm spot. Deliver overlapping pulses until mild to moderate erythema achieved
Nd:YAG (CoolTouch II; ICN Pharmaceuticals, Costa Mesa, CA)	1320	Photo-damage; acne scarring	Energy 12–16 J/cm^2, 10-mm spot, DCD before, during, and after
Diode (Smooth Beam, ICN Photonics, Costa Mesa, CA)	1450	Photo-damage; acne and acne scarring	12–14 J/cm^2, 6-mm spot (pulse duration is standard), DCD before, during, and after
Er:glass (Aramis-Quantel laser; Quantel Medical, Clermont-Ferrand, France)	1,540	Photo-damage	3 pulses per shot, 10 J per pulse, fluence 30 J/cm^2, 4-mm spot, slightly overlapping pulses, no visible changes occur
Fractional laser (Fraxel re:store™ Reliant Technologies, Palo Alto, CA)	1500	Photo-damage; acne and acne scarring	Treatment level 8–11 to obtain 23–32% coverage, energy level 50–70 mJ, approximately 8 passes to deliver total of 3–4 kJ
Intense pulsed light (Lumenis One, Lumenis, Santa Clara, CA)	500–1200	Photo-damage, including poikiloderma of Civatte; acne	560-nm filter, fluence 16–18 J/cm^2 with thin layer of gel. Double pulse with 3–4-ms pulse duration and delay of 10 ms. Parameters may vary for other systems
LED (GentleWaves, Virginia Beach, VA)	Predominantly 590	Periorbital rhytides	Total output of 0.1 J/cm^2 per treatment has been reported

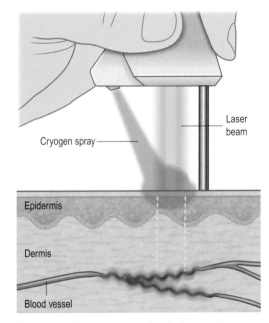

Figure 8-18 Cryogen spray cooling device technique. The handpiece should be held perpendicular to the skin to ensure alignment of the cryogen spray and laser pulse

More conservative parameters are used. Consider reducing fluence by 10–20%, increasing spot size, or, if using Fraxel re:store™, decreasing the number of MTZs. Conversely, more aggressive treatment settings may be required to treat the ear, nose, and alar creases.

Device-specific technique

The most popular PDL system (Candela) is equipped with a cryogen cooling device. The handpiece is held perpendicular to the skin and stamped over the target areas. Acne lesions may be treated individually, or the entire face from forehead to jaw line may be treated. The Q-switched Nd:YAG handpiece is held approximately 2 cm away from the skin, and moved in a "painting" fashion to cover the entire skin. Because the longer wavelength penetrates deeper, the Nd:YAG laser is always kept outside the periorbital rim to avoid eye damage, even if internal eye shields are worn. The diode systems use a "stamping" technique. The entire face, or affected areas, can be treated with nonoverlapping pulses.

The current Fraxel re:store™ laser protocol involves a topical anesthetic, followed by application

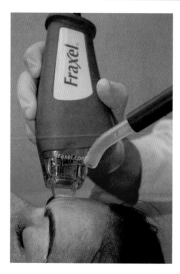

Figure 8-19 Fraxel re:store™ tracking system. Newer rolling tip fits old handpieces, eliminating need for blue dye. Cooled air tip used in conjunction with Fraxel re:store™

of a thin layer of LipoThene gel to the treatment area. Reflections from the lubricant are used to sense handpiece motion. The use of anesthetic or too much gel can impede treatment. The handpiece is held perpendicular to the skin, and rolled evenly along the skin (Fig. 8-19). Adjacent tracks should not be overlapping, and multiple passes are used to achieve the desired coverage. Superficial lesions such as lentigos are treated with lower energy levels, and deeper lesions such as acne scars with higher energy levels. Less auxillary cooling may be used to optimize the treatment of superficial targets. If more aggressive treatment is desired, treatment levels (corresponding to percentage coverage) are increased (see Fig. 8-11). After treatment, gel, smudges, and debris are removed from the handpiece window with a cotton swab.

Before treatment with IPL, a thin layer of coupling gel is applied to the skin. If there is not an attached cooling device, the handpiece glides across the gel, hovering over and never coming into direct contact with the skin. If there is an active cooling device, such as cooled crystal, the handpiece is pushed down over the gel and touches the skin; fluence should be lowered by 20%. Parameters are adjusted to achieve mild edema and mild to moderate erythema 10 min after treating a test spot.

PEARLS

Photo-aging may manifest differently in patients with a darker skin.

Dyspigmentation is the major limiting factor.

Consider lowering fluence, using higher cutoff filters, and lowering treatment level (if applicable).

Cooling is imperative to protect pigmented epidermis, but overcooling itself can also result in dyspigmentation.

Considerations regarding ethnic skin

The advent of nonablative lasers makes ethnic skin (typically classified as types IV–VI, but also type III) a candidate for laser treatment – now more so than ever. The ethnic population is increasing, and ethnic skin accounts for more than 20% of all cosmetic procedures. Hispanics lead minority racial and ethnic groups in the number of procedures: Hispanics, 8%; African-Americans, 6%; Asians, 4%; and other non-Caucasians, 2%.

Photo-aging is mostly the result of UV light on the epidermis and dermis. UVB, long recognized as the culprit of cutaneous malignancies and photo-aging, penetrates white epidermis much more than black epidermis (29.4% versus 5.7%). UVA, which comprises 95% of total UV radiation and has recently been found to contribute to photo-aging, also penetrates white epidermis significantly more than black epidermis (55.5% versus 17.5%). The main site of UV filtration in white epidermis is the stratum corneum, whereas the major site of filtration in black epidermis is the malpighian layers, which contain melanin. Although skin of different ethnicities contains the same number of melanocytes, darker skin has larger melanosomes and more melanin, which is the main protective factor against photo-aging.

Because of these differences, not only does photo-aging occur later in most ethnic skin, but the manifestations also differ. Black skin develops mottled pigmentation, dermatosis papulosa nigra, and malar fat pad sagging. East and South-East Asians primarily complain of discrete pigmentary changes such as solar lentigenes, seborrheic keratoses, and sun-induced melasma.

Although protective, the presence of melanin makes it more difficult to treat photo-aging. Melanin absorption of laser energy can result in epidermal damage and decrease the amount of energy that reaches the intended dermal chromophores. Because the absorption coefficient of melanin decreases as wavelength increases (see Fig. 8-3), near-infrared and infrared wavelengths can best provide nonablative rejuvenation for darker skin types. Epidermal cooling is the most important part of treating ethnic skin; however, too much cooling can result in postinflammatory hyperpigmentation.

Studies of various lasers in ethnic skin report a low frequency of side-effects with nonablative laser and light sources. Using the 532-nm laser for the treatment of pigmentation and telangiectasia in type IV skin, the incidence of hyperpigmentation was 10% and that of hypopigmentation was 25%. These side-effects resolved after 2–6 months. Using the same laser, in patients with skin types III and IV, there was a 5% incidence of postinflammatory hyperpigmentation, which resolved in 4–6 weeks. Using longer pulsed PDLs (585 nm, 3.5-ms pulse duration) for acne scarring, no side-effects were reported. The IPL has been used in Japanese patients (skin types IV and V) without any dyspigmentation. Another Asian study of the IPL reported only one case of hypopigmentation. Higher cut-off filters are recommended to protect epidermal melanin, but may impede results when treating rhytides. The 1320-nm laser has been used safely in type IV skin, although five cases of central facial blistering were reported with the 1320-nm Nd:YAG laser; the authors believed that this was due to the long cryogen duration of 60 ms. Others have also reported increased dyspigmentation with longer cryogen spurts.

Both the LED and Fraxel re:store™ have been used in type IV skin, without side-effects. Any postinflammatory hyperpigmentation associated with Fraxel re:store™ laser may be related to MTZ density, so lower treatment levels are recommended.

Post-treatment care

There are usually not any adverse events, and virtually all patients can return to work the same day. Any side-effects are generally limited to transient edema, purpura, erythema, dyspigmentation, and, very rarely, blistering or scarring (Table 8-3). Pain or a "deep heat" sensation will diminish in 1–2 h. Cooling gels and sheets can be used to minimize erythema and edema, and to alleviate any postprocedure discomfort (Fig. 8-20).

All patients should be counseled to use sunblock regularly to prevent repigmentation and postinflammatory hyperpigmentaton. There is no increased photosensitivity related to non-ablative laser treatment. Make-up may be applied immediately after treatment. Topical retinoids and acids may be temporarily stopped for up to 2 weeks to avoid epidermal inflammation. There are no activity restrictions.

Patients should be reminded that the collagen remodeling response is delayed and that maximal regeneration occurs 30–90 days after treatment. Patients may like the immediate post-treatment look, which is attributable mainly to edema, and can be advised that this end-result is possible after multiple treatments. Maintenance therapy can be performed three to four times per year.

Most of the side-effects reported with "non-ablative lasers" are associated with the treatment of pigmented lesions or hair removal. When the same devices are used to achieve nonablative rejuvenation and to treat acne, lower fluences are used, so the incidence of adverse events is also lower. Still, a brief review of possible side-effects follows.

Table 8-3 Adverse events associated with nonablative lasers

Adverse event	Comments
Pain	Depends on device, more so with deep-infrared devices that target water
Erythema	Usually clears in hours, but can last several days. This is expected endpoint with Fraxel re:store™
Edema	Usually clears within 24 h. May last longer with Fraxel re:store™
Purpura	Most commonly occurs with PDL. Transient purpura may be obtained when treating telangiectasia. For acne and photo-aging, lower fluence or lengthen pulse duration
Crusting	Indicates too much epidermal heating
Blistering	Indicates too much epidermal heating; may result in scarring
Infection	Query patient as to history of prior HSV infection. Consider *Staphylococcus aureus* infection if epidermis is inadvertently ablated
Dyspigmentation	Most common in darker skin types. Correct amount of epidermal cooling should be used
Textural scarring	Rare

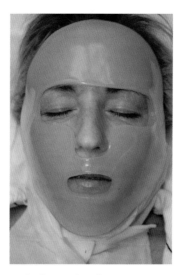

Figure 8-20 Cooling masks offer post-treatment comfort. Masks can be refrigerated and reused at home

Pain

Pain is common during treatment. Each pulse can cause a stinging or heated sensation. The pain can be likened to that of a snapped rubber band. Topical anesthetics and practices to increase tolerability are discussed above. When treating acne, there may be more pain during initial treatments, but as acne counts and inflammation are reduced, there is less associated pain with laser treatment.

There is usually no pain post-treatment. Any remaining warm sensation generally subsides within 1–2 h. Cooling gels and sheets, ice packs, cold water soaks, simple occlusion with petrolatum, or other dressings alleviate pain. Pain medication should not be needed.

Erythema and edema

Any erythema or edema subsides within 24 h. In a study of 150 patients treated with a KTP or 1064-nm Nd:YAG laser, only four developed erythema and edema that lasted for 2–3 days. These patients had severe rosacea with a strong vasoactive component, and a history of being sensitive to heat. With subsequent treatment, the amount of erythema and edema diminished, presumably because there were fewer vessels after each treatment. In addition, it has been suggested that nonsteroidal drugs may increase the risk of purpura, scarring, and hyperpigmentation.

The exception is nonablative fractional devices, which are regularly associated with erythema and edema. Post-treatment edema can be mild to severe, and usually resolves in 3-4 days. Particularly when periocular areas are treated (Fig. 8-21), patients should be forewarned about swelling and ways to prevent it: sleeping upright, lower sodium intake, ice application, and ibuprofen. A few patients may feel more comfortable with the administration of oral prednisone for 3 days. The effect of steroids has not been studied, and it is plausible that their anti-inflammatory action may inhibit the desired wound healing effect. Patients may experience minor exfoliation or dryness that is readily abated with moisturizers. Overall, side-effects are few (see Table 8-3) and postoperative care is generally not needed.

Purpura

Purpura is usually encountered only after using a vascular-specific laser, particularly with the PDL. The longer pulse durations used for dermal heating are less likely to cause photo-acoustic shattering of capillary walls and extravasation of red blood cells. Any bruising will be apparent immediately after therapy, and may last for 2 weeks.

Pigmentary changes

Patients with darker skin are at higher risk for pigmentary changes, especially if a sun-exposed area is treated. All patients should be counseled to wear sunblock for at least several months. Most dyspigmentation becomes visible within 30–90 days and should resolve spontaneously over several months. Infrequently, pigmentary changes may not become evident until months after treatment. With IPL, darkening of ephilides and lentigos for 7–10 days is considered a normal response.

Hyperpigmentation results from heat-induced melanin production by epidermal and follicular melanocytes. After ablative resurfacing, it can reportedly last for up to 18 months. In darker patients receiving aggressive treatment, some mild hyperpigmentation may be anticipated; these patients may use hydroquinone, tretinoin, and sunblock, not only after treatment, but also 1 month before treatment. One study of 57 patients with Asian skin being treated with a 1450-nm diode laser for scarring recorded a hyperpigmentation rate of 39%. When the duration of the cryogen spray was reduced from 50 to 40 ms, there was a lower incidence and severity of hyperpigmentation. In two other studies with the 1450-nm diode, reduction of cryogen spurt duration from 60 to 50 ms also resulted in less hyperpigmentation, suggesting that aggressive cooling can induce postinflammatory hyperpigmentation. If treating melasma, hormonal supplements should be discontinued when possible. Hydroquinone cream is available up to 4% in standard prescriptions, but can be compounded at speciality pharmacies to higher concentrations.

Hypopigmentation results from heat destruction of melanocytes at the dermal–epidermal junction. Damage from shockwaves, the physical effects of thermal expansion, and extreme temperature gradients within the cells may be involved.

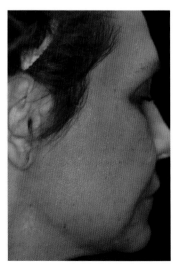

Figure 8-21 Immediate post-treatment erythema and edema is common with Fraxel re:store™

Hypopigmentation is rarely reported in association with nonablative laser therapy, but can sometimes be permanent.

Blistering or crusting

Blistering or crusting occurs only when the epidermis is damaged, and should not arise when the proper technique and parameters are used for nonablative rejuvenation or the treatment of acne scars. Possible errors that may result in epidermal ablation include excessive fluence, small spot size or pulse duration, too many passes, excessive melanin absorption, and insufficient epidermal cooling. If there is a superficial burn, the ablated skin should be treated with emollients, as if the patient had undergone ablative resurfacing.

Scarring

Textural scarring, atrophic or hypertrophic, is extremely rare with nonablative laser therapy. However, excessive damage to the dermis may lead to scarring, and can be prevented by using devices associated with shallow penetration or epidermal cooling. Postoperative wound infections can also contribute to scarring.

Infection

HSV infection has been reviewed above. Bacterial infections with *Staphylococcus epidermidis* or *Staphylococcus aureus*, or candidal infections, are generally not an issue, unless the epidermis is compromised inadvertently. Systems employing a contact cooling device may be a source of cross-infection between patients.

Directions for the future

Nonablative lasers are the result of technology meeting patient demands for "lunchtime" treatments. The ability to use light to treat acne, especially recalcitrant acne and acne scarring, is a great addition to the dermatologist's armamentarium. Fractionated laser delivery may maximize tissue response relative to tissue injury, and other fractional lasers will surely follow. Nonablative resurfacing is relatively new and, although results may be mild and sometimes inconsistent, new developments and protocols will improve efficacy. The current lasers and protocols are already welcomed by patients seeking minimally invasive procedures with an outstanding safety profile.

Further reading

Alam M, Hsu TS, Dover JS, Wrone DA, Arndt KA. Nonablative laser and light treatments: histology and tissue effects – a review. Lasers Surg Med 2003;33(1):30–39.

Alexiades-Armenakas M. Long pulsed dye laser-mediated photodynamic therapy combined with topical therapy for mild to severe comedonal, inflammatory, or cystic acne. J Drugs Dermatol 2006;5:45–55.

Alster TS, Lupton JR. Are all infrared lasers equally effective in skin rejuvenation? Semin Cutan Med Surg 2002;21:274–279.

American Society for Aesthetic Plastic Surgery. Survey data. 2005. Available at: http://www.surgery.org/press/news-release.php?iid=325 (accessed July 2007).

American Society for Dermatologic Surgery. Membership survey data. 2005. Available at: www.aboutskinsurgery.com/old/Media/Articles/ASDS2003StatsReport.pdf (accessed March 2005).

Behroozan DS, Goldberg LH, Glaich AS, et al. Fractional photothermolysis for treatment of poikiloderma of Civatte. Dermatol Surg 2006;32(2):298–301.

Behroozan DS, Goldberg LH, Dai T, et al. Fractional photothermolysis for treatment of surgical scars: a case report. J Cosmet Laser Ther 2006;8(1):35–38.

Bellew SG, Lee C, Weiss M, et al. Improvement of atrophic acne scars with a 1320 nm Nd:YAG laser: retrospective study. Dermatol Surg 2005;31:1218–1222.

Bene NI, Weiss MA, Beasley KL, et al. Comparison of histologic features of 1550 nm fractional resurfacing and microlens array scattering of 1440 nm. Laser Surg Med 2006;S18:26.

Bernstein EF. A pilot investigation comparing low-energy, double pass 1450 nm laser treatment of acne to conventional single-pass, high-energy treatment. Lasers Surg Med 2007;39(2):193–198.

Bhardwaj SS, Rohrer TE, Arndt K. Lasers and light therapy for acne vulgaris. Semin Cutan Med Surg 2005;24:107–112.

Bhatia AC, Dover JS, Arndt KA, et al. Patient satisfaction and reported long-term therapeutic efficacy associated with 1320 nm Nd:YAG laser treatment of acne scarring and photoaging. Dermatol Surg 2006;32:346–352.

Bogle MA, Dover JS, Arndt KA, et al. Evaluation of the 1540 nm erbium:glass laser in the treatment of inflammatory facial acne. Dermatol Surg 2007;33:810–817.

Carniol PJ, Vynatheya J, Carniol E. Evaluation of acne scar treatment with a 1450 nm midinfrared laser and 30% trichloroacetic acid peels. Arch Facial Plast Surg 2005;7:251–255.

Chan HH, Lam LK, Wong DS, et al. Use of the 1320 nm Nd:YAG laser for wrinkle reduction and the treatment of atrophic acne scarring in Asians. Lasers Surg Med 2004;34:98–103.

Chiu RJ, Kridel RW. Fractionated photothermolysis: the Fraxel 1550 nm glass fiber laser treatment. Facial Plast Surg Clin North Am 2007;15(2):229–237.

Chrastil B, Glaich AS, Goldberg LH, Friedman PH. A novel treatment for disseminated superficial actinic porokeratosis. Arch Dermatol 2007;143:1450–1452.

Chua S, Ang P, Khoo LSW, et al. Nonablative 1450 nm diode laser in the treatment of facial atrophic acne scars in type IV to V Asian skin: a prospective clinical study. Dermatol Surg 2004;30(10):1287–1291.

Chung JH, Lee SH, Youn CS, et al. Cutaneous photodamage in Koreans: influence of sex, sun exposure, smoking, and skin color. Arch Dermatol 2001;137:1043–1051.

Dierickx C. Laser hair removal: scientific principles and practical aspects. Santa Clara: Lumenis, 2002.

Doshi SN, Alster TS. 1450 nm long-pulsed diode laser for nonablative skin rejuvenation. Dermatol Surg 2005;31:1223–1226.

Effron C, Briden ME, Green BA. Enhancing cosmetic outcomes by combining superficial glycolic acid (alpha-hydroxy acid) peels with nonablative lasers, intense pulsed light, and trichloracetic acid peels. Cutis 2007;79(Suppl 1):4–8.

Fatemi A, Weiss MA, Weiss RA. Short-term histologic effects of nonablative resurfacing: results with a dynamically cooled millisecond-domain 1320 nm Nd:YAG laser. Dermatol Surg 2002;28:172–176.

Fisher GH, Geronemus RG. Short-term side effects of fractional photothermolysis. Dermatol Surg 2005;31(Pt 2):1245–1249.

Fisher G, Voorhees J. Molecular mechanisms of photoaging and its prevention by retinoid acid: ultraviolet irradiation induces MAP kinase signal transduction cascades that induce AP-1 regulated matrix metalloproteinases that degrade human skin in vitro. J Invest Dermatol 1998;3:61–68.

Fisher GJ, Wang ZQ, Datta SC, et al. Pathophysiology of premature skin aging induced by ultraviolet light. N Engl J Med 1997;337:1419–1428.

Fisher G, Datta S, Wang Z, et al. c-Jun-dependent inhibition of cutaneous procollagen transcription following ultraviolet irradiation is reversed by all-trans retinoid acid. J Clin Invest 2000;106: 663–670.

Fournier N, Dahan S, Barneon G, et al. Nonablative remodeling: clinical, histologic, ultrasound imaging, and profilometric evaluation of a 1540 nm Er:glass laser. Dermatol Surg 2001;27:799–806.

Fournier N, Lagarde JM, Turlier V, et al. A 35-month profilometric and clinical evaluation of nonablative remodeling using a 1540 nm Er:glass laser. J Cosmet Laser Ther 2004;6:126–130.

Friedman PM, Skover GR, Payonk G, et al. Quantitative evaluation of nonablative laser technology. Semin Cutan Med Surg 2002;21(4):266–273.

Friedman PM, Jih MH, Skover GR, et al. Treatment of atrophic facial acne scars with the 1064 nm Q-switched Nd:YAG laser: six month follow-up study. Arch Dermatol 2004;140:1337–1341.

Fulchiero GJ, Parham-Vetter PC, Obagi S. Subscision and 1320 nm Nd:YAG nonablative laser resurfacing for the treatment of acne scars: a simultaneous split-face single patient trial. Dermatol Surg 2004;30:1356–1360.

Geronemus RG. Fractional photothermolysis: current and future applications. Lasers Surg Med 2006;38:169–176.

Glaich AS, Friedman PM, Jih MH, Goldberg LH. Treatment of inflammatory facial acne vulgaris with combination 595-nm pulsed-dye laser with dynamic-cooling-device and 1450-nm diode laser. Lasers Surg Med 2006;38:177–180.

Glaich AS, Goldberg LH, Dai T, et al. Fractional photothermolysis for the treatment of telangiectatic matting: a case report. J Cosmet Laser Ther 2007;9(2):101–103.

Glaich AS, Goldberg LH, Friedman RH, et al. Fractional photothermolysis for the treatment of postinflammatory erythema resulting from acne vulgaris. Dermatol Surg 2007;33:1–5.

Glaich AS, Goldberg LH, Dai T, et al. Fractional re-surfacing: a new therapeutic modality for Becker's nevus. Arch Dermatol 2007;143:1488–1490.

Glaich AS, Rahman Z, Goldberg LH, et al. Fractional photothermolysis for the treatment of hypopigmented scars: a pilot study. Dermatol Surg 2007;33:289–294.

Goh SH. The treatment of visible signs of senescence: the Asian experience. Br J Dermatol 1990;122(Suppl 35):105–119.

Goldberg DJ. Nonablative subsurface remodeling: clinical and histologic evaluation of a 1320 nm Nd:YAG laser. J Cutan Laser Ther 1999;1:153–157.

Goldberg DJ. Full-face nonablative dermal remodeling with a 1320 nm Nd:YAG laser. Dermatol Surg 2000;26:915–918.

Goldberg D. Laser treatment of benign pigmented lesions. eMedicine. Available at: http://www.emedicine.com/derm./topic517.htm (accessed July 21, 2006).

Goldberg DJ, Cutler KB. Nonablative treatment of rhytids with intense pulsed light. Lasers Surg Med 2000;26:196–200.

Goldberg DJ, Silapunt S. Histologic evaluation of a Q-switched Nd:YAG laser in the nonablative treatment of wrinkles. Dermatol Surg 2001;27: 744–746.

Goldberg DJ, Whitworth J. Laser skin resurfacing with the Q-switched Nd:YAG laser. Dermatol Surg 1997;23:903–907.

Goldman MP, Weiss RA. Treatment of poikiloderma of Civatte on the neck with an intense pulsed light source. Plast Reconstr Surg 2001;107(6): 1376–1381.

Handley JM. Adverse events associated with nonablative cutaneous visible and infrared laser treatment. J Am Acad Dermatol 2006;55:482–489.

Hantash BM, Bedi VP, Sudireddy V, et al. Laser-induced transepidermal elimination of dermal content by fractional photothermolysis. J Biomed Opt 2006;11(4):041115.

Hardaway CA, Ross EV, Barnette DJ, Paithankar DY. Non-ablative cutaneous remodeling with a 1.45 microm mid-infrared diode laser: phase I. J Cosmet Laser Ther 2002;4(1):3–8.

Huzaira M, Anderson RR, Sink K, Manstein D. Intradermal focusing of near-infrared optical pulses: a new approach for non-ablative laser therapy. Lasers Surg Med 2003;32(Suppl 15):17–38.

Jih MH, Friedman PM, Goldberg LH, et al. The 1450 nm diode laser for facial inflammatory acne vulgaris: dose response and 12-month follow-up study. J Am Acad Dermatol 2006;55:80–87.

Kaidbey KH, Agin PP, Sayre RM, et al. Photoprotection by melanin – a comparison of black and Caucasian skin. J Am Acad Dermatol 1979;1:249–260.

Kaufmann R, Hibst R. Pulsed erbium:YAG laser ablation in cutaneous surgery. Lasers Surg Med 1996;19:324–330.

Khan MH, Sink RK, Manstein D, Eimerl D, Anderson RR. Intradermally focused infrared laser pulses: thermal effects at defined tissue depths. Lasers Surg Med 2005;36:270–280.

Kligman AM, Zheng P, Lavker RM. The anatomy and pathogenesis of wrinkles. Br J Dermatol 1985;113:37–42.

Kono T, Nozaki M, Chan HH, et al. A retrospective study looking at the long-term complications of Q-switched ruby laser in the treatment of nevus of Ota. Lasers Surg Med 2001;29:156–159.

Kono T, Chan HH, Groff WF, et al. Prospective direct comparison study of fractional resurfacing using different fluences and densities for skin rejuvenation in Asians. Lasers Surg Med 2007;39(4):311–314.

Kuo T, Speyer MT, Ries WR, et al. Collagen thermal damage and collagen synthesis after cutaneous laser resurfacing. Lasers Surg Med 1998;23:66–71.

Lanigan SW. Incidence of side effects after laser hair removal. J Am Acad Dermatol 2003;49:882–886.

Laubach HJ, Tannous Z, Anderson RR, et al. Skin responses to fractional photothermolysis. Lasers Surg Med 2006;38(2):142–149.

Lee MW. Combination 532-nm and 1064-nm lasers for noninvasive skin rejuvenation and toning. Arch Dermatol 2003;139:1265–1276.

Lipper GM, Perez M. Nonablative acne scar reduction after a series of treatments with a short-pulsed 1064 nm neodymium:YAG laser. Dermatol Surg 2006;32:998–1006.

Lloyd JR, Mirkov M. Selective photothermolysis of the sebaceous glands for acne treatment. Lasers Surg Med 2002;31:115–120.

Lupton JR, Williams CM, Alster TS. Nonablative laser skin resurfacing using a 1540 nm erbium glass laser: a clinical and histologic analysis. Dermatol Surg 2002;28:833–835.

Majaron B, Svaasand LO, Aguilar G, Nelson JS. Intermittent cryogen spray cooling for optimal heat extraction during dermatologic laser treatment. Phys Med Biol 2002;47:3275–3288.

Manstein D, Herron GS, Sink RK, et al. Fractional photothermolysis: a new concept for cutaneous remodeling using microscopic patterns of thermal injury. Lasers Surg Med 2004;34:426–438.

McBurney EI. Side effects and complications of laser therapy. Dermatol Clin 2002;20:165–176.

Mordon S, Capon A, Creussy C, et al. In vivo experimental evaluation of skin remodeling by using an Er:glass laser with contact cooling. Lasers Surg Med 2000;27:1–9.

Munavalli GS, Weiss RA, Halder RM. Photoaging and nonablative photorejuvenation in ethnic skin. Dermatol Surg 2005;31(Pt 2):1250–1260.

Nelson JS, Kimel S. Safety of cryogen spray cooling during pulsed laser treatment of selected dermatoses. Lasers Surg Med 2000;26:2–3.

Nelson JS, Milner TE, Anvari B, et al. Dynamic epidermal cooling during pulsed laser treatment of port-wine stain. A new methodology with preliminary clinical evaluation. Arch Dermatol 1995;131:695–700.

Nelson JS, Majaron B, Kelly KM. Active skin cooling in conjunction with laser dermatologic surgery. Semin Cutan Med Surg 2000;19:253–266.

Nelson JS, Majaron B, Kelly KM. What is nonablative photorejuvenation of human skin? Semin Cutan Med Surg 2002;21(4):238–250.

Nernstein EF, Chen YQ, Kopp JB, et al. Long-term sun exposure alters the collagen of the papillary dermis: comparison of sun-protected and photoaged skin by Northern analysis, immunohistochemical staining, and confocal laser scanning microscopy. J Am Acad Dermatol 1996;34:209–218.

Nestor MS. Prophylaxis for and treatment of uncomplicated skin and skin structure infections in laser and cosmetic surgery. J Drugs Dermatol 2005;4(Suppl):20–25.

Nikolaou VA, Stratigos AJ, Dover JS. Nonablative skin rejuvenation. J Cosmet Dermatol 2005;4:301–307.

Oringer JS, Kang S, Hamilton T, et al. Treatment of acne vulgaris with a pulsed dye laser: a randomized controlled trial. JAMA 2004;291(23):2834–2839.

Orringer JS, Voorhees JJ, Hamilton T, et al. Dermal matrix remodeling after nonablative laser therapy. J Am Acad Dermatol 2005;53:775–782.

Paithankar DY, Ross EV, Saleh BA, et al. Acne treatment with a 1450 nm wavelength laser and cryogen spray cooling. Lasers Surg Med 2002;31:106–114.

Patel N, Clement M. Selective nonablative treatment of acne scarring with 585nm flashlamp pulsed dye laser. Dermatol Surg 2002;28:942–945.

Pereira AN, Eduardo Cde P, Matson E, Marques MM. Effect of low-power laser irradiation on cell growth and procollagen synthesis of cultured fibroblasts. Lasers Surg Med 2002;31:263–267.

Ratner D, Viron A, Puvion E. Pilot ultrastructural evaluation of human pre-auricular skin before and after high-energy pulsed carbon dioxide laser treatment. Arch Dermatol 1998;134:582–587.

Rokhsar CK, Fitzpatrick RE. The treatment of melasma with fractional photothermolysis: a pilot study. Dernatol Surg 2005;31(12):1645–1650.

Ross EV, Zelickson BD. Biophysics of nonablative dermal remodeling. Semin Cutan Med Surg 2002;21:251–265.

Ross EV, Aajben FP, Hsia J, et al. Nonablative skin remodeling: selective dermal heating with a mid-infrared laser and contact cooling combination. Lasers Surg Med 2000;26:186–195.

Sadick NS, Weiss R. Intense pulsed-light photo-rejuvenation. Semin Cutan Med Surg 2002;21: 280–287.

Seaton ED, Charakida A, Mouser PE, et al. Pulsed-dye laser treatment for inflammatory acne vulgaris; randomized controlled trial. Lancet 2003;362:1347–1352.

Seaton ED, Mouser PD, Charakida A, et al. Investigation of the mechanism of action of nonablative pulsed-dye laser therapy in photorejuvenation and inflammatory acne vulgaris. Br J Dermatol 2006;155:748–755.

Tannous ZS, Astner S. Utilizing fractional resurfacing in the treatment of therapy-resistant melasma. J Cosmet Laser Ther 2005;7:39–43.

Tanzi EL, Alster TS. Treatment of transverse neck line with a 1450 nm diode laser. Lasers Surg Med 2002;30(Suppl):33.

Tanzi EL, Alster TS. Treatment of facial rhytides with a nonablative 1450 nm diode laser: a controlled clinical and histologic study. Dermatol Surg 2003;29:124–128.

Tanzi EL, Alster TS. Cutaneous laser surgery in darker skin types. Cutis 2003;73:21–30.

Tanzi EL, Alster TS. Comparison of a 1450 nm diode laser and a 1320 nm Nd:YAG laser in the treatment of atrophic facial scars: a prospective clinical and histologic study. Dermatol Surg 2004;30: 152–157.

Taylor SC. Skin of color: biology, structure, function, and implications for dermatologic disease. J Am Acad Dermatol 2002;46(Suppl):541–562.

Thomsen SL, Ellard J, Schwartz JA, et al. Chronology of healing events in pulsed CO_2 laser skin resurfacing in fuzzy rat. In: Anderson RR, Bartels KE, Bass LS, et al, eds. Lasers in Surgery: Advanced Characterization, Therapeutics, and Systems VII, Prac SPIE 3245. 1998:347–343.

Trelles MA, Allones I, Luna R. Facial rejuvenation with a nonablative 1320 nm Nd:YAG laser: a preliminary clinical and histologic evaluation. Dermatol Surg 2001;27:111–116.

Vinck EM, Cagne BJ, Cornelissen MF, et al. Increased fibroblast proliferation induced by light emitting diode and low power laser irradiation. Lasers Med Sci 2003;18:95–99.

Weiss RA, Goldman MP, Weiss MA. Treatment of poikiloderma of Civatte with an intense pulsed light source. Dermatol Surg 2000;26:823–827.

Weiss RA, McDaniel DH, Geronemus RG, et al. Clinical trial of a novel non-thermal LED array for reversal of photoaging: clinical, histologic, and surface profilometric results. Lasers Surg Med 2005;36(2):85–91.

Yaghmai D, Garden JM, Bakus AD, et al. Comparison of a 1064 nm laser and a 1320 nm laser for the nonablative treatment of acne scars. Dermatol Surg 2005;31:903–909.

Zelickson BD, Kilmer SL, Bernstein E, et al. Pulsed dye laser therapy for sun damaged skin. Lasers Surg Med 1999;25(3):229–236.

Zelickson B, Altshuler G, Erofeev A, et al. Comparative evaluation of Palomar Starlux 1540 Fractional™ and Reliant Fraxel™ devices for treatment of photo-damaged skin. Laser Surg Med 2006;S18:27.

Skin tightening with radiofrequency and other devices

Chapter 9

Carolyn I. Jacob and Amy Forman Taub

Key Points

Devices currently available that tighten the skin include:
- Carbon dioxide lasers
- Er:YAG lasers
- Infrared lasers (ReFirme ST, Titan, LuxDeepIR Fractional)
- Radiofrequency devices (Thermage NXT, Accent)
- PanG System

Introduction

Rapid advances in skin rejuvenation treatments have characterized the new millennium, with patient demand and improved technology driving the development of treatments that require little or no recovery time. Multiple devices for reducing wrinkles and improving skin texture have been developed. To date, none has been approved by the US Food and Drug Administration (FDA) for skin tightening per se, but many are used to achieve this effect. In this chapter we outline these technologies and explore their place among the armamentarium of facial rejuvenation. For definitions and key words, see Box 9-1.

To meet the demands of aging baby boomers who desire an ever-youthful appearance, many devices and therapies have been developed. In 1995, 10600-nm carbon dioxide lasers became available commercially. They provide immediate tissue tightening along with thermal ablation of the epidermis. In 1997 erbium:YAG (Er:YAG) lasers were developed to produce skin rejuvenation through shallow epidermal ablation and provide less dermal heating. Although effective, these ablative lasers require 7–14 days of healing and may produce erythema lasting for weeks to months.

To improve efficacy, but decrease healing time (compared with fully ablative lasers), a fractionated 1550-nm erbium:doped laser (Fraxel; Reliant Technologies, Mountain View, CA) was developed. The Fraxel has been shown to elicit some improvement in skin texture and acne scars after several treatments. It does, however produce 3–5 days of erythema, edema, and peeling after each treatment, and more aggressive treatments lead to a longer healing time.

A similar device (StarLux; Palomar Medical Technologies, Burlington, MA), at 1540 nm, may also lead to skin improvement. A greater variation on the fractionated Er:YAG laser at 1440 nm allows microwounding of the epidermis at 100–300 μm (Affirm; Cynosure, Westford, MA). The Affirm uses "combined apex pulse" technology with microbeams that create 1000 coagulated zones 100–300 μm deep with each 10-mm spot. This may lead to improvement of elastosis with only moderate erythema after each treatment.

More recently, adaptations in CO_2 10600-nm and Er:YAG 2940-nm lasers to include fractionated delivery of pulses has shown efficacy in treating dyspigmentation and fine lines, but no studies evaluating tissue tightening have been done to date. In addition, a fractionated 2790-nm erbium:yttrium–scandium–gallium–garnet (Er:YSGG) laser with a water absorption coefficient that lies between that of Er:YAG and CO_2 lasers has been developed (Pearl; Cutera, Brisbane, CA). The purpose of this laser is to provide fractionated vaporization of the upper epidermis while heating the dermis more than a traditional Er:YAG laser. Studies are currently pending.

An infrared (IR) fractionated laser (LuxDeepIR Fractional; Palomar, Burlington, MA) using a wavelength range of 850–1350 nm has led to clinical improvement and skin tightening on facial and nonfacial sites without epidermal ablation.

At the end of the 20th century, nonablative lasers were proven to provide dermal neocollagenesis while protecting the epidermis. These less invasive lasers improve facial rhytides by 0–75%, but subjective evaluation and data showing actual skin tightening are lacking. These technologies often require multiple, time-consuming treatment sessions, use highly delicate optics, and can be costly to acquire and maintain. In addition, results from nonablative lasers can be subtle, and results may vary significantly from patient to patient in both magnitude and duration of effect. These include long-pulsed neodymium : yttrium–aluminum–garnet (Nd:YAG) (1064 nm) lasers (Gemini, Iridex Corporation, Mountain View, CA – formerly Lyra, Laserscope; XeoGenesis, Cutera Corporation, Brisbane CA; GentleYAG; Candela Corporation, Wayland, MA), the 1450-nm Er: YAG laser (Smoothbeam; Candela Corporation), and the 1320-nm CoolTouch (CoolTouch Corporation, Roseville, CA).

A novel nonablative laser, the Titan (Cutera, Brisbane, CA), consists of an IR device emitting a broadband spectrum of light of 1100–1800 nm (Fig. 9-1), and delivering heat to the dermis. Epidermal protection occurs by contact cooling before, during, and after the heating phase of each exposure. This generates energy of up to 50 J/cm^2 and targets the dermis at a depth of 1–3 mm (Fig. 9-2), which is more superficial than that with radiofrequency (RF) devices. The heating of the water in the dermis produces immediate conformational collagen changes that result in a larger volume and long-term upregulation of fibroblasts

to produce more collagen over time (Figs 9-3 & 9-4). Heating of the papillary dermis has been shown to create fibroblastic changes and thickening of collagen after 3 months in animal studies.

A separate, nonlaser, technology using electrical energy for tissue tightening was introduced at the beginning of this century. Known as RF tissue tightening, this technology can be used as an alternative, or complement, to nonablative laser technologies. Earlier RF technologies were low-energy modifications of the traditional ablative RF electrosurgery units that were used with limited success for cosmetic purposes to improve the surface of the skin. A nonlaser RF device delivering much higher energy was developed to remodel and tighten collagen in the deeper dermis and subcutaneous tissue, to improve lax or aging skin.

The ThermaCool TC™ (now termed ThermageNXT; Thermage, Hayward, CA) device uses a form of monopolar radiofrequency (MRF) energy to create a uniform field of dermal and even subdermal heating, while contact cooling protects the epidermis. This device can safely deliver higher energy fluences to a greater tissue volume than nonablative lasers. In November 2002, The ThermaCool TC™ received FDA approval for the reduction of periorbital rhytides, and is used for tightening the skin of the forehead to improve brow positioning and reduce upper lid dermatochalasis. In addition, other areas including the cheek, jawline, submentum, abdomen, eyelids, hands, and thighs have been treated with success. Studies into the effectiveness of the ThermaCool TC™ in the treatment of acne are under way, as is the use of the device to reduce fat in areas such as the submentum.

Subsequent to the development of the ThermaCool device, other RF devices emerged. Bipolar radiofrequency (BRF) and optical energy were combined to form ELOS (electro-optical

BOX 9-1	
Definitions and key words	
LASER	light amplification by stimulated emission of radiation
Radiofrequency	electrical current used to create thermal injury in skin
MRF	monopolar radiofrequency
BRF	bipolar radiofrequency
IR	infrared
ELOS	electro-optical synergy
Nd:YAG	neodymium : yttrium–aluminum–garnet

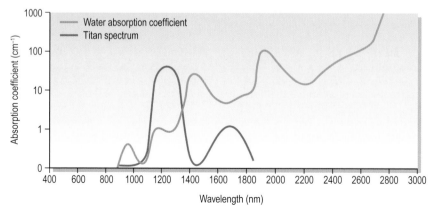

Figure 9-1 The Titan absorption spectrum

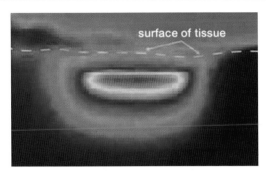

Figure 9-2 The Titan heating profile, depicting depth of dermal heating

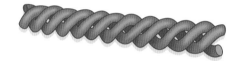

Figure 9-3 Schematic of collagen fiber strand before heating

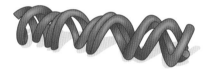

Figure 9-4 Schematic of contracted collagen strand following application of heat

synergy) technology. When combining RF and optical light/laser sources, it was noted that lower levels of both energies could be used, potentially reducing the risk of side-effects associated with either optical or RF treatment alone.

The first device, the Aurora, used BRF and intense pulsed light (IPL). Then, a combination of BRF and diode laser (ELOS, Polaris WR™; Syneron Medical, Yokneam, Israel) was created to deliver RF and 900-nm diode laser energy sequentially through a bipolar electrode tip with epidermal cooling.

A newer combination of BRF and 700–2000-nm IR laser light has been developed to tighten skin and treat wrinkles (ReFirme™ Skin Tightening; Syneron Medical). Preliminary studies showed a median wrinkle clearance rate of 50% in 31 patients treated two to five times at 3–4-week intervals. Most recently another device combining 910-nm diode laser with RF was released, called the Matrix IR; this is currently being evaluated for efficacy with regard to perioral, periorbital, and nasolabial fold rhytides.

A variation on using BRF with IR light and mechanical suction-based massage has been studied for the tightening of the skin on the body and improvement of cellulite (Velasmooth; Syneron Medical). Twice-weekly treatments are performed with the device for 3–4 months to achieve results.

Recently, a device using both BRF and unipolar RF was designed (Accent; Alma Lasers, Buffalo Grove, IL). The BRF is used for volumetric heating, while the unipolar handpiece is for deep penetration into the dermis. The concept is to create tightening of fibrous septa, induce fat cell apoptosis, and enhance local circulation and drainage of fat components to the lymphatic system. This device is currently under investigation for the reduction of cellulite on the body.

Pure electrical stimulation of the facial muscles has also been shown to provide improvement in skin laxity by training the muscles supporting the skin (PanG Lift; Pan Germinal Systems, Clearwater, FL). Biweekly treatments along with further maintenance treatments have been shown to tighten facial and neck skin.

This chapter reviews the current modalities for tissue tightening including nonablative long-pulsed Nd:YAG lasers, nonablative broadband technology, RF devices, and electrical stimulation.

Literature review

Nonablative lasers and pure light sources (without RF) (Table 9-1)

1064-nm Nd:YAG laser

The study by Lee (2003) using the Gemini (Iridex Corporation – previously Lyra, Laserscope) 1064-nm Nd:YAG laser revealed subtle and gradual improvements in wrinkles, skin laxity, and overall appearance supported by histological evidence of collagen remodeling. A 28% improvement in skin tone/tightening was seen after six treatments at the 6-month follow-up.

In studies using the GentleYAG™ device, Dayan and colleagues (2003) found an approximately 12% reduction in Fitzpatrick scores for coarse wrinkles, a 17% reduction for skin laxity, and a 20% overall improvement after seven or more treatments. Taylor & Prokopenko (2006) studied seven patients and reported a 30% median improvement (range 0–42%) in wrinkles and skin laxity, and approximately 15% improvement in texture, pores, and pigmentation. Key (2007) found that a single high-fluence treatment with the long-pulse Nd:YAG laser gave an overall 47% improvement in a split-face study. The evaluation judged improvement in forehead lines, brow positions, periorbital lines, eyelid position, malar

Table 9-1 Studies of infrared broadband light sources for skin tightening

Reference[a]	Device[b]	Fluence (J/cm²)	Local anesthesia	Treatment target	Efficacy	Adverse effects	Follow-up (months)
Ruiz-Esparza (2006) (n=25)	IR 1100–1800 nm (1–3)	20–40	For first 5 patients	Forehead, lower face and neck	Immediate improvement in 22 patients, persisted during follow-up; all patients satisfied	Small burns	Up to 12
Taub et al (2006) (n=42)	IR 1100–1800 nm (2)	30–38	Sometimes	Face, neck, abdomen	Improvement moderate or higher in 52.4% of patients	Transient minor swelling and erythema; rare blister	4
Negishi et al (2006) (n=21)	IR 110–1800 nm (unknown)	32–38	None	Forehead and cheeks	Mean 10.4% improvement of nasolabial fold depth after 3 treatments	None noted	

Values in parentheses are [a]number of patients and [b]number of treatments

cheek and jowl positioning, nasolabial fold depth, and fold extension.

1100–1800-nm Broadband light source

Chua et al (2007) treated patients with the IR 1100–1800-nm broadband Titan, using three passes of 28–40 J/cm² at monthly intervals for 3 months. This resulted in 57% of patients with moderate to good improvement 6 months after treatment. The manageable complication of superficial blistering arose in seven patients in whom higher fluences were used (36–40 J/cm²). Taub and coworkers (2006) used the device on 42 patients who received at least two treatments consisting of two passes and four to eight sculpting passes at fluences ranging from 30 to 38 J/cm² and an average of 150 to 250 pulses per treatment. They found greater than 26% improvement in 52% of patients treated. Negishi et al (2006) studied 21 Asian women aged 31–59 years who were treated three times with the Titan at fluences ranging from 32 to 38 J/cm². PRIMOS technology (the name PRIMOS was given after an internal award at Beiersdorf AG (Nivea), and stands for Phaseshift Rapid In vivo Measurement Of Skin – a contactless, optical, three-dimensional measuring device that uses a digital stripe projection based on micro-mirrors which allows for fast and highly precise data acquisition, with ranges up to micrometers, for objective evaluation of the roughness, volume, and dimensions of wrinkles or scars) was used to determine improvement in the depth of nasolabial folds (NLFs). Of the 15 patients analyzed at 1 month after three treatments, 93% showed a reduction in NLF depth. Of the 12 patients analyzed at 3 months after three treatments, 75% showed a reduction in

NLF depth. The percentage improvement in NLF depth ranged from 10.2% to 30.2%. Twenty-five patients (23 women and 2 men) were treated by Ruiz-Esparza (2006) at different facial sites; 20 had only one treatment. Fluences ranged from 20 to 40 J/cm². Review of photographs revealed demonstrable changes in 22 of 25 patients in at least one of the areas treated that persisted through the full 12-month follow-up period. Patients with higher fluences and higher pulses appeared to have greater responses.

Radiofrequency Studies (Table 9-2)

Monopolar radiofrequency – Thermage ThermaCool

To obtain FDA clearance for the aesthetic application of the ThermaCool TC™, Fitzpatrick et al (2003) performed a 6-month study to evaluate the device's efficacy and safety. Eighty-six subjects received a single treatment with the ThermaCool TC™ on the forehead and temple area using the 1.0-cm² thermatip. On average, patients were treated on 68 cm² of tissue with a single pass at settings ranging from 65 to 95 J/cm². Twenty-two patients received a nerve block just superior to the eyebrows immediately before treatment. Independent scoring of blinded photographs taken 6 months after treatment resulted in Fitzpatrick wrinkle score improvement of at least 1 point in 83.2% (99 of 119) of treated periorbital areas. Additionally, 14.3% (17 of 119) of treated areas had no change, and 2.5% (3 of 119) worsened. Photographic analysis revealed an eyebrow lift of at least 0.5 mm in 61.5% (40 or 65) of patients after 6 months. Some 50 per cent (41 of 82) of subjects were satisfied or very satisfied

Table 9-2 Studies of the use of radiofrequency for skin tightening

Reference[a]	Fluence (J/cm²)	Areas treated	Efficacy	Adverse effects	Follow-up (months)
Iyer et al (2003) (n=40)	–	Face, anterior neck	70% of patients noticed significant improvement in skin laxity and texture at 3 months	Moderate pain during treatment; 3 patients experienced superficial blistering	1, 2, 3
Ruiz-Esparza & Gomez (2003) (n=15)	52 (only for 2 patients treated with 1-cm² tip)	Face	14 patients responded; 50% of patients had ≥50% improvement in nasolabial folds; 60% had 50% improvement in cheek contour; 27% had ≥50% improvement in mandibular line; 65% had ≥50% improvement in marionette lines	Minimal discomfort during treatment in all patients; superficial burn (n=1)	6–14
Fitzpatrick et al (2003) (n=86)	58–140	Periorbital wrinkles, brow position	Fitzpatrick wrinkle scores improved by 1 point or more in 83.2% of patients; 50% of patients satisfied to very satisfied; 61.5% of eyebrows lifted by 0.5 mm	Minimal erythema, edema, second-degree burn; small residual scar at 6 months in 3 patients	6
Hsu & Kaminer (2003) (n=16)	–	Cheeks, jawline, upper neck	5 of 15 patients contacted were satisfied with results	Mild, transient erythema and edema	6
Narins (2003) (n=17)	125–144	Brow, jowls, nasolabial folds, puppet lines	Gradual tightening	Mild, temporary erythema	4
Alster & Tanzi (2004) (n=50)	97–144 (cheeks) 74–110 (neck)	Mild to moderate skin laxity in neck and cheek	Significant improvement in most patients; patient satisfaction was similar to observed clinical improvement	Mild and temporary edema, erythema, rare dysesthesia	6
Bassichis et al (2004) (n=24)	–	Upper third of face; brow elevation; forehead, temporal regions	Objective data showed nonuniform (asymmetric) improvement; patient satisfaction low; 72.7% said they would not have the procedure again; results not predictable	Pain during treatment; redness	4–14 weeks
Finzi & Spangler (2005) (n=25)	62–91	Cheek, neck, submentum, multipass vector	Moderate or better improvement in majority	Erythema and edema	12 weeks
Kushikata et al (2005) (n=85, Asians)	74–124	Cheek, jowls	Objective ratings showed 89% had >50% improvement in jowl appearance, 89% had >50% improvement in depth of marionette lines and nasolabial folds, 83.8% had >50% improvement in other facial wrinkles at 6 months	Edema (3), burn (1), blister (1)	6
Taylor & Prokopenko (2006) (n=7)	73.5	Face: laxity, wrinkles, pores, pigmentation, texture	≈16% median improvement in wrinkles and skin laxity; ≈16% improvement in texture, pores, and pigmentation; patients satisfied; improvement maintained 2–6 months	None	2–6

[a]Values in parentheses are number of patients

with their treatment outcome. The incidence of side-effects was low and consisted of edema (14% immediately) and erythema (36% immediately). By 1 month, no subject had signs of edema, and only three (4%) had lingering signs of erythema. Rare second-degree burns occurred in 21 firings of 5858 RF exposures, indicating a burn risk of 0.4% per application. Three patients had small areas of residual scarring 6 months after treatment. The authors concluded that a single treatment with the ThermaCool TC™ reduced periorbital wrinkles, produced lasting brow elevation, and improved eyelid aesthetics, and that the safety profile of this device, used by physicians with no previous experience with its operation, was impressive.

In another study, Hsu & Kaminer (2003) evaluated 16 patients treated with a single pass on the cheeks, jawline, and/or upper neck. Treatment levels averaged 113.8 J/cm^2 on the cheeks, decreasing to 99-7 J/cm^2 on the neck. In follow-up phone interviews, 36% of patients who were treated at all three sites reported satisfactory results, compared with 25% of patients who were treated at only one or two sites. In addition, satisfied patients were those treated with higher energies. This study had three important findings:

- Higher treatment fluences generally led to improved or more consistent results.
- The greater the surface area treated, the better the results.
- Younger age is a predictor of increased efficacy with the Thermage procedure.

These findings have direct implications for refining treatment algorithm guidelines. The goal of treatment is to determine the needs of the patient. When treating the face, the physician can essentially look at the face as two distinct areas: upper and lower face. There may be some benefit to treating the entire face in one session, but it is possible to treat either the forehead region or the cheek–jawline region alone. Both treatment zones include treatment of the periorbital area (crow's feet).

Alster & Tanzi (2004) evaluated cheek laxity in 30 patients and neck laxity in 20 patients after one treatment with the ThermaCool TC™. Patients were pretreated with 5–10 mg of oral diazepam as well as topical anesthetic cream (LMX 5% cream; Ferndale Laboratories, Ferndale, MI). The cheek treatment area extended from the nasolabial folds to the preauricular margin and down to the mandibular ridge. Treatment of the neck extended from the mandibular ridge to the mid-neck. Fluences ranged from 97 to 144 J/cm^2 on the cheeks and from 74 to 134 J/cm^2 on the neck. Mild post-treatment erythema was seen in all patients and persisted for up to 12 h after the procedure. Some 56% of subjects complained of

soreness at the treated sites; the soreness resolved with oral nonsteroidal anti-inflammatory medication. Erythematous papules that resolved over 24 h were observed in three patients. One patient developed dysesthesia along the mandible that resolved over 5 days. No blistering or scarring was observed. A quartile grading system was used and independent assessment noted improvement in 28 of 30 patients treated on the cheeks and in 17 of 20 patients treated on the neck. The five subjects who demonstrated no clinical improvement were all older than 62 years. At 6 months, the mean clinical improvement score was 1.53 on the cheeks and 1.27 on the neck (scale: 1, 25–50% improvement; 2, 51–75% improvement). On a scale of 1–10, the average patient satisfaction score was 6.3 for cheek treatment and 5.4 for neck treatment.

In a study by Ruiz-Esparza & Gomez (2003), 15 patients ranging in age from 41 to 68 years were treated with one pass on the preauricular area using investigational tip designs. Five patients were treated with a 0.25-cm bipolar electrode, eight with a "window frame" bipolar electrode, and two with a 1-cm monopolar electrode. Independent evaluators graded nasolabial softening to be at least 50% improved in half of the patients. Cheek contour was 50% improved in 60% of patients, and marionette lines improved by 50% or more in 65% of patients. The mandibular line improved by 50% or more in only 27% of patients. One patient did not have any improvement. Results were typically seen after 12 weeks, but one patient developed results after only 1 week.

Kushikata et al (2005) tested the device on Asian skin and found good improvement at 3 months, with increased results at the 6-month evaluation.

Newer techniques have developed over the years to improve patient outcomes. Finzi & Spangler (2005) suggested a technique coined "multipass vector" or "mpave" to treat facial and neck laxity. They treated 25 patients with multipass vectors of four to five passes targeted over areas of skin that would most improve facial laxity. The majority of patients demonstrated a moderate or better improvement of skin laxity, and stacked pulses in the submental region were shown to reduce fat. Histologically, multiple passes at lower energies have been shown to create increased collagen fibril changes with increasing passes. Changes seen after five multiple passes (122 J) were shown by Kist et al (2006) to be similar to those detected after much more painful, single-pass, high-energy treatments. A review by Weiss et al (2006) evaluated the safety of MRF treatment in 600 patients and showed that most patients experienced erythema and edema lasting for less than 24 h. Tenderness occurred in three patients, lasting for 2–3 weeks. There were rare depressions with the 1-cm² tip that resolved over 3.5 months. The newer treatment tips and algorithms have increased safety and efficacy.

Bipolar radiofrequency and light sources – ELOS technology (Table 9-3)

Aurora SR

Bitter & Mulholland (2002) used the original ELOS technology using IPL with ranges of 580–980 nm plus BRF for skin rejuvenation. They found a 70% improvement in erythema and telangiectasia, and 78% improvement in hyperpigmentation, along with 60% average wrinkle reduction. The device, however, was not evaluated for tightening of the skin.

Polaris WR

The second generation of ELOS technology used a 900-nm diode together with BRF to treat facial rhytides and skin laxity. Doshi & Alster (2005) evaluated this combination BRF and diode device (Polaris WR) and found that three treatments given at 3-week intervals resulted in significant improvement in facial and neck rhytides, and a modest improvement in skin laxity in the majority of patients. Kulick (2005) treated 15 patients with three full-face treatments at energies ranging from 50 to 100 J/cm² RF and 15 J/cm² for the optical laser component. In the eight patients who completed the study an average 25% reduction in wrinkles was found. Hammes et al (2006) treated 24 subjects with periorbital and perioral wrinkles six times at 4-week intervals. Each treatment consisted of two passes and the follow-up period was 3 months after the final treatment. Some 58% of patients reported a notable reduction in wrinkles. Alexiades-Armenakas (2006) studied the combination of treatment with BRF and diode, followed immediately by BRF and IPL. Patients received one to five treatments at monthly intervals. The mean improvement per treatment for rhytides was 9-6% and for laxity 9.9%, and for overall treatment was 20.4% and 22.6% respectively. Other categories of improvement included elastosis, dyschromia, erythema, texture, and keratosis.

ReFirme™ ST

Sleightholm & Bartholomeusz (2007) treated 31 patients with skin laxity and facial wrinkles with two to five treatments at 3–4-week intervals with combined IR (700–2000 nm, 10 W/cm²) and RF energies (50–100 J/cm³). The median wrinkle clearance was 50% and the median patient satisfaction rate was 7.0 on a 10-point scale. Adverse effects included mild transient erythema or edema that resolved within 2–4 h.

Table 9-3 Studies of the use of ELOS technology for skin tightening

Reference[a]	Device	Fluence	Application/study group	Results
Bitter & Mulholland (2002) (n=100)	Aurora SR	Optical 28–34 J/cm², RF 20 J/cm³	Skin rejuvenation; skin types II–IV	Improvement in erythema and telangiectasia (70%), and in lentigines and other hyperpigmentation (78%); average wrinkle reduction 60%
Doshi & Alster (2005) (n=20)	Polaris WR 900 nm	Optical 15–50 J/cm², RF 40–100 J/cm³	Rhytides and skin laxity; skin types I–VI	Significant improvement in facial and neck rhytides; modest improvement in skin laxity in majority of patients
Kulick (2005) (n=8)	900 nm	Optical 15 J/cm², RF 50–100 J/cm³	Wrinkles	3 treatments 25% reduction in skin wrinkles; patient discomfort was an issue
Hammes et al (2006) (n=24)	900 nm	Optical 50 J/cm², RF 100 J/cm³	Wrinkles (6 treatments per month)	Improvement score of at least 1 (scale 0–3); little discomfort
Alexiades-Armenakas (2006) (n=28)	900 nm + RF, followed by IPL (500–1200 nm) + RF	Optical 20 J/cm², RF 50–80 J/cm³ (10 passes, decreasing diode fluence, increasing RF to maximum of 100 J/cm³, optical 20–30 J/cm², RF 18–22 J/cm³)	Rhytides, laxity, photo-aging (1–5 treatments per month)	20.4% rhytides, 22.6% laxity, overall 25.6%

[a]Values in parentheses are number of patients

VelaSmooth

Tissue tightening using BRF plus IR light (700–1500 nm) and mechanical suction-based massage was performed on 20 women by Alster & Tanzi (2005). They found that after eight biweekly sessions, 90% of patients noticed clinical improvement averaging 1.82 on a 4-point scale.

Bipolar and monopolar radiofrequency – Alma Accent

Other uses for MRF have been studied, including its use in improving the appearance of cellulite. Emilia del Pino et al (2006) treated 26 women with cellulite on the buttocks and/or thighs with the monopolar portion of the Accent device only. Two treatment sessions (three passes) performed 15 days apart were performed. Subjects were evaluated with ultrasound imaging 15 days after the last treatment from the stratum corneum to Camper's fascia, and from the stratum corneum to the muscle. Some 68% of patients had a contraction of the volume of approximately 20%. Further studies using the bipolar and monopolar devices sequentially are under way.

Muscle stimulation – PanG lift

Biweekly treatments with an electrical facial muscle stimulator for 10 weeks led to moderate (26–50%) lifting of the cheeks and jowls, eyebrows, and neck (Taub 2006). Further maintenance treatments monthly, after 12 months, led to a good to marked (51–100%) improvement.

Patient evaluation: examination and history

Key Points

- The best candidates include younger patients, patients with mild laxity, and those with mild to moderate amounts of facial adipose.
- Some devices cannot be used on darker skinned patients.

The nonablative tissue-tightening devices are capable of providing improvement, but patient selection is key. These treatments are not meant to be a replacement for rhytidectomy when the patient has severely lax skin, nor should it be promoted as such. Millimeters, not centimeters, of improvement are expected, and may require more than one treatment. Patients with coarse wrinkles (Fitzpatrick skin type IV) are not candidates as the devices will not (in their current state at publication) remove dynamic muscle movement lines or deep rhytides from sun damage.

The best candidates for these procedures are patients who have good skin texture, usually between the ages of 35 and 65 years, without excessive or minimal facial adipose. They may have early jowling, meilolabial fold draping, eyelid and neck laxity. Medium-quality skin thickness and laxity, due more to dermatochalasis than to subcutaneous fat volume weighing down the area, seems to respond best. Patients being evaluated for forehead/brow treatment with the Titan IR device should have mobility of the brow with gentle fingertip pressure of a minimum of 2 mm in order for the treatment to be effective clinically.

For body treatments, minor crêping and skin laxity of the abdomen, anterior thighs, and upper inner arms seem to respond best. Patients with defined striae may have some improvement of laxity, but the striae themselves will still be present.

As with any laser or IPL, skin chromophores play a role in outcome and restrictions of use. Long-pulsed 1064-nm Nd:YAG lasers can be used on most skin types, but lower fluences and longer pulse durations must be used. These devices may cause loss of hair, especially with skin types V and VI. Patients with skin types I–IV can be treated safely when staying within treatment parameters, but tightening modalities have not been tested on skin type VI.

With RF (monopolar or bipolar), all skin types can be treated effectively, as dermal heating while simultaneously cooling the epidermis with the devices has been shown not to cause hypo- or hyper-pigmentation when used within treatment parameters. BRF plus IPL should be used cautiously on skin types V–VI owing to the absorption of IPL wavelengths by melanin.

The key in the approach to the aging patient is to try to analyze the person's features to determine which procedures or combination of procedures will produce the desired effect, and to make sure that these are prioritized for the patient's desires. It is a good idea to ask the patient to look in a hand mirror and ask them to point to areas that they find objectionable. Sometimes they will pull back their cheeks and say, "This is what I want," in which case tissue tightening of the lower face could be a good solution as long as the patient understands that the result will not be as tight or perfect as when they tug on it. In addition, occasionally someone who can't afford multiple procedures will point to a pre-jowl sulcus as their objectionable area. It may be the lack of volume in the perioral area that is causing this more than laxity; the patient should be given the option of choosing fillers over tightening, or a combination of the two, and an understanding of how they differ.

There are no pretreatment tests that are required before performing most laser, broadband IR light, or RF tissue tightening. Some key historical points, however, could include a history of typical wound healing and the presence of any diseases that might interfere with collagen production. Patients with skin that is extremely sun damaged, those who smoke and/or who actively pursue tanning, and people with metabolic or collagen disorders are not the best candidates. It would be best either to avoid such treatment in these patients, or to counsel that they may require more treatments or have a lesser response than expected for others.

It is important to have an excellent concept of the three-dimensional aspects of the face and neck, and how various (including other) treatment modalities, such as lasers, fillers, and neuromodulating injectables, could affect, contribute to, or be replaced by the proposed tightening procedure. The ideal patient for tissue tightening is one with lax skin but not much fat. At the same time, anyone with concave cheeks or a very thin face might best be avoided. By tightening the skin, this "gaunt" appearance may age them still more, yielding tighter skin but an undesirable overall effect. Those patients would be better served first by filler substances, and then re-evaluated for tissue tightening.

Remind the patient that they will continue to age, breaking down collagen as well as being subjected to the forces of gravity. It is also important to make sure that they take responsibility for skin care, including high-grade cosmeceutical or pharmaceutical preparations known to stimulate collagen synthesis, as well as practicing excellent sun protection to protect the investment they have made in their skin.

Mechanisms of action and treatment application

The devices discussed in this chapter are shown in Box 9-2.

Nonablative lasers and pure light sources (without RF)

Nd:YAG 1064 nm

Nd:YAG lasers, with a wavelength of 1064 nm are used to cause heat-induced injury to the dermis resulting in collagen production and improved quality of the skin. The absorption coefficient of melanin for 1064-nm radiation is lower than that for shorter wavelengths, so patients with dark skin can be treated with minimal risk of pigmentation abnormalities.

Gemini

The 1064-nm component of the Gemini laser (Fig. 9-5) can be used with one of two handpieces: a variable size or "versastat" handpiece with a treatment beam ranging from 1.5 to 5 mm in diameter, or a 10-mm handpiece. Both use a sapphire

---

BOX 9-2

Devices

Nonablative lasers and pure light sources (without RF)

- Nd:YAG 1064-nm laser

—Gemini (formerly Lyra, Laserscope) (Iridex Corporation, Mountain View, CA)

—GentleYAG™ (Candela Corporation, Wayland, MA)

—Genesis (component of Xeo CoolGlide) (Cutera, Brisbane, CA)

- Broadband 1100–1800-nm light source

—Titan (Cutera, Brisbane, CA)

Monopolar radiofrequency devices

- ThermaCool (Thermage, Hayward, CA)

Bipolar radiofrequency (BRF) devices – ELOS Technology (Syneron Medical, Yokneam, Israel)

- Aurora (BRF + 580–980 nm IPL)

- Polaris (BRF + 900-nm diode laser)

- ReFirme ST™ (BRF + 700–2000-nm infrared light)

- Velasmooth (BRF + 700–1000-nm infrared light + vacuum pressure)

Combined radiofrequency devices – monopolar and bipolar

- Accent (Alma Lasers, Buffalo Grove, IL)

Electrical stimulation

- PanG (PanG Corporation, Clearwater, FL)

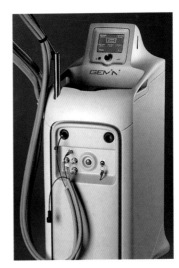

Figure 9-5 The Gemini laser

window through which water at about 2–6°C circulates, allowing continuous contact cooling. The 10-mm handpiece is typically used for treating wrinkles and tightening skin. The reflective optics of the handpiece walls bounce photons reflected from the skin back into the tissue (photon recycling). As a result of this photon recycling, the total energy applied to the tissue is estimated to be increased approximately 1.5 times.

Prior to treatment, patients should remove all make-up. Use of a topical anesthetic is optional. Immediately before treatment, chilled ultrasound gel is applied to the treatment area to allow for gliding the cooling tip over the surface of the skin. Laser goggles or external treatment shields are worn by the patient. The entire surface of the face should be treated in order to achieve some skin tightening. This may be done in cosmetic units (forehead and temples, then left cheek, then right cheek, then chin) if desired. Depending on skin type, severity of rhytides, and anatomic area, pulses from 30 to 65 ms at 24–30 J/cm^2 are used. Lighter skin types can tolerate higher fluences, but bony areas can be more sensitive and may require a decrease in fluence. The face should be treated in a brushstroke-like manner, being careful to treat in nonoverlapping pulses, and to keep complete contact of the handpiece with the skin. Men should not be treated in the beard area to avoid risk of hair loss. Treatments can be repeated every 4–6 weeks, for three to six treatments. Studies show greater efficacy with more treatments.

GentleYAG™

Fluences for the GentleYAG are selected on the basis of patient tolerability. Some patients chose to use a topical anesthetic such as a mixture of 20% benzocaine, 10% lidocaine, and 4% tetracaine 20 min prior to treatment. Patients can be treated multiple times on a monthly basis or via multiple passes in a single treatment. For multiple visit treatments, parameters include a 10-mm handpiece, 50-ms pulse duration, and 22 J/cm^2. These patients are treated seven or more times on a monthly basis.

Two studies have shown higher response rates with higher fluences and higher tissue peak temperatures attained with pulse stacking. The multiple-pass single treatment parameters include 10-mm spot size, 50-ms pulse duration, 50 J/cm^2 with dynamic cooling of 40 ms delay and 20 ms duration with a total of three passes. Alternatively, a 10-mm spot size, 50-ms pulse duration, and fluences of 40 J/cm^2 for the cheek and 20–30 J/cm^2 for the thinner-skinned forehead can be used. Each area is treated with three sets of two stacked pulses, 1.5 s apart. The cosmetic units can each be treated with one set of stacked pulses; it is then recommended to start at the beginning area and repeat the process. These patients may need topical anesthesia and/or mild anxiolytics such as diazepam and analgesics such as oxycodone and acetaminophen. If oral medications are used, the patient should arrive 30 min before treatment, and should have transportation and assistance home.

Genesis 1064 laser

This treatment uses a defocused "painting" technique with a 5-mm handpiece and a fluence of 13–15 J/cm^2, 300-ms pulse duration, and up to 10 Hz repetition rate. Typically the handpiece is held approximately 2 cm above and perpendicular to the skin, and the handpiece is kept moving in sweeping motions to cover the entire area gradually over time. Typically 3000 to 10 000 pulses are required, depending on the size of the area treated. Topical anesthetic is not needed, because, when performed properly, only a warm sensation occurs. After the treatment there is usually erythema in the treated area; occasionally edema may be present, and can last for a few days. This procedure is usually performed three to five times at intervals of 3–5 weeks for maximal improvement.

1100–1800nm Broadband light source

Titan

This device (Fig. 9-6) can be utilized on all skin types. Another advantage is that patients with titanium or other implants or pacemakers, for whom a RF device could pose a hazard, may be safely treated with the Titan device. Pregnant women should not be treated with this device due to the lack of data on its effect.

There is no particular pretreatment strategy for the Titan device. Sun avoidance is, of course, desirable, but increased melanin does not appear to affect the treatment settings or outcome. It would be advantageous to have a patient on high-grade cosmeceuticals or pharmaceutical topical preparations that are maximized to stimulate

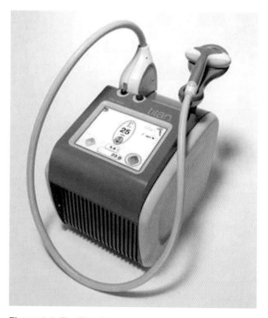

Figure 9-6 The Titan laser

collagen renewal (e.g. retinoids, peptides, and/or growth factors).

If a browlift is the desired effect, pretreatment botulinum toxin is recommended. Often patients who choose tightening devices for this area do so because of a fear or an aversion to toxin, or a preference for a procedure that is longer lasting. Discussion with these patients that pretreatment may increase the efficacy of the procedure is important and often does convince them to use it. It is believed that relaxation of the wrinkle-causing and depressor muscles of the forehead, both during the procedure and for a few months afterwards, leads to a better result. The treatment should be done approximately 2 weeks before the first procedure, to obtain maximal effect of the botulinum toxin for the longest period of time.

No anesthetic, topical or oral, is utilized. Only occasionally, for a very apprehensive patient, a mild anxiolytic such as alprazolam or tramadol may be utilized. It is important to seek patient feedback during treatment. Specifically, each pulse should feel warm and almost somewhat uncomfortable, without being painful. Not every pulse will fall into this ideal range, but the goal is that most of the pulses should.

There are different recommendations for protocols from different sources. However, the authors recommend the following:

- For the lower two-thirds of the face, begin on one cheek. Treat from the temple to the neck, one to two fingerbreadths below the jawline.
- If the neck is to be treated then include that, but do the lower part of the neck separately.
- It is important not to do a pass over the entire face and then to return and do another. This is because the skin cools off too much between the first pulse on one lateral cheek and the last pulse on the medial part of the other cheek.
- As the stimulation of collagen production depends on both temperature and time, it is essential to heat the targeted skin for a sufficient length of time.
- Complete three to four passes over one cheek from the temple to two fingerbreadths below the jawline. For the third and fourth passes do not include the central cheek.
- Then perform vector passes. Determine the vectors by placing your second and third fingers on the skin (usually at the temple, the preauricular area, the lateral neck, and the area lateral to the nasolabial fold) and pulling to see whether the skin elevates to a desired clinical endpoint.
- Then proceed to treat this area repeatedly. Typically this would result in a "C" pass (draw an open C from temple to jowl with two fingerbreadths). There are usually approximately six to eight passes over this area.

- Then do an inverted L (lateral to the nasolabial fold) and along the malar area for four to eight passes, followed by four to eight passes over the two rows of the upper neck.
- By now you should be able to feel the skin firming – this is similar to when you put liquid jello mix into the refrigerator and come back later and see if it has formed a solid gel.
- You should also see some of the desired clinical effects you are looking for: elevated malar pad, reduced jowl laxity, flattening of the nasolabial fold, and overall reduction of redundancy of skin, along with much more resistance to the two probing vector fingers.
- In addition, you should be able to see a clear difference between the one half of the face and the other, either by sitting the patient up, or by looking at them from above their head (a great place to locate yourself for treatment as this is an excellent vantage point to observe the three-dimensional aspects of the face).

At this point there is no cookbook. The skin is heated to a point where it is quite moldable. Place pulses where you think you will get the best effect and watch, as a couple of well placed pulses at this point make a difference. This is a good point to sit the patient up and give them a mirror. When they see the difference between the two sides, you are helping them to realize some of the immediate effects of the device. This is important as the long-term effects may take months to appear (Figs 9-7 & 9-8).

Treatment of the neck (Figs 9-9 & 9-10) and forehead is more straightforward:

- Perform four passes over each half and then do "vectors"– on the neck this is the lateral neck, and on the forehead the area above the eyebrows for women (to get an arch), or all across for men.
- If there is a large area over the jowl or under the chin, do repeated passes over and over to try to shrink the tissue. Be careful, though, and monitor for discomfort as this stacking of pulses can cause overheating, and the jawline is one of the most common areas for overheating as the bone underneath seems to amplify the heat.

In terms of settings, most treatments on the face should be between 32 and 38 J. You may find that over the course of the treatment, as the skin heats up, you need to decrease the setting because of patient discomfort. Do not forget to reset it when you advance to another vector area or another area of the face. For the neck, the forehead, and right on the jawline, you may need to use lower settings (e.g. 28–32 J), owing to the thinness of the skin, the presence of bone, and the sensitivity of the areas.

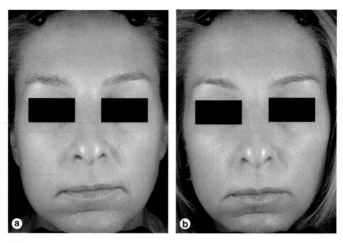

Figure 9-7 Cheek and jawline contour in a 41-year-old woman (A) before and (B) after two Titan treatments. Courtesy of Amy Forman Taub MD

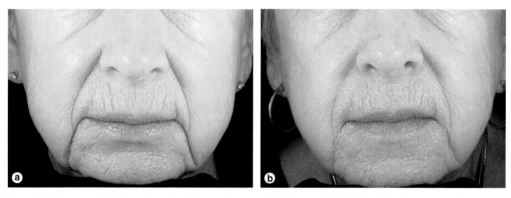

Figure 9-8 Cheek and jawline contour in a 70-year-old woman (A) before and (B) after two Titan treatments. Courtesy of Amy Forman Taub MD

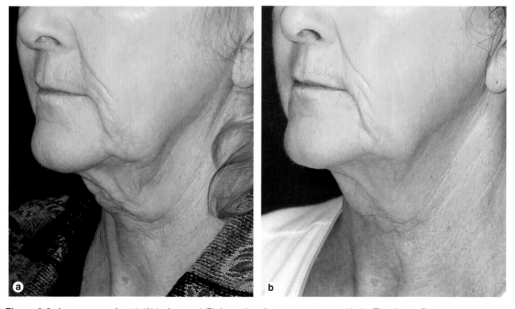

Figure 9-9 Appearance of neck (A) before and (B) 6 months after one treatment with the Titan laser. Courtesy of Lisa Bunin MD

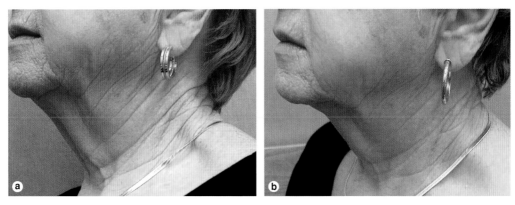

Figure 9-10 Neck of a 70-year-old woman (A) before and (B) after two treatments with the Titan laser. Courtesy of Amy Forman Taub MD

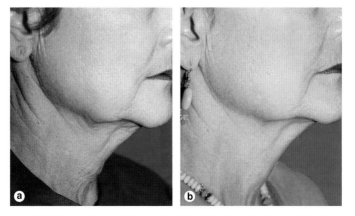

Figure 9-11 (A) Before and (B) after treatment of the neck with the Titan laser. Courtesy of Lisa Bunin MD

There is no postoperative care other than to resume the skin care regimen that was prescribed beforehand, and for the patient to report immediately if any untoward effect should occur. Adverse events are limited to blisters or burns. Causes of this could include an inappropriately high fluence, pulse stacking, or excessive sedation or anesthesia that blunts the patient's ability to report pain. Experienced practitioners usually have a side-effect incidence of well below 1%. In one white paper of the experiences of five early adopter physicians on more than 1000 patients there was only one complication, and that was in the first month of device use. However, it is certainly possible to burn and scar patients with inappropriate protocols.

Any breakage of the skin should be examined as quickly as possible and treated with occlusion and ointment, either antibacterial or petroleum based. As long as uninfected, most wounds heal best in a moist wound healing environment, and this should be explained to the patient for best compliance with the regimen. If skin breakage occurs, call and/or evaluate the patient frequently until there is satisfactory conclusion of the complication. If there is any increase in pain, redness, or oozing, consider infection with bacteria or virus, and culture and treat appropriately. If the patient was pretreated with an antiherpetic drug, you may consider extending that treatment for as long as the skin remains de-epithelialized.

The expected rate of apparent change 6 months after a series of two or three tissue-tightening procedures 1–2 months apart with adequate protocols should approach 90% (Fig. 9-11). However, the degree of improvement can probably be expected to be about 35% mild, 35% moderate, and 20% marked. Nobody really knows the length of improvement, as no long-term studies have been completed. Based on "conventional wisdom" and anecdotal reports, it appears that 1–2 years is a reasonable expectation.

One of the advantages of this procedure is its noninvasiveness and lack of downtime. Most patients understand the need for maintenance treatments and eagerly pursue them when they see the benefits they receive from the treatment.

Monopolar radiofrequency devices (Table 9-4)

Thermage ThermaCool

The ThermaCool TC™ RF device (Fig. 9-12) has four key components: a RF generator, a handpiece, a cooling module, and disposable treatment tips. RF energy production follows the principle of Ohm's law (Box 9-3), which states that the impedance to the movement of electrons creates heat relative to the amount of current and time.

The RF generator supplies a 6-MHz alternating current across a specially modified monopolar electrode to deliver volumetric heat to tissue in a targeted manner. A disposable return pad connected to the patient's flank creates a path of travel for the RF signal. The generator is regulated by a Pentium™ chip-based internal computer that processes feedback, including the temperature of the tip interface with the skin, application force, amount of tissue surface area contact, and real-time impedance of the skin. This information is gathered by a microprocessor in the handpiece and relayed to the generator via a high-speed fiberoptic link.

A unique capacitively coupled electrode disperses energy uniformly across the very thin (one-thousandth of an inch) dielectric material on the treatment tip, thereby creating a uniform electric field (Fig. 9-13). The RF generator operates at 6 MHz, which changes the polarity of an electrical field in biologic tissue six million times per second. The charged particles of the tissue within the electric field change orientation at that same frequency, and the dermal tissue's natural resistance (expressed in Ohm's law as Z) to the movement of electrons generates heat. This friction from electron movement creates volumetrically distributed deep dermal heating.

Before, during, and after delivery of the RF energy, a cryogen spray delivered onto the inner surface of the treatment tip membrane provides cooling to protect the dermis from overheating and subsequent damage. The treatment tip continually monitors heat transmission from the skin via thermisters mounted on the inside of the dielectric membrane. The cryogen spray also provides cooling to the upper portion of the dermis. This creates a reverse thermal gradient through the dermis and results in volumetric heating and tightening of deep dermal and even subdermal tissues (Fig. 9-14). The depth of this heating is dependent upon the geometry of the treatment tip and the duration of cooling. Various sizes of treatment tips are available, including 0.25, 1.0, 1.5, and 3 cm^2, and are used for different purposes. Newer designs will allow for further variations in treatment parameters, target even deeper heating delivery, and provide more vigorous epidermal protection.

Each treatment cycle consists of three phases: precooling, cooling and treatment, and post-cooling. A treatment cycle lasts for about 6 s with the initial generation of treatment tips and about 2 s with recently developed "fast" treatment tips. In addition, with the new "fast" treatment tips, the handpiece microprocessor aborts the treatment pulse to protect against burning if all four corners of the tip are not in complete contact with the skin.

The initial feasibility study of this RF device coupled with a concurrent epidermal cooling system utilized a three-dimensional Monte Carlo simulation mathematical model to gauge the theoretical temperature distribution within human skin. The results showed that this treatment tip design produces volumetric heating deep within the dermis yet protects the superficial skin layers from thermal injury. This creates a much greater temperature rise below the surface than in the epidermis. The depth of the RF field in tissue varies with the surface area of the treatment tip electrode design. The larger the tip electrode surface area, the deeper the heat produced. The amount

Manufacturer	Product	Technology	Power	FDA approval
Syneron	Aurora/SR/SRA	ELOS bipolar RF, visible and IR light	Pulsed light 10–40 J/cm^2, RF 5–25 J/cm^3, light 580–1200 nm (SR) 470–1200 nm (SRA)	Yes
Syneron	Polaris/WR	ELOS bipolar RF, diode light	IR 15–50 J/cm^2, RF 40–100 J/cm^3, light 900 nm	Yes
Syneron	ReFirme ST	ELOS bipolar RF, IR light	IR 10 W, RF 120 J/cm^3, light 700–2000 nm	Yes
Syneron	VelaSmooth	ELOS bipolar RF, IR light and suction; skin impedance control	IR up to 20 W, RF up to 20 W, light 700–2000 nm; vacuum, pulsed	Class II medical device
Thermage	ThermaCool, NXT	Unipolar RF	Up to 400 W	Approved for treatment of rhytides
Alma Lasers	Accent	Bipolar RF, unipolar RF	Up to 220 W	

Table 9-4 Comparison of radiofrequency device technology

ThermaCool®**NXT**

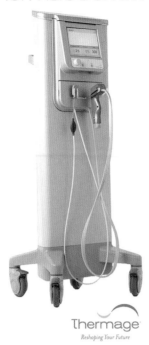

Thermage
Reshaping Your Future

Figure 9-12 The Thermage ThermaCool NXT™ device. Photograph courtesy of Thermage

---

BOX 9-3

Ohm's law

Energy (joules) $= I^2 \times Z \times t$

Where I is the current (amps), Z is impedance (ohms), and t is time (seconds)

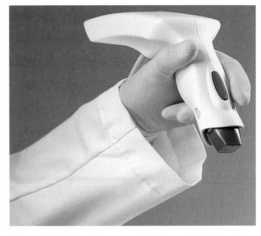

Figure 9-13 The unique capacitively coupled electrode treatment tip. Photograph courtesy of Thermage

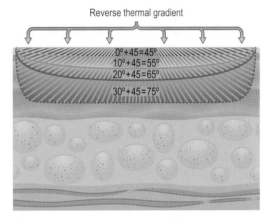

Reverse thermal gradient

$0° + 45 = 45°$
$10° + 45 = 55°$
$20° + 45 = 65°$
$30° + 45 = 75°$

Figure 9-14 The reverse thermal gradient created via simultaneous cooling of the epidermis and heating of the dermis. Photograph courtesy of Thermage

---

of heat generated depends on the impedance of the tissue being treated with each pulse and on the selected treatment setting. The depth of the protected tissue zone at the surface is controlled by the cooling time and intensity. Thus, the degree and depth of heat generated in the tissue can be customized by changing the size and geometry of the tip electrode, the amount of energy delivered (which is directly correlated to tissue impedance), and the cooling parameters designated for a given energy setting. These heating, cooling, and energy parameters are programmed into a small EPROM (Erasable Programmable Read Only Memory) chip located within each disposable treatment tip, with manufacturer-optimized parameters automatically upgraded without active user intervention or generator software upgrade.

In vivo studies have shown that this volumetric RF tissue heating creates a dual effect. Primary changes to collagen occur as heat disrupts hydrogen bonds, altering the molecular structure of the triple helix collagen molecule and resulting in collagen contraction. Secondary to the immediate thermal contraction of collagen, a more gradual contraction due to wound healing is predicted to occur over time as collagen regenerates, leading to a thicker remodeled dermis. Animal studies have documented that the ThermaCool TC™ device can achieve dermal collagen heating as shallow as the papillary dermis or as deep as the subcutaneous fat. Additional animal studies examined 1-cm² treatment tips with 2- and 6-s cycle times, described as "fast" and "standard" treatment tips respectively. Lactate dehydrogenase (LDH) and heat shock protein (HSP) stainings were used to determine the depth of action for these two treatment tips. Results showed that the depth of treatment was the same for both the "fast" and the "standard" tips. This was observed histochemically when the enzyme (LDH) or protein (HSP) was inactivated. Of note, LDH was deactivated at approximately the same treatment level for both tips even though the cooling and heating times and intensities were different (Karl Pope, Thermage, personal communication).

These reliable LDH and HSP heating depth results confirm the heating profile postulated by Zelickson et al (2004), who used transmission electron microscopy to evaluate ex vivo bovine tendon immediately after treatment with the ThermaCool TC™ at various energy and cooling settings. Results showed collagen fibrils with increased diameter and loss of distinct borders as deep as 6 mm. Higher energy settings produced deeper and more extensive collagen changes.

In a clinical study involving in vivo human skin, a similar pattern of immediate collagen fibril contraction was observed. In this same Zelickson study of intact abdominal tissue, Northern blot analysis demonstrated increased steady-state expression of collagen type I mRNA in treated tissue, evidence that wound healing is initiated by the single treatment. The secondary collagen synthesis in response to collagen injury is purported to occur over several (2–6) months. In another study fibroplasia and signs of increased collagen formation were noted in the papillary dermis, and less frequently in the reticular dermis. Histologic specimens taken 4 months after treatment demonstrate epidermal and papillary dermal thickening as well as shrinkage of sebaceous glands (Fig. 9-15).

Expected benefits

The ThermaCool TC™ is capable of tightening skin and improving contours. The physician must analyze the patient's three-dimensional facial structure to assess areas that will benefit most from tightening. Typically, this includes the forehead/brow area, as well as the mid cheek, jawline, and submental region.

Once this analysis has been done and the treatment plan created, therapy can be initiated. By varying the fluences used and the number of passes in each area of the face, the physician can preferentially tighten some areas, reduce the prominence of others (i.e. jowls), and improve the overall shape and appearance of the face.

Major determinants

The three variables that seem to determine how much benefit a patient will obtain from the ThermaCool TC™ are:

1 Individual patient extent of photo-aging, as well as age
2 Treatment fluences
3 Number of passes.

Early data suggest that younger patients (aged less than 60–65 years) will do best, as will those with mild to moderate amounts of skin laxity. Moderate fluences (titrated to patient comfort) covering a broad surface area of skin also appear to promote better results, as does the use of multiple (three to seven or more) carefully placed passes. The role of multiple treatments is not yet understood adequately.

Patient interviews

Patients scheduled for treatment must have good general health, and must not have a pacemaker. It is recommended that pregnant women not be treated. It is also important to assess the following pretreatment:

• Have you had a rhytidectomy? Patients with thin, overpulled skin from previous surgery may benefit less.

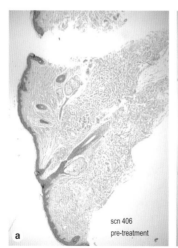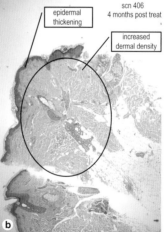

Figure 9-15 Human skin (A) before and (B) 4 months after treatment with the ThermaCool TC™, showing epidermal thickening as well as increased dermal density. Photograph courtesy of Thermage

- Do you have a low pain tolerance? The measure of heat felt during the procedure is important in determining treatment levels. Patients with a very low pain tolerance and no supplemental anesthesia may not be able to reach appropriate treatment levels, and may not achieve maximal benefit from the treatment.
- Do you have any important social events coming up? Rarely, patients will have edema lasting for several days. It is important they schedule the procedure at a time when they have no social obligations.
- What are your expectations? Patients expecting quality results following facelift or browlift need to be assessed carefully and counseled before treatment. Although in many patients the results are remarkable, this is not always the case. Patients who have lofty expectations may be disappointed, and this should be discussed with the patient before the treatment is started.

Equipment

Treatment equipment includes the ThermaCool TC™ device, return patient pad, coupling fluid, treatment grid, and an individual treatment tip(s). Anesthesia such as lorazepam or meperidine/hydroxyzine may be used if desired for anxious patients, or for those having large areas (such as the abdomen) treated. Remember that you want patient feedback, as this is a guideline for safe treatment.

Treatment algorithm

After preoperative photography, the treatment grid is applied with the ink side on the skin and the use of alcohol swabs to the back side of the grid paper, thoroughly wetting the paper. This allows transfer of the ink to the area to be treated (Fig. 9-16). The grid is used to ensure even placement of the treatment pulses and to prevent unintentional overlap, guiding the operator for direction of passes. The adhesive return pad is applied to the patient's left flank to ensure a travel conduit for the RF energy and to complete the circuit. It is important that the return pad be placed in this same location on all patients, because impedance readings can change when the pad is moved to other locations (Thermage, personal communication). The return pad is attached to the machine, and a new treatment tip is placed into the handpiece.

Early treatments (2001–2002) with the Thermage device were done with a single pass at relatively low fluences, using the so-called "slow tip" (1 cm², 6-s cycle). With the newer "fast" treatment tips, the rapid cooling allows for lower fluences to achieve a higher degree of dermal heating than with the standard slow tip. Therefore, lower

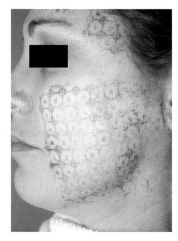

Figure 9-16 Placement of the ThermaCool temporary ink grid

fluences are needed to avoid overheating the epidermis and creating a superficial injury, burn, or blister.

As the understanding of RF tissue physics has improved, so has the comfort level by increasing both fluence per pulse and the number of passes over the same tissue area. A key breakthrough has occurred with the addition of selectively placed multiple passes to the treatment algorithm.

Periorbital rejuvenation

Treatment for periorbital improvement should extend across the entire forehead, down to the temples and the crow's feet area (Fig. 9-17). Initially, a "fine tune" series of one to three treatment firings is performed to tune the device to the patient's skin – which reads the impedance, in ohms, at the site. A generous amount of coupling gel is applied to ensure complete contact between the treatment tip and the skin. The gel can be added or reapplied as needed during the treatment session. After the fine tuning, actual treatment firings may begin after choosing the energy level based on the patient's heat sensation feedback.

Using a scale of 0–4, with 0 being no sensation, 1 being slightly warm, 2 being warm but tolerable, 3 being slightly hot but tolerable, and 4 being intolerably hot, patients are asked to rate the sensation, with a goal of 2–2.5. With the 3.0-cm² tip, settings on the forehead for the first pass are in the 356–357.5 range (67–85 J), and 355.0–356.5 (56–73 J) for the temples. It is critical to reduce treatment fluences over the temporal region (lateral to the frontalis muscle) as there may be an increase in side-effects (subcutaneous depressions or superficial burning) when settings producing over 96 J are used in this thin tissue area (Fig. 9-18), although this side-effect has not been seen using the 3.0-cm² tips at recommended settings. Extending treatment to the lateral periorbital

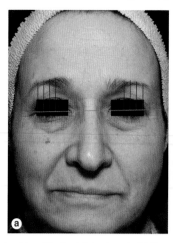
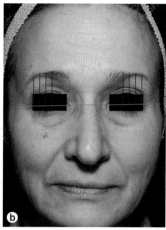

Figure 9-17 Example of browlift after RF treatment. (A) Pretreatment, (B) 4 weeks post-treatment: average lift 3.42 mm (right) and 3.41 mm (left). Photograph courtesy of Thermage

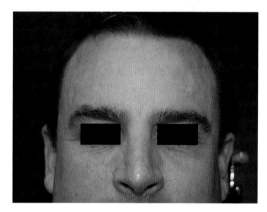

Figure 9-18 Subtle indentations 4 weeks after high-energy treatment on lateral forehead. They resolved spontaneously after 5 months

region can have a significant impact on periorbital rhytides, providing substantial local rejuvenation and tissue tightening that can affect adjacent areas.

With the treatment tip, pain sensation is a crescendo of warmth ending in a brief "spike" of heat. Differing patient tolerances to this sensation may inhibit higher treatment levels. The sensation appears to be stronger over the temporal area, where the frontalis muscle is absent, and this is yet another reason for dropping the treatment setting to adjust to patient comfort.

Treatment recommendations utilize multiple passes on the forehead over the brows. The second pass is performed at a slightly lower setting than the first pass, and only over the central two-thirds of the forehead where there is frontalis muscle deep to the treatment tip. Placement of the second and further passes is critical over "lifting points," from the medial to lateral portion of the brow extending up to the hairline. Typically 75 to 150 treatment pulses are used to cover the entire forehead and temples. This number may

vary based on the size of the patient's forehead (men tend to have larger foreheads) and on the number of passes used.

Eyelid treatment

Two different treatment handpieces are used when treating the eyelid area. The 0.25-cm^2 treatment tip is used for the upper eyelid covering the globe, and the 1.5-cm^2 tip for the upper eyelid over the orbital rim and the lower eyelid, lateral canthus, crow's feet area, and infrabrow temple. Skin marking should be employed by cutting a small section of 0.25-cm^2 skin-marking paper that corresponds to the shape and size of the patient's upper eyelid, measuring from the lash margin to no more than three rows above the margin, using alcohol pads on the noninked side of the paper. The remaining areas should be marked with the 1.50-cm^2 skin-marking paper. Plastic ocular shields must be used to protect the patient's globe. After application of one or two drops of ocular anesthetic, such as tetracaine ophthalmic solution, the shield is placed under the eyelids in one eye as per the manufacturer's instructions; the other eye may simply be closed and covered with gauze to be treated later. The return pad should be placed on a well vascularized area, such as the lower back or side.

Treatment delivery should begin at a low setting, such as 32.0 for the 0.25-cm^2 tip and 62.0 for the 1.5-cm^2 tip. To determine the patient's heat tolerance, apply a generous amount of coupling fluid to the area and deliver one or two applications of energy to the targeted treatment area. Titrate the setting based on the patient's heat sensation feedback to achieve a level of 2–2.5 on the 0–4 scale. The first pass should include the entire upper eyelid area marked with the 0.25-cm^2 grid, placing the thermatip directly in the center of each square of the grid. Be sure to keep the

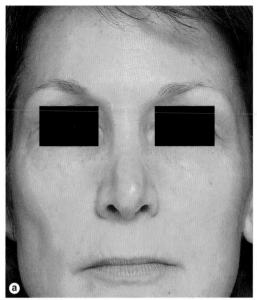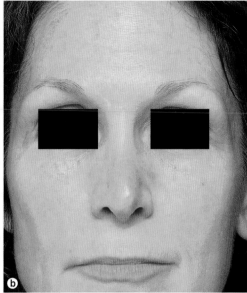

Figure 9-19 (A) Before and (B) after eyelid treatment with ThermaCool™

tip perpendicular to the skin with full tip-to-skin contact, and regularly apply generous amounts of coupling fluid. The second pass should be performed with the tip directly over the intersections of the grid. Subsequent passes similar to the first and second passes may be repeated. The average number of pulses per patient in the clinical studies was 205. Some slight erythema and/or edema may develop in the course of the treatment.

Switch to the 1.5-cm² tip and continue over the grid-marked areas of the upper eyelid (brow portion), lower eyelid, and temporal areas. Perform the first pass within the square, and the second pass over the circles of the grid. Perform subsequent passes by alternating square and circle treatments. Mild edema may or may not accompany treatment, but you should treat in multiple passes over the areas until some visible tightening has occurred. When the first eye area is complete, remove the eye shield and repeat the procedure on the other eye area (Fig. 9-19).

Treatment of the lower face

It is currently recommended to treat the entire cheek, jawline, and neck area as one cosmetic unit, beginning at the malar prominence and periorbital/crow's feet area, extending medially toward the nasolabial folds, laterally toward the preauricular area, and inferiorly to the mandible. The jawline, upper one-third of the neck, and submental region are included as well. One or two pulses on each side of the cutaneous upper lip may also be of benefit, but should be performed at low fluences. It is recommended that treatment pulses be placed lateral and inferior to the bony orbital rim.

Results have improved substantially when multiple passes are used. The skin is made taut, creating a trampoline-like effect, by putting tension on the skin to be treated with the nontreating hand. It is important for the treatment tip to meet some resistance when it is placed on the skin to allow equal contact throughout the surface of the electrode. It can also be useful gently to pull the skin off of the jawline and neck superiorly, to move this skin off the sensitive (and challengingly convex) mandibular region.

After the grid markings have been placed, a 3.0-cm² treatment tip is attached. Treatment settings for the first pass are usually in the 355.0–356.0 range for the entire lower face (Fig. 9-20 A,B). One side of the face can be performed at a time to compare treated versus untreated sides. A second pass at 354.0–355.0 (depending on patient tolerance) is performed in the periorbital region, the lateral cheek, and preauricular region, as well as the jawline, submental region, and upper neck. The medial upper cheek is avoided with this second pass (Fig. 9-20C,D). A third pass can then be performed in an L-shaped pattern, including the malar area and nasolabial folds (Fig. 9-20E,F), and this can be followed by a subsequent passes in areas that require maximal contraction, usually over the jawline in sweeping upward vectors towards the lateral malar area. Some physicians use an overlapping pattern by treating one square and then an adjacent circle on the grid in a zigzag fashion. This must be done at low fluences to prevent excessive dermal heating or ineffective epidermal cooling. After five to seven passes, a visible tightening of the skin can often be observed.

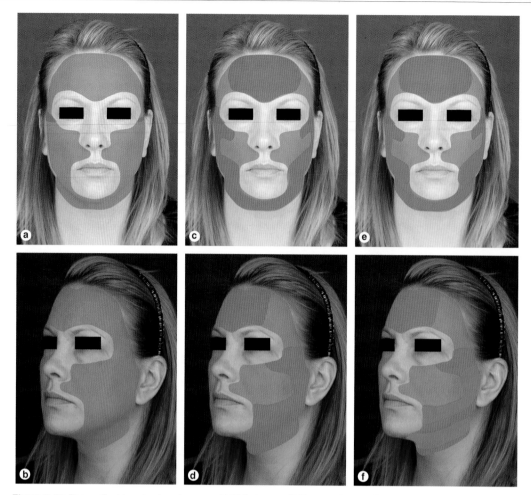

Figure 9-20 ThermaCool face treatment passes: (A,B) first pass; (C,D) second pass; (E,F) third pass

There are differing theories as to the mechanism of action of the third through sixth or seventh passes; they include:

- Tissue tightening in the x (horizontal) and y (vertical) plane along the cutaneous surface
- Melting of fat and tissue tightening in the z-axis, perpendicular to the skin, which pulls tissue in toward the bony underlying structures
- A combination of the two (Fig. 9-21).

This z-axis effect appears to be an important element of the results seen in treatment of the lower face (Fig. 9-22). Whether this comes from additional tightening in the x and y planes, or from a direct third-dimension effect on subdermal fat and collagen of the fibrous septae, remains to be determined. However, treating physicians can use these z-axis changes to their advantage. The third pass can therefore be carefully placed in areas where maximal z-axis improvement is needed.

This would include the jowl and submental region. Additionally, further x- and y-axis changes can be produced with this third pass, and should include the preauricular region to create a "vector" of pull laterally. The fourth and subsequent passes are used to augment the results of the third pass, and in many cases to achieve visible tissue tightening and contour changes at the time of the procedure.

Body treatments

Abdomen   The 3.0-cm^2 grid is placed on the upper and lower abdomen with the central area at the umbilicus. Treatment settings are approximately 353.0 (98 J), and passes are performed in a square/circle (50% overlap) alternating fashion. After two full passes (which would equate to four full passes owing to the overlap), vector passes can be performed on the lower abdomen, upwards and inwards toward the umbilicus, and on the upper abdomen upwards and outward from the umbilicus. Several passes can be performed in this fashion to a total of 600 to 900 pulses total (Fig. 9-23).

Anterior or posterior thighs   Using the 3.0-cm² grid, mark the anterior thigh beginning just above the knee (or popliteal fossa posteriorly) and extending upwards. A 50% overlap alternating pattern can be performed for two passes, followed by upward and outward vectors at a setting of approximately 350–355, for a total of four to five passes and 500 pulses for each leg (Fig. 9-24).

Inner thighs   Perform 3.0-cm² markings at the interior upper thighs and use 50% overlapping passes three times, and vectors upwards for a fourth pass at a setting of 352.5.

Buttocks   Mark the patient while standing and use overlapping passes, moving distal to proximal at a setting of 355. Some immediate overlapping pulses (called "stacking") can be allowed in the medial lower buttock square in order to round and tighten the area. Approximately 1200 pulses are used.

Post-treatment guidelines

After treatment, the ink grid is gently wiped off with the aid of coupling gel or a gentle cleanser. Alcohol swabs should be avoided as they may cause irritation to the newly treated skin. The patient is counseled to use sunblock containing a UVA block, such as zinc oxide or titanium dioxide, for 7–10 days and to avoid direct sun exposure as UV rays can increase levels of metalloproteinases, leading to potential collagen and elastic tissue degradation.

Troubleshooting

The ThermaCool TC™ device is equipped with sensors and mechanisms to detect whether excessive or inadequate pressure is being applied during treatment pulses. The machine also aborts any

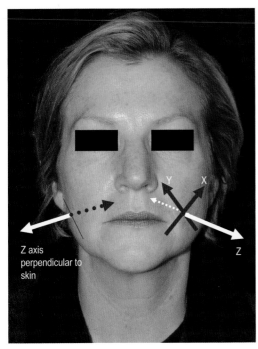

Figure 9-21 ThermaCool *x*, *y*, and *z* planes of tissue contraction

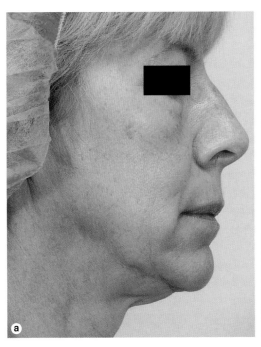
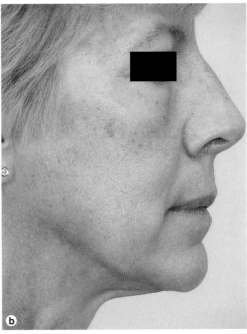

Figure 9-22 (A) Before and (B) after cheek and submental treatment with ThermaCool™

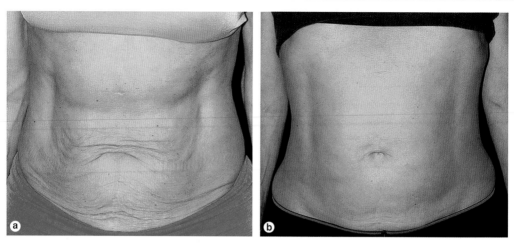

Figure 9-23 (A) Before and (B) after abdominal treatment with ThermaCool™

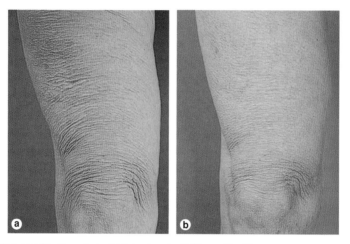

Figure 9-24 (A) Before and (B) after anterior thigh treatment with ThermaCool™

treatment pulse if all four corners of the treatment tip are not in contact with the skin. Sensors also alert the physician to excess temperature in the skin, as well as giving information about the status of the cryogen module.

It is also essential to observe the impedance readings while treating different areas. Any site with an impedance less than 100 ohms should not receive further passes, as the risk of overheating and possible blister formation is increased.

Side-effects, complications, and alternative approaches

Adverse effects from the device include, but are not limited to:

- discomfort during treatment and afterwards
- mild to moderate edema lasting for several days

- bruising from nerve blocks
- depressions from aggressive treatment and/or multiple passes
- blistering
- scarring
- no improvement in treated areas.

Treatment of the lower face can lead to mild to moderate edema of the jawline and neck, which usually resolves in 7–14 days, and occasional tenderness along the preauricular or mandibular area, which can be managed by ibuprofen. Small 0.5–1-cm nodules can also rarely be seen. These usually resolve without treatment or sequelae within 2–4 weeks.

As sagging of tissues is a fundamental part of the aging process, nearly all patients who are candidates for other forms of facial rejuvenation are also candidates for the Thermage procedure. RF tissue tightening is not a substitute for the wide array of nonablative lasers, but rather a companion to them. There may be some overlap, for example, in remodeling of the dermis achieved by nonablative lasers and the Thermage device. However, only the ThermaCool TC™ can produce tightening of dermal collagen in the x and y axes, and the z-axis changes discussed above are not seen with any of the other nonablative options available.

Bipolar radiofrequency devices – ELOS technology (Table 9-4)

Mechanism of action

Synergy between electrical energy and light, termed electro-optical synergy (ELOS) provides benefit in the following manner. The light-based component delivers optical energy that is absorbed by specific chromophores in the skin, such as melanin, hemoglobin, or water, and is converted to heat, according to the principle of selective photothermolysis. The bipolar RF component produces a thermal effect that is dependent on the electrical conductivity of the tissue. It generates heat from a current of ions that acts according to the physical principle of impedance: that electrical current will always follow the path of least resistance. Electrical current will always follow the path of highest conductivity (lower impedance); therefore, it does not penetrate matter of low conductivity such as bone. Impedance is also inversely correlated with heat. Higher temperatures produce a lower impedance and therefore direct the flow of current. Preheating with the light-based component will lower the impedance, thereby directing the bipolar RF to the heated target. In addition, precooling of the skin will increase the impedance of the skin and direct electrical current to a greater depth of penetration while protecting the epidermis.

The ELOS system consists of a bipolar RF generator and a flashlamp pulsed light delivered through a contact sapphire light-guide, with the bipolar RF energy delivered through electrodes embedded in the system applicator and brought into contact with the skin surface. The RF component of ELOS systems is a bipolar configuration with two electrodes affixed on opposite sides of the rectangular sapphire light-guide. Electrical current is passed between two electrodes and is limited by the area between the electrodes.

The penetration depth of electrical current can be calculated as half the distance between electrodes. The pulses of optical and RF are initiated at the same time. The device contains an active dermal monitoring system that measures changes in the skin impedance, which is adjustable by the user to provide an integrated safety mechanism (impedance safety limit) to prevent overheating of the dermis. A thermoelectric cooling handpiece provides contact cooling at a temperature of approximately 5°C before, during, and after energy delivery.

Aurora/SR – skin rejuvenation

Skin type must be determined before treatment with IPL/SR (skin rejuvenation) technology. Patients with skin types I–IV can be treated safely. The Aurora had two handpieces, one for skin rejuvenation, now termed SR, and one for hair removal. The SR uses IPL of 580–980 nm for optical energy. The SRA handpiece, which is newer, uses IPL of 470–980 nm. RF energy settings range from 5 to 25 J/cm^3, whereas light energies range from 1 to 45 J/cm^2. The handpiece is 12 × 25 mm, which is large enough to allow treatment of the entire face within a matter of minutes. The optical energy is absorbed by pigmented and vascular lesions, and RF heating of the dermis leads to neocollagenesis.

Polaris

The Polaris device contains three handpieces, one for wrinkle reduction, now termed WR, one for hair removal, and one for leg veins. It uses a 900-nm diode laser for optical energy. The fluence for the WR can be as high as 50 J/cm^2, and the RF energy can be up to 100 J/cm^3. The handpiece is an 8 × 12-mm rectangle and can deliver up to two pulses per second. Typically three passes are used per treatment, and patients are treated three to six times at 3–4-week intervals. RF energy ranges from 40 to 100 J/cm^3, with optical energy ranging from 15 to 50 J/cm^2. Optical energy settings are based on skin type and distribution of target chromophores. Darker skin types require less optical energy so as to not damage normal melanin chromophores. The greater the depth of wrinkles, the higher the RF setting used. Most patients have mild erythema and/or edema after treatment; this resolves in 24 h.

ReFirme ST™

The patient's face should be clear of all make-up. One side of the face is fully treated before starting the other to provide a reference point so that the tightening endpoint can be seen when the patient is sitting up. The lower face and submental area should be treated with RF intensities of 80–120 J/cm^3, with 10-J/cm^3 increments, and IR energy fixed at 10 W/cm^2.

A vector area is chosen to produce tightening in the desired area. Markings can be made with a white eyeliner pencil to identify rows of tissue representing vectors to be tightened. Ultrasound gel is used to ensure contact and gliding with the handpiece. Cooling intensity should be "normal" to "strong," equivalent to 10°C or 5°C respectively. No anesthesia is used.

The first pass should cover the complete treatment area with 30–50% overlap. Consecutive passes should be performed on vector zones of 20 to 30 pulses, each with 30–50% overlap, until sustained endpoint of tightening and mild edema is seen, often accompanied by erythema. Typically four to seven passes are done within several seconds of each other to achieve a temperature of 60°C. The forehead and bony prominences should be treated with RF at 90–120J/cm^3 and two to five passes (Table 9-5). Consecutive passes should be performed repeatedly until endpoint tightening is seen, before similar treatment is performed on the other side of the face or other body area. If any of the pulses cause discomfort or excessive response from the patient (i.e. pain), reduce the energy level and, if necessary, change the cooling level to strong. Stack pulsing is to be avoided to prevent burns.

Two to five treatment sessions at 3–4-week intervals are recommended (Fig. 9-25). More may be needed for more severely aged skin. One touch-up session may be needed every 6 months, according to individual response, due to natural processes of aging (Fig. 9-26). Combination of ST treatment with SR/SRA or VelaSmooth is possible in the same session. If following SR/SRA treatment, perform only the vector zones for tightening.

Treatments off face, such as the thighs (Fig. 9-27) or abdomen (Fig. 9-28), can also be performed in a similar overlapping and repeated pass pattern. Ongoing studies of off-face treatment algorithms are under way.

VelaSmooth

A series of treatments, along with maintenance treatments, are the protocol for patients using the VelaSmooth. Typically 14 to 16 treatments are done over 7–8 weeks, with monthly maintenance. Before treatment, patients are advised to exfoliate the skin and come to the office with clean, dry skin. Hair may hinder the movement of the applicator and overheat the treatment area. Prior shaving is advised. Patients should (when medically acceptable) avoid anticoagulants, such

Table 9-5 Treatment parameters

Fitzpatrick skin type	Area	RF energy (J/cm^3)	Cooling	Typical passes per area
I–VI	Lower face, under chin	100–120	Normal	4–7
I–VI	Forehead, bony areas	90–120	Normal/strong	2–5

Settings are general guidelines only, and should be adjusted following individual responses to test spots. The IR energy is up to 10W/cm^2. The operator-controlled parameters are: FR intensity of 30–120J/cm^3, with 10-J/cm^3 increments; cooling intensity can be normal or strong, equivalent to 10°C and 5°C respectively.

Zone	Area	No. of passes
1	Nasolabial region	5 to 7
2	Temporal region	2 to 4
3	Preauricular	2 to 4
4	Jowl	5 to 7
5	Periorbital	2 to 4
6	Medial forehead	2 to 4
7	Submental	5 to 7
8	Submandible	5 to 7

Indication	Recommended zones
General facial laxity	1,2,3
Mid face laxity/nasolabial fold	1,3
Lateral browlift – lower eyelid	2,5
Medial browlift – lower and upper eyelid	2,6
Lower face – jowl laxity/marionettes	3,4
Lower eyelid – eyelid laxity	5*
Neck laxity	3,4,7,8

* Area should be treated with Matrix IR if possible

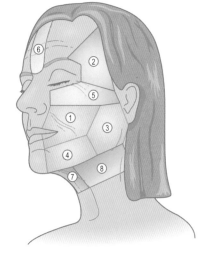

Figure 9-25 ReFirm ST™ facial and neck passes. An algorithm for treatment.

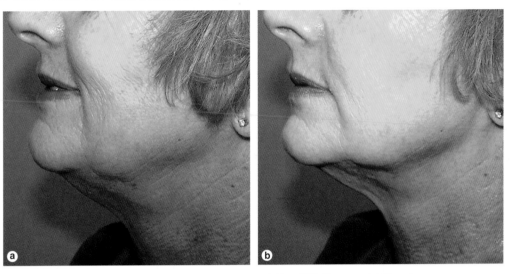

Figure 9-26 (A) Before and (B) after treatment of the neck with ReFirm ST™. Courtesy of J. Shaoul MD

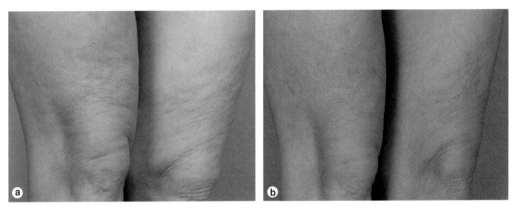

Figure 9-27 (A) Before and (B) after leg treatment with ReFirm ST™. Courtesy of Ron Russo MD

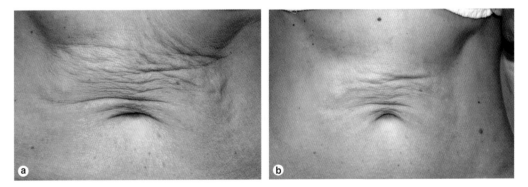

Figure 9-28 (A) Before and (B) immediately after one abdominal treatment with ReFirm ST™. Courtesy of Peterson Pierre MD

as aspirin, ibuprofen, vitamin E, garlic, ginseng, gingko, feverfew, and saw palmetto, which may increase chances of bruising.

Treatment times vary from 45 to 60 min, depending on the size of the area to be treated. Preoperative photos are recommended, as are photos at every fourth session, and at maintenance sessions to assess clinical response. Treatment areas are marked with a white or yellow marker, while the patient is standing, as cellulite or contour may change characteristics when the patient is lying down.

Large anatomic areas are treated with the body (large) applicator. Settings are approximately 20Ws RF, 20W IR light, and 200 millibar vacuum (750 mmHg negative pressure). The vacuum mode is set at intensity level 1 for one to two sessions, and increased to intensity levels 2 or 3 during subsequent sessions, according to the patient's skin response and comfort. Vacuum levels for sensitive areas, such as the abdomen, inner thigh, and over loose skin areas, should be increased according to the patient's tolerance. Set the RF at intensity level 2. This may be increased to level 3 as the treatment progresses or in subsequent sessions, if the patient feels comfortable and skin response allows. The IR level is set at 1–3, according to the vacuum level, so that the total of the two levels does not exceed 4. Use lower IR levels for very dark or tanned skin, or over dark hair or tattoos.

VelaSpray Ease lotion is used on the skin to ensure coupling and conductivity of the handpiece. The lotion should be rubbed well into the skin, leaving a coating thickness of less than 1 mm. Replenish the spray only if it becomes difficult to move the applicator over the treated area, or when the IR and RF indicators blink constantly. The applicator should be placed perpendicular to the treatment area and minimal pressure applied. When pressing the applicator's trigger, the skin will be lifted by the suction and drawn into the applicator chamber. If you hear air being sucked into the applicator chamber, this indicates that the applicator is not positioned properly on the skin. Stretching of the curved skin areas with the free hand can aid in proper applicator positioning.

Treatment patterns vary, but one method is to perform two passes, overlapping in a cross-hatched pattern, at a vacuum setting of 1. For the third and fourth passes, the vacuum setting is increased to 2–3, and cross-hatching is again performed. Subsequent passes are done over focal areas using two to six stacked pulses (about 5 s), with 50% overlap using the vacuum setting at 3, IR at 3, and RF at 3.

The small treatment head is used for areas such as the neck and arms. Similar settings and cross-hatching is performed for four passes. Focal areas are treated with stacked pulses, approximately 3 to 15 of them, with 50% overlap, vacuum setting 2–3, IR of 1, and RF of 3. Vacuum setting for the neck should not be higher than 1. Avoid bony areas such as the thyroid cartilage. Arms should be treated along the triceps from the axilla to the elbow, while the patient is lying on their back with the elbows are above the head. The outer portion of the arm can be treated with the arm placed alongside the body. The stacking should be performed to achieve persistent radiant warmth, which may be accompanied by erythema and some edema. The warmth should last for 5–10 min. This is the endpoint indicator to stop treatment over that area.

After treatment, if the heat sensation is excessive, the areas can be cooled with ice packs. In case of any side-effect, such as a burn, stop treatment, and apply cooling and appropriate creams. Further treatment should be performed at reduced settings. Transient skin texture improvement and tightening may be apparent after each session. Long-term skin texture improvement and skin tightening, as well as circumference reduction can be seen in early sessions as well; however, monthly maintenance is required to maintain the effect achieved (Figs 9-29 & 9-30).

Combined monopolar and bipolar radiofrequency

Accent RF System

Facial treatments are performed weekly for 4 weeks. Sequential treatment with the bipolar handpiece followed by the unipolar handpiece is performed on the face. Treatment settings are chosen to reach therapeutic temperatures of 39–41°C. With the bipolar handpiece, energies of 55–100W are used with passes of 20 s each, followed

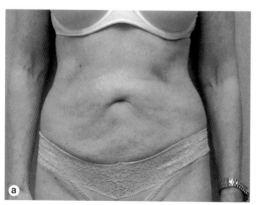
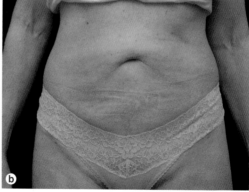

Figure 9-29 (A) Before and (B) after abdominal treatment with VelaSmooth. Courtesy of Amy Forman Taub MD

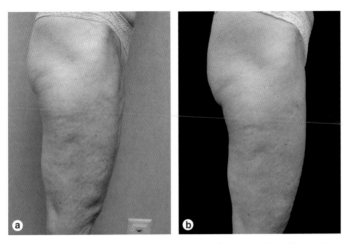

Figure 9-30 (A) Before and (B) after thigh treatment with VelaSmooth. Courtesy of Amy Forman Taub MD

by three passes of 20s to maintain therapeutic temperature for 1min. The unipolar handpiece is used at 110–130W to reach therapeutic temperature with passes of 20s each, followed by three passes of 20s to maintain temperature for 1min. Treatment on the neck is done at lower energies or 55–80W with the bipolar handpiece, and 80–110W with the unipolar handpiece, in a similar fashion to that on the face (Michael Gold MD, personal communication, 2007).

Electrical stimulation

PanG™ Lift

The PanG™ Lift is a noninvasive procedure using facial muscle tightening, ultrasonic microdermabrasion, and low-frequency ultrasound energy to deliver skin care products into the dermis. These three combined treatments allow for treatment of all the component layers of the face that contribute to the aging process – specifically the epidermis, dermis, subcutaneous layer, and muscle. Treatments for the PanG™ Lift protocol are performed biweekly, at least 1day apart. Typically 20 Myofacial™ treatments are performed (twice weekly) followed by either a SonoPeel™ (once weekly for the first 6weeks) or a SonoFacial™ (once weekly for the first 4weeks).

The resistive Myofacial™ therapy employs high-voltage electrical current from the M.E.D.U.C.E.™ medical ultrasonic generator to stimulate the prime elevating facial muscles. The generator receives standard 110-V electrical energy from a regular outlet. The voltage is converted to high-frequency, high-voltage alternating current. The facial muscle elevators consist of the frontalis, the zygomaticus major and minor, the suprahyoid muscles, and the platysma. The goal is to strengthen, hypertrophy, tone, and shorten these muscles to elevate the soft tissue envelope

and reposition the skin. This can occur only when the overlying soft tissue envelope is still attached by the dermal facial connecting fibers and retaining ligaments of the face. If the skin is too loose and there is not reasonable attachment, the hypertrophic effects on the prime elevators will not have a significant elevating effect.

The MyoFacial™ system generator produces a specific and proprietary, premodulated, alternating waveform and current to recruit full fiber contraction of the elevator muscles. The procedure is performed in sets of three to six, with 10 to 14 repetitions per set, with maximal current and fiber contraction with resistive tensile loads. Prior to the resistive portion of treatment, all muscle groups of the face are treated, without resistance and at lower currents to allow augmented blood flow to all muscles. This also causes increased skin blood flow, lasting for approximately 4–6h.

There are three phases to MyoFacial treatment: nonresistive MyoFacial, isotonic resistive MyoFacial hypertrophy, and maintenance MyoFacials. The nonresistive MyoFacial is performed during the first 2–3 weeks (first four to six sessions). There is no MyoFacial resistive apparatus used and thus no tensile force on the myofilaments. During these nonresistive MyoFacials, there is strong electrical stimulation and contraction of the facial musculature. This allows the patient to become acclimated to the therapy without undue injury to the facial muscles. The treatment steps are as follows:

1 Protect the hair with a band, and cleanse the face with a mild alcohol-based cleanser to remove oil and dirt.
2 Put fresh water in a bowl and have gauze and ultrasonic gel near the ultrasound generator.
3 Have blue-tinted MyoFacial conductive gel in a clear plastic 6-oz cup and a tongue depressor.

4 Turn on the M.E.D.U.C.E.™ and begin programming in the MyoFacial parameters.
5 Press the fish-shaped icon, which is the proprietary MyoFacial premodulated waveform.
6 Press the Hz button three times so that the green light on the MyoFacial panel moves down to the fourth and last position on the panel denoted by the Hz-Hz label. This setting will enable the necessary sinusoidal, premodulated wave pattern of the MyoFacial. Ensure the premodulated waveform is set to "continuous."
7 Move up to the timer icon. Press the following sequence: no. 2 then the triangle sign, no. 2 then the triangle, then press the diamond with the horizontal line in the middle.
8 The times will now begin to count in seconds.
9 Place both electrodes in the gel, approximately 1 inch apart and so that half of the shaft of the MyoFacial probe is submerged in the gel. Make sure the MyoFacial probes do not touch each other or the sides of the cup, as this contact will deactivate the electrical charge required for treatment.
10 With the MyoFacial probes in the gel, press the Amperage Icon on the MyoFacial M.E.D.U.C.E. contact panel. The current can be programmed only with the probes in the gel. Move up the current to the desired amperage. Allow the current to reach the desired level. The current level used will vary depending upon the tolerance of the patient, the specific facial muscle elevator being treated, and how many weeks into the program the patient is. The following current levels are good starting points, from which you can adjust specific levels:

- Frontalis 25 mA
- Orbicularis 20 mA
- Zygomaticus 30 mA
- Digastric 35 mA
- Platysma 40 mA.

11 With the desired current entered for the MyoFacial treatment of the particular facial region, remove the MyoFacial probes from the gel in a scooping fashion. Ensure that there is a small collection of gel on the end of the MyoFacial probe. There will be two audible beeps from the device when the probes are clear of the gel. There must be sufficient gel on the skin at the probe–skin interface, or there will be excessive epidermal resistance to the passage of electrical current and localized pain or a burn may ensue.
12 Keep the probes separate from each other. Check once again the desired current level and adjust if necessary.
13 The electrical current levels will be determined by patient sensitivity. Always begin at lower amperage levels (18–25 mA) and then increase the voltage up toward and then above the guidelines above.

After the first 3 weeks, the resistor is applied to the patient. The resistor is comprised of a Velcro strap, wrapped around the patient, an outrigger, applied to the resistor through the Velcro attachment, and resistance bands attached to the patient's face (Fig. 9-31). The degree of inferior soft tissue

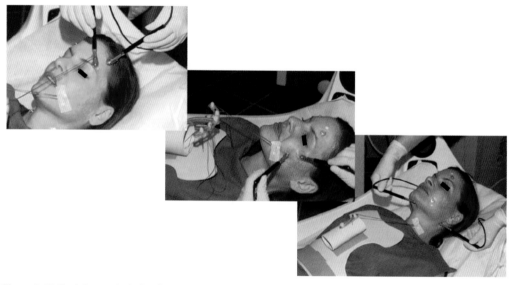

Figure 9-31 Resistive myofacial PanG treatment. Photographs depict the device and proper application of the treatment wands

translocation of the brow, cheek, and neck is assessed, as this will be the degree of tensile load and stretch that must be applied to the facial elevators to place the myofibrils and their contractile filaments on optimal stretch. The bands are affixed to the skin using the electrode tabs and Hypafix adhesive tape strips, creating a resistive force when the electrodes are applied to the skin. Twice-weekly 45-min resistance training sessions are performed with isotonic, eccentric, and concentric contractions of the facial muscles of elevation.

The SonoPeel™ procedure consists of ultrasound of high frequency and energy from the M.E.D.U.C.E.™ medical ultrasonic generator. The electricity is sent to a handpiece that contains piezoelectric crystals, an amplifier, and a horn. The crystals are made of barium sulfate. As the alternating electrical current from the generator is passed across the magneto-strictive stacks, there is a displacement of ions and an alternating expansion and contraction of the crystals with the alternating current. Thus, through the crystals, the electrical energy is converted into mechanical energy in the form of deformation.

The amount of deformation of the stacks is predictable and constant, measuring from 5 to 25 μm. The average deformation, or oscillatory amplitude of deflection during the SonoPeel measures 20 μm with a frequency of 30 000 Hz. The amplifier unit boosts the ultrasound signal and waves, while the directional horn funnels the ultrasound signal down the CaviFacial accuator, or the blade. This blade is fastened to the handpiece. The oscillation of this titanium blade leads to peeling of the stratum corneum. The epidermis is protected by a continual stream of normal saline, which optimizes cavitation on the stratum corneum and cools the epidermal surface. The ultrasound wave creates expansion and rarefaction forces within the water droplets lying on the epidermis. With each cycle, the air micro-bubbles get larger until their size exceeds the forces keeping them together and they implode. This process is called cavitation. The heat released disrupts the bonds and forces that hold in the stratum corneum keratinocytes together, and they are cleaved off the deeper layers of the epidermis, producing the peel. Excessive resistance, however, can lead to intense thermal energy and possible skin burns. The entire process takes 10–15 min.

The SonoFacial™ is a dermal skin care product delivery procedure that is instituted after two to three SonoPeels. It uses low-frequency ultrasonic energy and cavitation to optimize dermal penetration of skin care products. The frequency of ultrasound used results in a heating of the target tissue, vasodilatation, increased permeability, and altered cell membrane function. The products, in the form of serums, are mixed in clear ultrasound gel and applied to the face. The handpiece is then

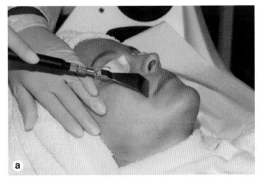

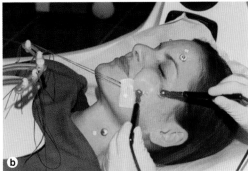

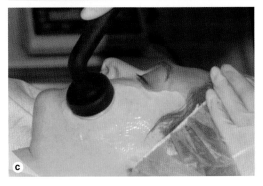

Figure 9-32 PanG Lift treatments: (A) the SonoPeel; (B) the Myofacial; (C) the SonoFacial

turned on and set at 2.1 W/cm^2. The procedure takes approximately 20 min. All three components of this treatment comprise the PanG Lift program (Fig. 9-32).

Maintenance treatments are recommended for the PanG™ Lift program. These are typically done every 3–5 weeks and consist of either the Myofacial™ treatment alone to stimulate the muscles, or the Myofacial™ along with the SonoPeel™ and the SonoFacial to maintain the health of the overlying skin (Fig. 9-33).

The PanG™ Lift program also consists of one optional treatment with botulinum toxin (if desired), either at the beginning of treatment or after the fifth week to allow the patient to see the results from the lift alone. This amplifies the results, as the botulinum toxin relaxes the depressor muscles, which tend to oppose the lifting muscles.

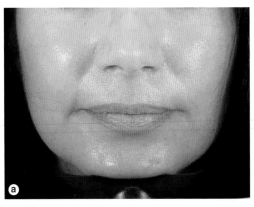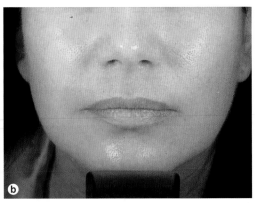

Figure 9-33 (A) Before and (B) after PanG facial treatment. Courtesy of Amy Forman Taub MD

PEARLS

Choose patients with mild to moderate laxity only.

Explain limitations and expectations to patients.

Multiple passes with any device results in better outcomes.

Directions for the future and conclusions

Recent years have brought about a plethora of new technologies for the remodeling of human skin. With these technologies come numerous new devices and treatment protocols. We are only beginning to understand and modify algorithms to achieve consistent maximal clinical results. Further research into the methodology of collagen tightening, and collagen and elastic tissue remodeling, is warranted. It is hoped that, with time and knowledge, the above-mentioned devices and their treatment applications will create reproducible skin-tightening benefits for all patients.

Further reading

Alexiades-Armenakas M. Rhytides, laxity, and photoaging treated with a combination of radiofrequency, diode laser and pulsed light and assessed with a comprehensive grading scale. J Drugs Dermatol 2006;5(8):731–738.

Alster TS, Tanzi E. Improvement of neck and cheek laxity with a nonablative radiofrequency device: a lifting experience. Dermatol Surg 2004;30(Pt 1): 503–507.

Alster TS, Tanzi EL. Cellulite treatment using a novel combination radiofrequency, infrared light, and mechanical tissue manipulation device. J Cosmet Laser Ther 2005;7(2):81–85.

Anderson RR, Parish JA. Selective photothermolysis: precise microsurgery by selective absorption of pulsed radiation. Science 1983;220:524–527.

Bassichis BA, Dayan S, Thomas JR. Use of a nonablative radiofrequency device to rejuvenate the upper one-third of the face. Otolaryngol Head Neck Surg. 2004;130(4):397–406.

Bitter P Jr, Mulholland S. Report of a new technique for enhanced non-invasive skin rejuvenation using a dual mode pulsed light and radio-frequency energy source: selective radiothermolysis. J Cosmet Dermatol 2002;1:142–143.

Chua, SH, Ang P, Khoo L, Goh CL. Nonablative infrared skin tightening in type IV to V Asian skin: a prospective clinical study. Dermatol Surg 2007;33:146–151.

Dayan SH, Vartanian AJ, Menaker G, et al. Nonablative laser resurfacing using the long-pulse (1064nm) Nd:YAG laser. Arch Facial Plast Surg 2003;5:310–315.

Doshi SN, Alster TS. Combined diode laser and radiofrequency energy for rhytides and skin laxity: investigation of a novel device. Cosmet Laser Ther 2005;7:11–15.

Duck FA. Physical Properties of Tissue. New York: Academic Press, 1990.

Emilia del Pino M, Rosado RH, Azuela A, et al. Effect of controlled volumetric tissue heating with radiofrequency on cellulite and the subcutaneous tissue of the buttocks and thighs. J Drugs Dermatol 2006;5(8):714–722.

Finzi E, Spangler A. Multipasss vector (mpave) technique with nonablative radiofrequency to treat facial and neck laxity. Dermatol Surg 2005;31(Pt 1): 916–922.

Fitzpatrick R, Geronemus R, Goldberg D, et al. Multicenter study of noninvasive radiofrequency for periorbital tissue tightening. Lasers Surg Med 2003;33(4):232–242.

Gabriel S, Lau RW, Gabriel C. The dielectric properties of biological tissues: III. Parametric models for the dielectric spectrum of tissue. Phys Med Biol 1996;41:2271–2293.

Hammes S, Greve B, Raulin C. Electro-optical synergy (ELOS) technology for nonablative skin rejuvenation: a preliminary prospective study. J Eur Acad Dermatol Venereol 2006;20(9):1070–1075.

Hsu TS, Kaminer MS. The use of non-ablative radio-frequency technology to tighten the lower face and neck. Semin Cutan Med Surg 2003;22:115–123.

Iyer S, Suthamjariya K, Fitzpatrick R. Using a radio-frequency energy device to treat the lower face: a treatment paradigm for a nonsurgical facelift. Cosmet Dermatol 2003;16:37–40.

Key D. Single-treatment skin tightening by radiofre-quency and long-pulsed, 1064-nm Nd:YAG laser compared. Lasers Surg Med 2007;39:169–175

Kist D, Burns AJ Sanner R, Counters J, Zelickson B. Ultrastructural evaluation of multiple pass low en-ergy versus single pass high energy radio-frequency treatment. Lasers Surg Med 2006;38(2):150–154.

Koike S, Ogawa R, Aoki R, Hyakusoku H. Intra-dermal change resulting from irradiation with broadband infrared light. J Jpn Soc Aesth Plast Surg 2006;28(2):39–41.

Kulick M. Evaluation of a combined laser–radiofrequency device (Polaris WR) for the nonablative treatment of facial wrinkles. J Cosmet Laser Ther 2005;7(2):87–92.

Kushikata N. Negishi K, Tezuka Y, Takeuchi K, Wakamatsu S. Non-ablative skin tightening with radiofrequency in Asian skin. Lasers Surg Med 2005;36(2):92–97.

Lee MW. Combination 532-nm and 1064-nm lasers for noninvasive skin rejuvenation and toning. Arch Dermatol 2003;139(10):1265–1276.

Mulholland RS. The PanG Lift: Non-surgical Facelift. Toronto: Beautiful Solutions, 2005.

Narins D, Narins R. Non-surgical radiofrequency facelift. J Drugs Dermatol 2003;2:495–500.

Negishi K, Takeuchi K, Nagao K, Kushikata N, Wakamatsu S. An objective evaluation on the effects of non-ablative skin tightening with a broadband infrared light device. American Society for Laser Medicine and Surgery presentation. April 2006, Boston, MA.

Ruiz-Esparza J. Painless, nonablative, immediate skin contraction induced by low-fluence irradiation with new infrared device: a report of 25 patients. Dermatol Surg 2006;32:601–610.

Ruiz-Esparza J, Gomez JB. The medical face lift: a noninvasive, nonsurgical approach to tissue tight-ening in facial skin using nonablative radiofrequency. Dermatol Surg 2003;29(4):325–332.

Sadick N. Combination radiofrequency and light energies: electro-optical synergy technology in esthetic medicine. Dermatol Surg 2005;31:1211–1217.

Sleightholm R, Bartholomeusz H. Skin tightening and treatment of facial rhytides with combined in-frared light and bipolar radiofrequency technology. Australian Journal of Cosmetic Surgery (in press).

Taub AF. Evaluation of a nonsurgical, muscle-stimulating system to elevate soft tissues of the face and neck. J Drugs Dermatol 2006;5(5):446–450.

Taub AF, Battle EF, Nikolaidis G. Multicenter clinical perspectives on a broadband infrared light device for skin tightening. J Drugs Dermatol 2006;5(8):771–778.

Taylor M, Prokopenko I. Split-face comparison of radiofrequency versus long pulse Nd:YAG treatment of facial laxity. J Cosmet Laser Ther 2006;8:17–22.

Weiss RA, Weiss MA. Early clinical results with a multiple synchronized pulse 1064nm laser for leg telangiectasias and reticular veins. Dermatol Surg 1999;25:399–402.

Weiss RA, Weiss MA, Munavalli G, Beasely KL. Monopolar radiofrequency facial tightening: a ret-rospective analysis of efficacy and safety in over 600 treatments. J Drugs Dermatol 2006;5(8):707–712.

Zelickson BD, Kist D, Bernstein E, et al. Histologi-cal and ultrastructural evaluation of the effects of a radio-frequency-based non-ablative dermal remodeling device: a pilot study. Arch Dermatol 2004;140(2):204–209.

Hair transplantation

10

Daniel Berg and Paul C. Cotterill

Introduction and history

Hair transplantation is a relatively new technique in the field of cosmetic surgery and cosmetic dermatology. Modern-day hair transplants can be credited in large part to Dr Norman Orientreich who, in the 1950s, transplanted 4-mm diameter hair-bearing grafts into the alopecic area of a patient with male-pattern hair loss. The commonly accepted theory of donor dominance was developed by Orientreich. Since that time the field of hair restoration surgery has evolved from rudimentary punch grafts, or plugs, to the current state of the art follicular unit transplantation employing microscopic dissection techniques.

In 1992, in response to the growing demand for education in the field of hair restoration surgery, the International Society of Hair Restoration Surgery was born to promote the dissemination of knowledge pertaining to hair and hair restoration surgery worldwide. The American Board, and eventually the International Board, of Hair Restoration Surgery came into existence 10 years ago as an examining body for physicians who routinely perform hair restoration surgery.

The performance of proper hair restoration surgery requires a thorough knowledge in key aspects of anatomy, pathology, diagnostic acumen, and surgical planning and execution. Hair restoration surgery is appropriate for both men and women with male- and female-pattern hair loss, hair loss from congenital abnormalities, and scarring resulting from trauma and burns; in addition hair can be transplanted from the scalp to other body parts and vice versa. Although techniques and results have advanced dramatically in the past 20 years, the basic principles remain unchanged:

- Surgical removal of skin containing hair follicles from an area of permanent hair growth (donor site)
- Preparation of the hair follicles and surrounding tissue (grafts)
- Insertion of the grafts into the thinning or bald recipient area.

The purpose of this chapter is to give the reader a solid foundation in the basic fundamentals of modern hair restoration principles and to act as a springboard for further investigation and learning in this growing field. It is important for the reader to be aware that there is a difficult learning curve with hair transplantation, because it can take up to a year to see results (and thus learn any lessons) from any individual surgery.

Causes of hair loss and indications for hair transplantation

General considerations

The vast majority of patients who are candidates for hair transplantation are patients of both sexes with androgenetic alopecia (pattern hair loss).

Because patients may present with other diagnoses, it is important to be familiar with the large spectrum of conditions that can also present with hair loss. To help with diagnosis and treatment, dermatologists have divided hair loss into scarring (cicatricial) and nonscarring forms. Causes of scarring alopecias include conditions such as lupus or lichen planopilaris, and nonscarring alopecias include alopecia areata, telogen effluvium, and androgenetic alopecia.

When deciding on whether a patient is a good candidate for hair transplantation, the following questions should be all answerable in the affirmative:

- Is there a predictable stable donor site from which to take the hair?
- Is the recipient site free of conditions that might either limit graft take (e.g. scar) or threaten graft survival (e.g. ongoing disease activity)?

Table 10-1 Causes of hair loss and suitability for transplantation

Diagnosis (cause of hair loss)	Predictable donor site?	Recipient site normal (graft take and long-term survival expected?)	Hair transplantation a good choice?
Androgenetic alopecia (men)	Yes	Yes	Usually
Androgenetic alopecia (women)	Often	Yes	Often
Telogen effluvium	No	No	No
Alopecia areata	No	No	No
Active inflammatory alopecia (e.g. discoid lupus)	No	No	No
Burnt-out scarring alopecia	Sometimes	Survival may be reduced because of scar, or disease may recur	In selected cases
Burn or other scar	Sometimes	Survival may be reduced because of scar	In selected cases

For example, alopecia areata may affect a potential donor site as well as the recipient site's ability to accept or maintain a transplanted graft. This is also true of scarring alopecias. Table 10-1 outlines some of the most common conditions causing hair loss and their suitability for hair transplantation.

In patients with a history of scarring alopecia that has been inactive for some time (at least 2 years) it may be possible to consider hair transplantation, but the patient must be warned that the scarring may decrease graft yield and that the disease may recur and destroy the grafts. With appropriate counseling, successful outcomes can be obtained in unusual conditions such as "en coup de sabre."

Androgenetic alopecia in men

Androgenetic alopecia (also called male-pattern hair loss, MPHL) in men is usually easy to diagnose based on its typical clinical presentation and lack of findings to suggest other causes. The natural progression in men has been classified by both Hamilton and Norwood. The Norwood classification (Fig. 10-1) does not include all common patterns of hair loss but serves as a guide when counseling patients for hair transplantation. Miniaturization is a common finding in areas affected by MPHL (Fig. 10-2) and is evidenced by progression through a stage of fine vellus hair prior to baldness.

Androgenetic alopecia in women

Androgenetic alopecia in women, commonly called female-pattern hair loss (FPHL), affects up to 50% of women by the age of 40 years. Due to greater societal expectations for women to have a full head of hair at all ages, psychological studies have shown women to be much more severely affected by their hair loss than men. The difficulty in both diagnosing and treating women with FPHL is that, owing to the more diffuse nature of the hair loss, without the total balding as seen with their male counterpart, other medical conditions can either mimic or present concurrently with

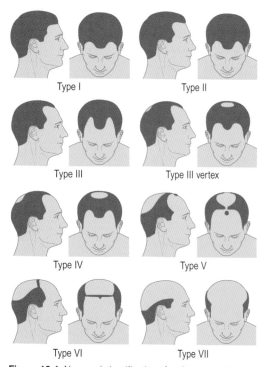

Type I   Type II

Type III   Type III vertex

Type IV   Type V

Type VI   Type VII

Figure 10-1 Norwood classification of male pattern alopecia

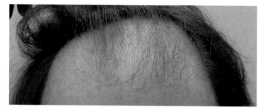

Figure 10-2 Patient with MPHL and miniaturization (decreased caliber) of the remaining few hairs in the anterior hairline area

FPHL, masking its early presentation (e.g. diffuse alopecia areata, acute/chronic telogen effluvium).

All of these factors can make diagnosis and treatment options much more difficult. It is important to rule out, and try to treat, significant

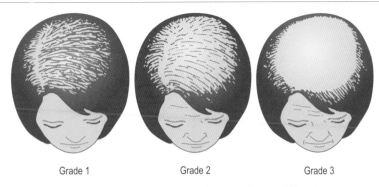

Grade 1   Grade 2   Grade 3

Figure 10-3 Ludwig classification of female pattern hair loss a) Type 1, b) Type 2, c) Type 3

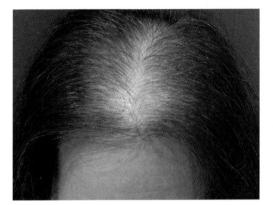

Figure 10-4 Typical presentation of female pattern thinning showing preservation of the frontal hairline and frontal accentuation of thinning in a "Christmas tree pattern"

- A search for causes of telogen effluvium: rapid weight loss, high fever, recent childbirth, certain medications.
- Routine lab exams to look for treatable causes of telogen effluvium: serum thyroid stimulating hormone, serum iron, serum ferritin, total iron binding capacity, complete blood count, free thyroxine.
- Biopsy, to exclude and help differentiate from chronic telogen effluvium, diffuse alopecia areata, and cicatricial hair loss (e.g. central centrifugal cicatricial alopecia). Tip: When performing a biopsy for scalp hair loss consider two 4-mm biopsies and request horizontal sectioning.

telogen effluvium if considering hair transplantation because telogen effluvium, especially if chronic, may lead to ongoing unstable hair loss in both the donor and recipient area – a recipe for an unhappy patient.

The most common clinical presentation of FPHL is maintenance of the frontal hair line, with diffuse thinning posteriorly as classically seen with Ludwig's three grades of thinning (Fig. 10-3). There is typically, but not always, complete or relative occipital sparing, which must be present if hair transplantation is to be considered. To aid in the diagnosis, Olsen has described a Christmas tree pattern of frontal thinning with frontal accentuation (Fig. 10-4). Other patterns of FPHL do exist.

Evaluative considerations for women are designed to rule out underlying causes of telogen effluvium, androgen excess, or other mimics of FPHL, and can include:

- Physical examination to look for signs of androgen excess: hirsutism, acne, menstrual irregularities, galactorrhea, and development of a husky voice and rapid thinning of frontotemporal recessions. If present, referral to a gynecologist/endocrinologist for androgen excess workup is suggested.

Alternative and medical treatment for androgenetic alopecia

Any patient considering hair transplantation for androgenetic alopecia should be made aware of options and alternative treatments. This includes medical treatment, as summarized in Table 10-2.

Discussion of the medical treatment of the spectrum of conditions causing hair loss is beyond the scope of this chapter. Nevertheless hair transplant surgeons should be familiar with the medical treatment of androgenetic alopecia in men and women. Medical treatment may serve as an alternative to, or adjunct treatment along with, hair transplantation.

Medical treatment of androgenetic alopecia in men

Topical minoxidil (Rogaine) and oral finasteride are the only drugs approved by the Food and Drug Administration (FDA) for MPHL. Although significant hair growth may be seen with both drugs, patients should be counseled more typically to expect a decrease in the rate of ongoing hair loss with these drugs. They should be informed that no change in hair density over time is likely evidence of success rather than failure.

Table 10-2 Alternatives to hair transplantation in patients with androgenetic alopecia

Therapy	Examples
FDA-approved medical therapy	Minoxidil, finasteride (men)
Non-FDA-approved medical therapy	Examples: dutasteride, antiandrogens (women)
Wigs	
Weaves	
Camouflage	Colored powders, sprays
Lasers	Require further studies for proof of efficacy

Minoxidil 5% is now available as a foam with a glycerin base and hence is prone to less irritation and better absorption on the scalp; it is more effective than the 2% preparation. The drug should be left on the scalp for at least 4 h to maximize absorption.

Finasteride (Propecia) is an inhibitor of type 2 5α-reductase, and in a dose of 1 mg per day has been shown to be effective in halting the progression of hair loss in men in studies lasting for up to 5 years. It acts by lowering levels of dihydrotestosterone (DHT). Side-effects are infrequent and include sexual side-effects such as impotence or decreased libido, although these occur at rates only slightly higher than with placebo, and respond to cessation of treatment. Patients taking finasteride have a roughly 50% decrease in serum levels of prostate-specific antigen (PSA); this should be taken into account when interpreting the results. Because finasteride is a long-term therapy for many patients, they should also be told about the Prostate Cancer Prevention Trial (Thomson et al 2003), which demonstrated an overall reduced risk of prostate cancer in men taking finasteride 5 mg per day, but a slightly increased incidence of higher grade tumors, which may possibly be attributed to the study methods. The significance of this is unclear for men taking the much lower 1-mg dose for hair loss.

Multiple off-label medications and herbal remedies are touted for treatment of MPHL, but lack randomized controlled trials to demonstrate efficacy. Of these, it is worth mentioning dutasteride (Avodart) because of its biologic basis of action that might suggest benefit in MPHL. Dutasteride is an inhibitor of both type 1 and 2 isoenzymes of 5α-reductase, and is more potent at reducing serum DHT levels than finasteride. It was FDA approved in 2002 for benign prostatic hypertrophy and is typically given as 0.5 mg once daily. It is well tolerated for that indication, with sexual side-effects (impotence, decreased libido, gynecomastia) being the main reported adverse events, all at a low single-digit percentage. Preliminary studies and case reports suggest a possible benefit over finasteride,

but in the absence of phase 3 studies specifically for hair loss, and because the long-term side-effects are less well documented, the authors do not currently prescribe this medication on a routine basis.

Medical treatment of androgenetic alopecia in women

The only FDA-approved treatment specifically for FPHL in women is minoxidil 2% solution. Studies have shown that 5% minoxidil is more effective, but because 5% minoxidil is associated with a 3% incidence of hypertrichosis many practitioners avoid it or use it once daily combined with the 2% solution. The 2% solution is applied with a dropper, 1 mL twice daily, to the dry scalp. Patients should use the medication for 12 months to determine individual efficacy.

Scalp irritation may occur. Patients may experience transient shedding after starting medication; this resolves after 4–6 weeks. Use of antiandrogens may be considered in women with FPHL; these include spironolactone 100–200 mg/day, finasteride 1–1.25 mg/day, cyproterone acetate combined with ethinylestradiol (e.g. the oral contraceptive pill Diane). Owing to possible feminization of a male fetus caused by medications with antiandrogen effects, women of childbearing potential should be counseled on the concurrent need for contraception. Studies on the efficacy of all of these medications show variable results and may depend on whether raised androgen levels are demonstrated; randomized trials are needed.

Assembling a team

Proper hair restoration is a team effort. The physician needs to determine his or her own goal as to a typical case size (i.e. number of grafts per session) that he or she is prepared to do. Staff requirements will be dependent on this decision. In all cases, there is a great need for well trained staff who will be efficient in preparing grafts and planting them.

Who does what and how many people are involved depends on the typical number of grafts transplanted by that surgeon. Surgeons who perform hair transplantation as 100% of their practice, and can complete two or three cases per day, may have a staff of eight or more nurses and/or technicians. In that setting, the only job of some technicians may be to dissect and trim grafts, while others may only plant the prepared grafts. For those performing only a few hair restoration procedures per month, attempting cases with very large numbers of grafts and a very large contingent of staff may be inadvisable.

Suggested staffing and task assignments, for a physician who performs only three to five cases per month (of up to 1500–2000 grafts per case) is illustrated in Table 10-3.

Table 10-3 Assembling a team

Five basic steps of a typical hair transplant	Who does what?
Anesthetizing of donor and recipient sites	Physician
Graft harvesting	Physician + 1 assistant
Graft preparation	2–4 assistants
Recipient site creation	Physician + 2 assistants
Graft implantation	2–3 assistants

With this division of labor the physician will have a total of two to four assistants. It is suggested that at least one of the surgical assistants be a registered nurse to help with more advanced tasks, including ongoing patient assessment and reinforcing anesthesia. However, the other assistants can be hair transplant technicians who have been trained in graft preparation and placement.

There is a large variety of practice styles in common use. In some practices, the physician removes only the donor tissue and allows the staff to make all the sites and plant the grafts (stick and place technique). In other offices, the physician, in addition, makes all the sites. In still others, the physician will remove the donor tissue, make all the recipient sites, and assist in planting all the grafts.

One of the major obstacles in being able to perform proper hair restoration is finding experienced staff. All team members must demonstrate excellent hand to eye coordination and also work well in a team atmosphere. The physician may end up training the assistant on site, but this is difficult unless there is a large case load and experienced staff already on hand. Initial training will start with a period of observation followed by a period of hands-on training. Often there may be a network of experienced hair transplant technicians in a geographic area that the physician can tap into. Regardless of staff hired or training methods used, the physician at all times is the team leader and is responsible on an ongoing basis for ensuring quality control of all aspects of graft preparation and planting.

Preoperative consultation

Key Points

- Take the time to assess properly for unrealistic expectations. This is especially important in the young male and all female patients. Hair loss carries on throughout a patient's life. Plan the hairline and areas to be treated, bearing in mind likely future thinning.
- Incorporate medical therapy, along with surgical therapy, into the overall treatment plan, where appropriate.

- The differential diagnosis is wider and more complex in women, owing to the more diffuse nature of thinning, and therefore necessitates a more involved workup with a more detailed history, physical examination, and a greater need for laboratory tests.

For all patients

A relevant history, physical examination, and appropriate tests should be performed to confirm a diagnosis that is amenable to hair transplanting (see above). The history and physical examination should also aim quickly to identify medical contraindications to elective surgery (e.g. severe bleeding disorders). An assessment of the psychologic impact of hair loss on the patient, as well as an assessment of the patient's expectations from treatment, are the next critical step. Alternative treatments should always be mentioned in the consultation. Photographs should be taken either at the consultation or on the morning of surgery (or both).

In competent hands, by far the most common cause of dissatisfaction with a modern hair transplant is unreasonable expectations. These may arise from an unreasonable patient, but are frequently due to a lack of understanding of both the possible natural progression of pattern hair loss and the limits of the procedure, given inherent limits on donor hair and other factors. Progressive hair loss is unpredictable in its extent and speed but is an unfortunate reality, well documented in surveys. Progressive loss of the "at risk" areas of the scalp must be planned for. Only the older patient with very stable or advanced baldness can escape this prognosis. The patient must understand that the results of a transplant will, in time, be viewed in the context of this natural history. This understanding provides the rationale for planning the initial session and allows the patient to see the need for further surgery in the future as a continuation of their care, rather than a bad outcome.

The surgeon should consider discussing all of the following points at consultation to reduce the risk of the patient with unreasonable expectations:

- Possible surgical complications should be reviewed.
- The patient should understand that the final density achievable by transplantation will not be the same as in their youth. Other options (e.g. a wig) may be a better choice for some patients, given this reality.
- Because of possible/expected progressive hair loss, the patient's final result is a "moving target." The results of adding hair will be reduced by ongoing loss of the surrounding "native" hair.

- Further transplant sessions may ultimately be required, either as a result of a desire for more density or because of ongoing recipient area hair loss.
- It is impossible to transplant densely the entire potentially thin/bald area ("There are 10 acres of land and 4 acres of seed"). Therefore, grafts must be used in areas that will both look natural and provide maximal cosmetic improvement without setting up the patient for an unnatural result in the future with further hair loss. The future pattern of hair loss must be anticipated as best as possible (easier in older patients). Some donor hair should be saved for possible use in the future. It is important to remember that hair loss is unwanted but natural looking, whereas a poorly planned transplant (e.g. placement of an unnaturally low hairline) will be both unwanted and unnatural.
- It takes 10–12 months to see the final results, perhaps longer in women.
- The donor site scar will be visible if the patient later decides to shave their head.
- Significant postoperative effluvium may occur (primarily in women) and this can lead to a thinner appearance in the recipient area for a few months or longer after the transplant. Patients who cannot accept this risk should not be transplanted.
- Patients are surprised to learn that hair transplantation does not replace the need for medical therapy of MPHL. Patients with less advanced stage of balding are counseled to begin or continue use of minoxidil and/or finasteride (in men) prior to transplantation, and to continue afterwards. There is evidence that finasteride is of benefit specifically in the setting of hair transplantation. The cosmetic benefit of the transplanted hair will be better and more durable if the native hair in the recipient area remains as long as possible, to help provide density.
- Representative photographs of other patients' results should be shown, to indicate the range of expected results – rather than just showing "best results."

For men

At the initial consultation for men there are key factors to consider with the patient in determining what hairline is best for the patient:

- The age and expectations of the patient. A patient in their early twenties may desire the lower, flatter, so-called "juvenile" hairline that they had in their teens. This is more similar to a female hairline and will not look appropriate as the patient matures. As men

age, it is normal for most men to have some degree of natural frontotemporal recession. The physician can make an educated guess as to the future extent of thinning based on the patient's age, extent of present hair loss, and family history. As the patient ages, the physician's guess gets better. Many physicians will not transplant patients until they are in their thirties, because of this concern.
- As noted above, the potential donor supply and eventual degree of balding are important factors to be assessed. Hair density in the donor region needs to be determined, to help estimate how much hair is available for transplant. It is usually wiser to start with transplanting the frontal scalp region, including the hairline. Most patients will have enough hair in their permanent hair-bearing fringe to treat at least the frontal scalp.
- Hair characteristics such as color, curl, caliber, wave, and contrast with scalp color all play a part in the eventual cosmetic outcome and should be noted at the consultation.

For women

Special care and attention is required when assessing a woman with FPHL for transplantation. Social norms dictate the expectation that women will always have a full head of thick hair. For this reason, any amount of thinning can cause more anxiety in women than in men. Women typically present with:

- a more diffuse thinning pattern involving large areas of the scalp
- no truly bald areas in which large numbers of grafts can be placed to achieve dramatic density improvement
- the spoken or unspoken desire for a return to their prehair-loss appearance.

For these reasons, women are much more likely than men to have expectations that exceed what can be delivered. Extra time and discussion is warranted with women to set appropriate expectations.

It is especially important to make the correct diagnosis in women. The majority of men with MPHL can be diagnosed almost instantly based on their history, hair loss pattern, and lack of other findings. The differential diagnosis in women can be more difficult. One of the authors requires women to be seen first by a dermatologist who can help make the diagnosis. It is especially important to emphasize in women the natural history regarding progressive hair loss. In women with FPHL, there are two peaks of hair loss (in the third and fifth decades), and women with earlier onset may end up with more severe hair loss eventually. This should be considered, especially when counseling a younger woman.

At the consultation it is especially important to assess the potential donor area to ensure that it is of sufficient density to support transplantation, as diffuse thinning of the donor area occurs more frequently in women. Finally, to reduce the risk of postoperative telogen or damage to existing hairs, a smaller size of session is warranted. This, of course, reduces the impact of the transplant on change in appearance and should be discussed realistically at the visit.

Women with FPHL who are the best candidates may be those who would be satisfied with increased thickening of their hair in key areas, for example just behind the hairline in a Ludwig 1 or 2 patient. Women who state that they are particularly bothered by the visibility of their anterior scalp when they look in the mirror may also be pleased with the reduction of this effect that should be achievable with hair transplantation.

Planning the surgery

In men

Because of the inherent ultimate limit on available donor hair it is impossible to transplant the complete bald scalp densely. Therefore, transplantation in men requires separate consideration of the hairline/anterior scalp and the vertex. These will be discussed separately.

The number of sessions required to achieve desired results will depend on:

- the size of planned recipient areas
- the size of sessions (i.e. number of grafts per session) to be undertaken
- the final density desired by both the patient and the surgeon
- the ongoing thinning that may occur in patients who still have existing hair in the recipient areas.

Good density in a fairly bald area (e.g. anterior scalp and hairline) and a satisfied patient can usually be obtained in one or two sessions, depending on session size. In general it is unwise to promise that the patient will never need a second (or even more sessions). It is wise, however, to try to achieve a good cosmetic result with at least reasonable density in the first session. With experience, the surgeon will be able to predict with more accuracy the number of sessions required for any given patient.

The anterior scalp and hairline

One of the most challenging aspects of hair transplantation is planning the hairline in a balding man. A properly placed and executed hairline is one of the most rewarding features of hair restoration

surgery, but also one of the areas where the inexperienced surgeon is most apt to get into trouble.

Positioning of the hairline should be agreed upon by both physician and patient at the consultation. It must be emphasized that the following description is only an introduction to hairline design; space does not permit the full explanation that this topic deserves. Important differences that can influence hairline design are seen between sexes, races, degree of thinning, age of initial transplantation, hair characteristics, and individual patient expectations. Several excellent publications have expanded on this critical topic of surgical planning and design (see Further Reading list: Shapiro 2004, Unger et al 2004, Ziering & Krenitsky 2003), and should be consulted by the novice.

To create a hairline the surgeon must appreciate key anatomic points and regions. The three main landmark points in hairline design are the mid

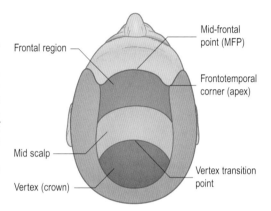

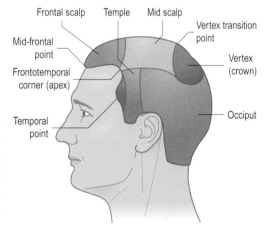

Figure 10-5 Important scalp zones and points. The mid-frontal point (MFP) is the lowest anterior mid-point of the frontal hairline. The apex is the corner of the frontotemporal junction, where the frontal hair meets the temple. The vertex transition point is the point on the scalp where the horizontal plane changes to vertical. This point is often used as the most posterior point when limiting transplantation to the frontal and mid scalp regions without committing to the vertex

frontal point (MFP), the apex, and the vertex transition point, which are illustrated in Figure 10-5.

To design the hairline/anterior scalp transplant, the surgeon should use the following steps in outlining the prospective hairline.

Step 1

The MFP can be the starting point for creation of the hairline. It is usually 7–11 cm above an imaginary horizontal line drawn across the glabella. Alternate guidelines for trying to define this point include: (a) identifying a point roughly four adult finger-breadths above the brows in the midline, or (b) identifying the point where the vertical plane of the forehead meets the horizontal plane of the scalp. These are only guidelines, and the surgeon

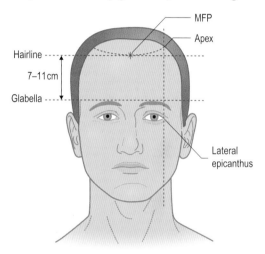

Figure 10-6 Designing the frontal hairline. The MFP is first chosen at 7–11 cm above an imaginary line drawn horizontally across the glabella. The apex is then chosen as the highest point on a line drawn vertically from the lateral epicanthus that will join up with a curved line drawn from the MFP

can consider going 1–2 cm above these if it looks natural, especially in someone with advanced hair loss. In general, a higher MFP is safer than one that is too low. Accommodation for a subtle widow's peak at the midline may also be made.

Step 2

The apex, or highest point of the frontotemporal recession, is then chosen. One technique is to draw an imaginary line vertically from the lateral epicanthus. The apex is placed at or medial to the intersection of this line and the line drawn from the MFP. It is a common mistake to try to fill in the frontotemporal recessions and make the apex too low. Figure 10-6 shows the positioning of the MFP and apex. Next, a curved line is drawn connecting the MFP and the apex. This line should be level with the ground or ascend slightly as it moves posteriorly (Fig. 10-7).

Step 3

Connect the apex to the lateral fringe by drawing a line running posteriorly from the apical point horizontal with the ground, to define the parietal hairline or part. If there is ongoing thinning, the physician needs to anticipate for future lowering so as not to be chasing a triangle of continuing hair loss in the future. It is a common mistake not to place insurance grafts into an area that, although not yet bald, will become hairless in the future (Fig. 10-8). This can be avoided to some degree by planning for further hair loss, and can ultimately be corrected by filling in the "gap" if sensible planning left some donor hair in reserve (Fig. 10-9).

If the degree of hair loss is such that the lateral temporal fringe has dropped, a new lateral fringe or "lateral hump" can be marked and filled in with grafts to allow the posterior portion of the new hairline to meet naturally with a lifted temporoparietal fringe (Fig. 10-10).

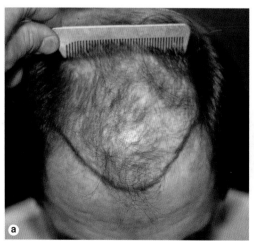

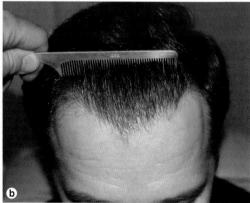

Figure 10-7 A typical hairline demonstrating the connection of the MFP and apex (A) before and (B) after transplantation

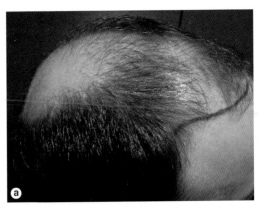

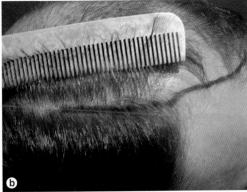

Figure 10-8 (A,B) Black line drawn to anticipate future area of loss. It is important to place insurance grafts into areas that, while not yet bald, will possibly be hairless in the future

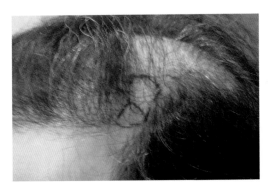

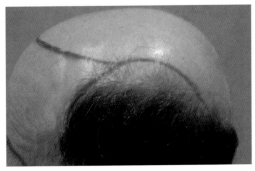

Figure 10-9 A patient who had several sessions of large grafts years ago now has a gap between the frontal and temporal hairline. This can be anticipated to some degree in original hairline design. It can be corrected if some donor hair has been left in "reserve"

Figure 10-10 Black line shows the lateral hump to be created in a patient in whom the temporoparietal fringe has receded

Step 4

Draw a posterior hairline that finishes the frontal to mid scalp area to be transplanted. This line should not go posterior to the vertex transition point. This is the point where the horizontal portion of the scalp changes to become vertical, and where the hair from the crown begins to take on a radiating direction or whorl.

This "posterior hairline" for the anterior and mid scalp can be finished in a curved or kidney-shaped pattern to mimic a natural balding crown, as shown in Figure 10-11.

Step 5

Ensure left to right symmetry of the planned hairline. Vertical measurements (e.g. at the midpupillary line and lateral canthus) should be roughly equal bilaterally. Further examples showing variations of the above technique are illustrated in Figures 10-12 & 10-13.

The concept of transplanting only the isolated frontal forelock may be considered in the very bald patient with little donor hair and large recipient area. It is also the safest way to treat the very young patient, by minimizing the use of grafts and placing them in an area that can be the basis of further transplantation in case of further hair loss. The outline of such a transplant is shown in Figure 10-14. This pattern is a reasonable design as it mimics a pattern of hair loss seen in natural MPHL, as shown in Figure 10-15. With this very conservative technique, a frontal central zone or island of hair is created without a connection to the lateral fringe, or only very sparsely filled in. Another option for the very bald patient is to reduce the amount of alopecic area by means of scalp reduction, which may entail scalp expansion, extension, or flap surgery. Although this technique has the ability to allow the patient to transplant more of the now reduced scalp, there are concerns of raising the lateral fringe to give an unnatural direction to existing hair direction, as well as a resulting scar that needs to be camouflaged. The reader is directed to Seery et al (2004) for a more detailed description of scalp reduction techniques.

The vertex (crown)

The vertex is a separate area, and should be considered so in planning and transplanting. Because the vertex baldness may progress with time, it is

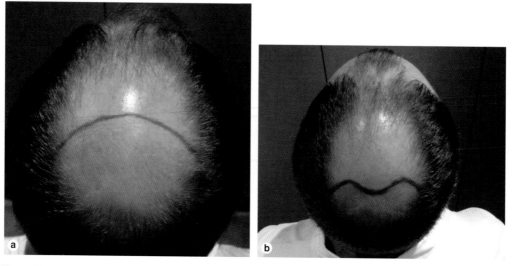

Figure 10-11 When only the frontal scalp is to be transplanted, the posterior hairline edge can finish in (A) a semi-rounded or (B) kidney shape

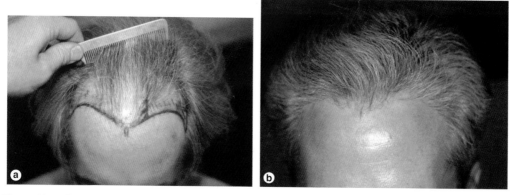

Figure 10-12 Example of a less common hairline design in a man (A) before and (B) after reconfiguration of the temporal area. This is a more advanced technique than in the other photos shown here of male hairline design

important to avoid transplanting densely in this area in a younger patient for fear of later revealing an unnatural island of hair surrounded by an increasing "moat" of baldness. This is especially problematic if the further grafts needed to fill in this expanding moat are needed later to transplant the more cosmetically important anterior scalp and hairline. For these reasons and those given below, it is the authors' view that a young male may be better served by creating a treatment plan that includes transplantation to the frontal scalp only, and the use of either finasteride and/or minoxidil to maintain the vertex hair until such time as the front is fully treated.

The decision of whether or not to transplant the vertex thus depends on many factors, including:

- *The age of the patient.* Some physicians never treat the vertex, and others do so only once the frontal scalp has been treated and the patient is at an age, over about 35 years, when a more accurate estimation of potential future balding can be made.
- *The amount of donor hair.* When transplanting the vertex, it is always best to leave an adequate amount of donor hair to ensure adequate coverage now or in the future for the frontal scalp and hairline. Dense transplantation of the vertex leads to the dual risk of: (a) an unnatural island of dense hair surrounded by an increasing moat of baldness; and (b) the depletion of donor site reserves, making it impossible to treat the more cosmetically important anterior scalp. If there is a limited amount of donor hair then transplantation should be limited to the anterior scalp.
- *Expectations of the patient.* When transplanting the vertex and reconstituting the whorl, it can be difficult to achieve the appearance of density that can be achieved when limiting treatment to the frontal scalp.

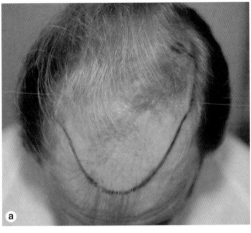

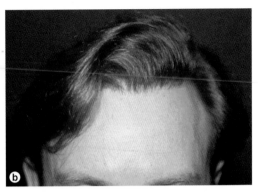

Figure 10-13 Another example of more common, typical hairline design in a male (A) before and (B) after surgery

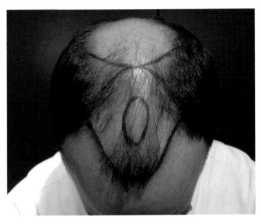

Figure 10-14 A frontal central zone or island of hair is marked for transplant with either no or much less dense transplanting planned laterally

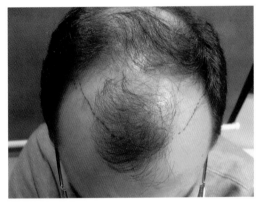

Figure 10-15 This patient, who has not had a transplant yet, demonstrates the natural existence of the frontal forelock in MPHL. A new transplanted hairline is planned (marked roughly on the scalp in pen)

The vertex, and especially at the center of the whorl with the hair radiating out in a 360° direction, will always appear thinner than the frontal hair, which all flows in a confluent direction.

Planning the surgery in women

Today's techniques, in which small follicular unit or multifollicular unit grafts can be placed between hairs without removing preexisting hairs, as was the case with the traditional 3.25–3.5-mm diameter punch transplants, has allowed many more women to be appropriate candidates for hair restoration (Figs 10-16 & 10-17).

For most women with Ludwig pattern hair loss, design of a new hairline is not necessary. Emphasis should be placed on thickening areas at and behind the hairline which are thin enough for scalp to show through when looking in the mirror. As there may be a higher risk of surgically induced postoperative telogen effluvium in women,

smaller sessions (of no more than 1000 grafts at a time) may be prudent in women. Patients should know that more sessions may be required if there is ongoing hair loss.

Key considerations in hair transplantation for FPHL are summarized in Table 10-4.

PEARLS

Transplantation in women

Wait 14–16 months for final assessment of growth. If assessed too early (at less than 1 year), full maturity is not present and full growth may not be appreciated.

Always warn about the possibility of postoperative telogen effluvium.

Suggest 5% minoxidil solution or 5% minoxidil foam. Pretreat and continue for at least 6 weeks after surgery.

Be available for reassurance.

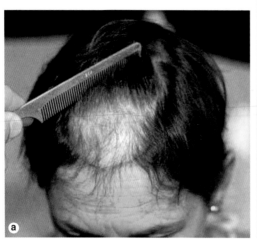

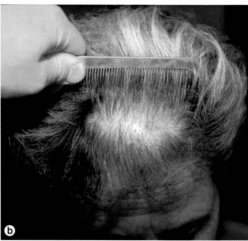

Figure 10-16 (A) Before and (B) after treatment of one session to the frontal scalp. Notice that in (B) the hair is permed and colored lighter in an attempt to make the transplanted hair look fuller with less contrast in color against the scalp

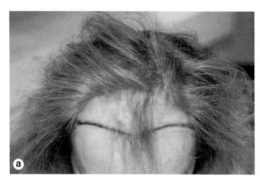

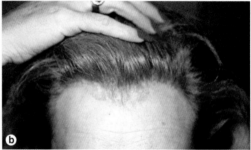

Figure 10-17 Example of reconstitution of lost frontal hairline into a more rounded feminine position (A) before and (B) after treatment. This is a less common presentation of FPHL

Table 10-4 Key considerations when transplanting women with FPHL	
Consideration	Reason
Perform a detailed history and physical exam	To rule out other causes of hair loss including concomitant telogen effluvium (contraindications)
Extensive discussion of expectations	Women must understand the risk of ongoing hair loss reducing the benefit of the transplant. Women less likely to be satisfied with "some" hair
Ensure adequate donor area density	Women with FPHL may have less density in donor site
Limit session size	May reduce risk of postoperative telogen
Select larger grafts behind hairline	Allow easier identification of transplanted hair
Limit density of packing of grafts	May reduce risk of postoperative telogen

Preoperative instructions

Many aspects of hair transplantation are common to most practitioners. Interestingly, the use or cessation of drugs in the perioperative period is a source of great variability in clinical practice, as was shown in a survey that noted that there was "no consensus about the withholding of agents that might increase bleeding; the use of pre- and postoperative analgesics; the use of topical and systemic antibiotics; the use of corticosteroids; or minoxidil" (Langtry et al 1998). Nevertheless, the authors offer the following preoperative suggestions.

One month before surgery

- Advise patients to arrange to take up to 1 week off work after surgery. This is because of the potential for postoperative swelling in the forehead region, which begins on day 2 or 3 and is noticeable for a few days. Rarely, the patient may have black, puffy eyes that can take a week to dissipate. If there is little preexisting hair in the recipient zone, the patient should be warned of the visibility of scabs on top of the grafts; these can take 7–12 days to clear.

- Blood tests – many, but certainly not all, physicians order a complete blood count and clotting profile, in addition to screening for hepatitis C, hepatitis B, and human immunodeficiency virus.
- To help reduce potential bleeding, anticoagulants and acetylsalicylic acid should be avoided for 1 week before surgery. Nonsteroidal anti-inflammatory drugs should be withheld for 48 h. In general alcohol, vitamin E supplements and *Ginkgo biloba* should also be avoided for up to a week before surgery.
- Patients should not cut their hair too short in order to insure that the donor site scar can be camouflaged immediately by existing hair.

The day of surgery

- Preoperative antistaphylococcal antibiotics are given by some practitioners 1–2 h in advance of surgery. This is most commonly a cephalosporin. In case of allergy or intolerance to this medication, substitutes such as Septra (trimethoprim–sulfamethoxazole) or clindamycin can be used. Postoperative antibiotics are continued by some.
- Some physicians suggest using 2% to 5% topical minoxidil solution applied directly on to the recipient area, starting 2 weeks prior to surgery and continuing for 1 month afterwards. Current studies suggest that, because of the vasodilatory action of minoxidil and propensity to cause extra bleeding during surgery, only the dose on the day of surgery needs to be stopped. Minoxidil has the theoretical benefit of potentially minimizing postoperative telogen and anagen effluvium.

Anesthesia for hair transplant surgery

Key Points

- Local anesthesia with oral sedation is the most commonly used form of anesthesia for hair transplantation.
- Nerve blocks (supraorbital, supratrochlear, occipital) may help with patient comfort and reduce the amount of local anesthetic needed.
- Surgeons must be knowledgeable about toxic levels of lidocaine and keep track of the total amount injected.
- Tumescent solutions with either saline or dilute lidocaine are helpful at both donor and recipient sites.

Hair transplantation can be successfully and comfortably done using local anesthesia in almost all cases. Intraoperative sedation may be used for the most painful portions of the procedure (e.g. during injection of local anesthetic), but most practitioners restrict their sedation to oral agents. Immediately before surgery a mild sedative such as oral diazepam (10–20 mg) or oral/sublingual lorazepam (1–2 mg) is typically administered, and can safely be given again in 4 h if necessary. In unusual instances, stronger sedation may be required. The clinical setting should meet all local and national regulatory guidelines for outpatient surgery with local anesthesia and the relevant level of sedation.

The most commonly used local anesthetics are lidocaine and bupivacaine. Epinephrine is routinely used to induce vasoconstriction in both the donor and recipient site, and to prolong the effect of the local anesthetic. It may be injected along with the local anesthetic or independently mixed at various concentrations. Standard lidocaine doses come as 0.5%, 1%, and 2%. Some surgeons feel that higher concentrations are more effective but this is based primarily on physician preference rather than evidence. Topical agents such as EMLA or lidocaine cream may be helpful as an adjunct to injectable anesthetics, but are likely unnecessary if other pain-reducing strategies are used.

Anatomic rationale for local anesthesia

The sensory nerve supply of the scalp travels to the hair-bearing scalp within the subcutaneous tissue layer from below via several named nerves (Fig. 10-18). The forehead and anterior scalp, for example, are supplied by the supratrochlear and supraorbital nerves which emerge at the level of the brow and travel superiorly. Because of this anatomy, injection of anesthesia anywhere on the scalp or forehead will cause anesthesia superior to the area injected. In addition, because of the anatomy, nerve blocks and ring blocks can be utilized to minimize the pain of injection in the blocked areas. Nerve blocks of the supratrochlear and supraorbital nerve, and less commonly the occipital nerve, are easily performed.

Dosages of local anesthesia

The maximal dose for lidocaine with epinephrine is roughly 7 mg/kg, although with tumescent anesthesia it increases to 35 mg/kg. The maximal dose of bupivacaine with epinephrine is considerably less at roughly 3 mg/kg. The patient's weight in kilograms, and a log of the total dose of lidocaine administered, should be kept through the case.

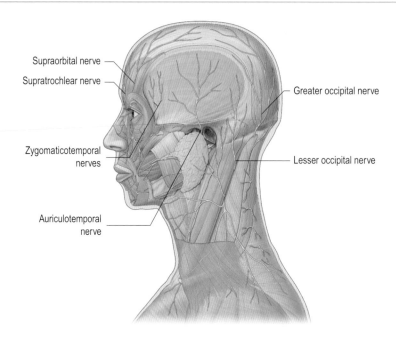

Supraorbital nerve

Supratrochlear nerve

Greater occipital nerve

Zygomaticotemporal nerves

Lesser occipital nerve

Auriculotemporal nerve

Figure 10-18 The nerve supply to the scalp travels in the skin inferior to superior. Any injection of anesthesia will thus generate anesthesia superior to the injection point. This logic underlies the use of nerve and ring blocks

Calculations of safe amounts of anesthesia can be made. For example, a 1% solution has 10 mg/mL lidocaine, so that 50 mL of 1% lidocaine contains 500 mg. Therefore, given a 7-mg/kg maximum dose, a 70-kg patient can safely receive 490 mg lidocaine with epinephrine (49 mL of 1% solution or 98 mL of 0.5% solution or 25 mL of 2% solution). Practitioners are expected to be able to prevent and treat the recognized toxicities of these agents.

Efforts should be made to employ techniques to minimize the amount of anesthetic used. Use of nerve blocks and ring blocks helps to reduce the total amount of anesthetic needed. Nerve blocks with marcaine are especially useful as they give prolonged anesthesia. Some practitioners mix marcaine with some of their lidocaine solutions for infiltration as well, but attention must be paid to possible additive toxicity. Reducing the concentration of lidocaine is helpful in reducing the total dose given to the patient. One of the authors uses 0.5% lidocaine with 1:200 000 epinephrine as a standard solution. This is commercially available and doubles the volume that can be given to a particular patient when compared with the more commonly used 1% lidocaine with 1:100 000 epinephrine. Tumescent anesthesia, allows large volumes of fluid to be infiltrated with minimal risk of toxicity.

Several techniques to reduce pain on infiltration of local anesthesia are noted below and summarized in Table 10-5. Practitioners can incorporate whichever techniques they feel helpful.

Donor site anesthesia

The donor site, usually in the occipital and sometimes temporal areas, is anesthetized first. Initial injections with either 1% or 0.5% lidocaine with epinephrine are placed along the area to be excised. This is followed by injection of tumescent anesthetic solution in volumes sufficient to tumesce the area to be excised, so that it feels firm along the length of the excision (Table 10-6).

Tumescence helps lift the skin and fat away from the occipital artery and nerve, minimizing possible transection of these structures, and also "stiffens" the tissue, minimizing follicular movement as the skin is excised and thereby reducing follicle transection. In addition, the use of the tumescent technique reduces bleeding from the donor site during the excision. Tumescent anesthesia lasts for hours – typically much longer than the duration of lidocaine in usual concentrations. It should be noted that normal saline can be substituted for tumescent anesthesia; it achieves the same physical benefits but without the anesthetic or hemostatic effects. Regardless of the type of anesthesia used, it is wise to allow 10–20 min for the anesthetic and epinephrine effect to take place.

Recipient site anesthesia

The recipient site is anesthetized after the donor site has been harvested. In some practices, the surgeon waits until the grafts have been prepared or nearly prepared prior to anesthetizing

Table 10-5 Tips to reduce pain of local anesthesia

Tip	Comment
Use nerve blocks where available	Supraorbital, Supratrochlear, Occipital
Use ring blocks on scalp	
Apply ice before injection	
Manipulate skin at needle entry site to distract pain fibers	Massage or vibration
Buffer local anesthetic	1 mL sodium bicarbonate (1 mEq/mL) added to 9 mL lidocaine
Use small-bore needles initially	30 G for initial injections. May use large gauge subsequently, so less difficulty pushing anesthesia
Inject from areas already anesthetized	Place needle into already anesthetized area and slowly push forward to areas not yet anesthetized
Use longer needles	1 inch or longer, so fewer needle sticks necessary
Use tumescent anesthesia	
Place needle into skin quickly and infiltrate slowly	Less pain in each case
Inject subcutaneously initially	Less pain than in the dermis

Table 10-6 Examples of tumescent anesthetic solutions for hair transplantation

To obtain: 0.1% lidocaine with 1:1 000 000 epinephrine	To obtain: 0.2% lidocaine with 1:500 000 epinephrine
Mix the following:	Mix the following:
• 100 mL normal saline	• 100 mL normal saline
• 10 mL 1% xylocaine plain	• 20 mL 1% xylocaine plain
• 1 mL sodium bicarbonate	• 1 mL sodium bicarbonate
• 0.1 mL epinephrine (1:1000)	• 0.2 mL epinephrine (1:1000)

anesthetized from the donor site anesthesia and needs no further injection.

Once the recipient area has been anesthetized with appropriate nerve blocks or ring blocks, further lidocaine with epinephrine or, less commonly epinephrine alone, may be injected painlessly throughout the recipient site to reinforce the anesthesia (lidocaine) and provide increased hemostasis (epinephrine). Many authors supplement the recipient site with injections of tumescent anesthesia. This technique may "swell" the subcutaneous tissue, allowing for decreased risk of transection of the supragaleal vascular plexus during recipient site creation. Tumescent anesthesia may also improve hemostasis in the recipient area.

Rationale for modern hair transplanting

Follicular units

In the early days of hair transplanting, grafts were excised using round punches of 3–4 mm in diameter containing large numbers of hairs. In the 1980s some surgeons would remove small pieces containing 1–3 hairs from these grafts to transplant in front of the hairline to decrease the abruptness of a punch-grafted hairline. Beginning in the 1980s it was recognized that hair commonly emerged from the human scalp in groupings of 1, 2, and 3 (and rarely 4 or 5) hairs surrounded by a common adventitia (Figs 10-19 & 10-20). These so-called "follicular units," or FUs, became the model for hair transplant surgeons who wished to achieve more natural results. The idea of removing donor hair by excision and dissecting out FUs with the aid of magnification (microscopy) revolutionized the field and became the new paradigm of modern hair transplantation.

Graft definitions and terminology

The basic unit of a hair transplant is a composite "graft" of epidermis, dermis, hair and follicle, and some surrounding soft tissue. Because of the shift

the recipient site. In other practices or with large sessions, transplanting the recipient site is begun while graft preparation is still not complete.

Anesthesia for the anterior scalp/hairline is initiated with bilateral nerve blocks of the supraorbital and supratrochlear nerves. An occipital nerve block may be helpful in some cases where the vertex will be transplanted. The injection site for an occipital block may be identified by identifying a depression in the skull 6.75 cm posterior to the insertion of the concha of the ear into the scalp above the mastoid. Use of bupivacaine for the nerve blocks is suggested as it produces anesthesia lasting for several hours.

A ring block using 0.5% or 1% lidocaine with epinephrine is then performed for the remaining areas of the scalp not anesthetized by the blocks. Ring blocks involve the injection initially of local anesthetic at points around the recipient area to create a circle of anesthesia within which further injection will then be painless. Long needles are then inserted into these already anesthetized points, and further anesthetic is slowly injected as the needle is advanced to create a ring of anesthesia linking the initial injection points in a ring around the recipient area. The portion of the recipient site in the posterior mid scalp is often

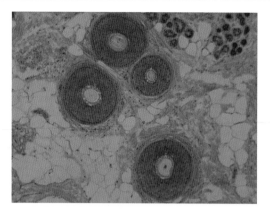

Figure 10-19 Horizontal sections of scalp show a 1- and a 3-haired follicular unit

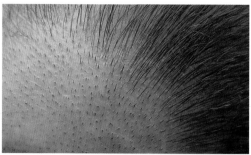

Figure 10-20 A section of shaved scalp showing the hairs emerging as 1-, 2-, 3-, and even 4-haired follicular units

in practice from round grafts obtained by a punch to FUs taken from an elliptical excision, a variety of confusing terminologies to describe grafts has evolved over the years. The terms noted in Table 10-7 are recommended by the authors to replace previous terms such as "minigraft" and "microgaft," which typically were used to describe small grafts obtained from punches or excisions without paying attention to preserving FUs or groupings of FUs.

It is important for physicians and patients to realize that it is difficult to compare results from modern hair transplant surgeries by simply considering the number of grafts transplanted. For example, a hair transplant using all FUs of 2000 grafts will move an average of 4000 hairs. At a different session or a case done by a different surgeon using some FUs and some multifollicular unit (MFU) grafts, the same number of hairs might be moved using 1400 grafts.

Donor site harvesting

Estimating the size of donor strip needed

Typically the donor site is harvested from the occipital and posterior temporal scalp from areas expected to maintain their hair indefinitely. It is possible mathematically to estimate the length of the necessary donor strip by knowing: (a) the density of FUs and thus grafts in the donor area, (b) the width and length of the proposed donor strip, (c) the density of grafting that will be attempted for each proposed recipient area, and (d) the total surface area to be transplanted.

Density of FUs in donor scalp

The average number of FUs per square centimeter on the nonbalding scalp is 100 FU/cm^2 (reported ranges between 60 and 140 FU/cm^2). Patients with less natural density will fall on the

Table 10-7 Recommended graft terminology	
Term	**Description**
Follicular unit (FU)	A grouping of 1, 2, 3, or 4 hairs surrounded by a common adventitia
Round graft (punch graft)	Grafts harvested using a punch of various sizes
Follicular unit graft (FUG)	A graft containing an intact follicular unit (1–4 hairs), usually dissected under magnification
Multifollicular unit (MFU) graft (MUG)	A graft containing 2 or more hairs that arise from adjacent FUs. These may have more hairs than FUs and thus provide more density per graft
Follicular unit pairing	The placement of more than 1 FUG or MUG into a single recipient site to obtain increased density
Follicular unit extraction (FUE)	A technique of harvesting FUGs individually from the donor site rather than from an excised strip

lower ends of the above ranges. In most patients, the majority of FUs are 2–hairs, with only about 20% arising as 1-haired FUs.

In most patients there are approximately 2–2.5 hairs per follicular unit in the nonbalding occipital scalp. The density of FUs/cm^2 can be calculated quite precisely for the individual patient after shaving a portion of the donor site and counting FUs in one or two 1-cm^2 areas with magnification, or more easily with a densitometer. With time, experienced practitioners can estimate the donor site density on inspection.

Width and length of the donor strip

The length of the donor strip can be increased to include the entire occipital scalp and posterior temples if needed for very large sessions, although for many transplant sessions only the occipital scalp needs to be harvested. The width of the donor strip is limited by the need to be able to close the excisional defect primarily, with minimal tension in order to minimize donor scarring. Although wider strips can be taken in many patients (especially on the first session), the authors recommend up to a 1.0-cm width in the occipital area as being virtually always safe (going up to 1.2 cm), with 0.8 cm as the width in the temporal areas. More conservative widths may be necessary in repeat transplants when excising through scar tissue.

Density of grafting in area to be transplanted

This is covered later in this chapter, but, for the beginning practitioner, aiming for an average density of 25–30 FU/cm^2 in a single session is reasonable for most areas of the bald scalp. It should be remembered that the normal nonbald scalp has hair density ranging from 60 to 140 FU/cm^2, and that hair at 50% of normal density may still appear as normal density to the observer. Therefore, final transplanted densities of 30–70 FU/cm^2 in any given area will give the illusion of very good density in most patients. Given the fact that donor sites are limited and that most patients will be happy with a final look that is thinner than original, densities of 25–30 FU/cm^2 in a single session are certainly likely to satisfy most patients.

The density needed to produce good results is also influenced by hair color and hair shaft diameter. With experience and a larger team, larger sessions and densities per session can be attempted, especially in critical areas such as the frontal tuft. Of course, transplanting areas with remaining terminal hair will require less density, and this can be estimated as well.

The total area to be transplanted in the session

This is decided at the consultation. For example, it is a common scenario in a man with moderate to more advanced balding to limit transplanting to the hairline and anterior scalp in the first session. The use of rulers or grids can estimate the surface area to be treated more precisely.

Sample calculation for a hypothetical case

Assume that one desires to transplant a bald scalp for a total of 60 cm^2 (e.g. hairline and anterior to mid scalp). The goal is to transplant an average of 25 FU/cm^2 density throughout. The donor strip will be 1 cm wide throughout. The patient has roughly 80 FU/cm^2 in the occipital area.

In this example, the number of FUs needed is: 60 cm^2 × 25 FU/cm^2 = 1500 FU. The length of a 1-cm wide strip needed to achieve this is: 1500 FU ÷ 80 FU/cm^2 = 18.75 cm in length. For more calculations, see Tables 10-8 & 10-9.

It should be noted that the number of total grafts will be less than the calculated FUs, if MFUs are to be used for some of the transplant. The calculations above should also be adjusted to account for:

- possible loss of grafts (e.g. by transection)
- the fact that some areas will require more density than others (e.g. higher densities to be transplanted in the frontal forelock area, or the patient's part side).

Table 10-8 Estimating the number of FUs needed based on planned density and area planned for treatment

Area to be transplanted (cm^2)	No. of FUs needed for average density of:		
	25 FU/cm^2	30 FU/cm^2	40 FU/cm^2
20	500	600	800
25	625	750	1000
30	750	900	1200
60	1500	1800	2400

Table 10-9 Estimating the length of a 1-cm wide donor strip based on the number of FUs needed and density of donor site

No. of FUs needed	Length (cm) of 1-cm wide strip with donor site density of:		
	60 FU/cm^2	80 FU/cm^2	100 FU/cm^2
800	13.3	10	8
1200	20	15	12
1500	25	18.75	15
2000	33	25	20

Table 10-10 Limits of safe occipital and temporal donor area

Boundary	Description
Anterior limit at temporal scalp	Line perpendicular drawn at level of external auditory canal
Superior limit at temporal scalp	6–7.0 cm above point where superior crus of pinna joins scalp
Superior limit at occipital scalp	Marked by horizontal line drawn from point 2 cm above where crus of ear meets posterior scalp
Inferior limit at midline of the occiput	Level of occipital notch

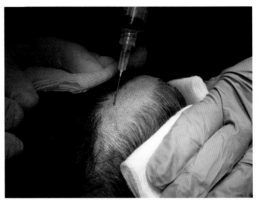

Figure 10-22 The donor site is tumesced until turgid to reduce follicle transection during excision, raise skin away from occipital vessels and nerves, and increase hemostasis

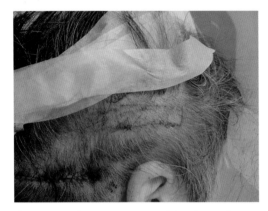

Figure 10-21 An extra, separate excision of a smaller strip at the temple is made after the initial occipital incision was felt to yield too few hairs for the planned recipient area. If needed, the temple incision is usually made as a connected extension of the occipital excision

Where to take the strip: the safe donor zone

The "safe" donor area is that portion of the occipital and temporal scalp that is not likely to lose hair with progression of the patient's MPHL or FPHL. Both the lower nuchal occipital hair and the superior occipital hair are at risk for loss with age. Excising a strip will cause two problems if that area proceeds to alopecia: (a) a visible scar once the hair no longer camouflages it, and (b) possible loss of the transplanted hairs in the recipient area.

Several guidelines for the safe area exist. A detailed family history may help guide the decision as well as the patient's age (younger patients being much harder to predict). An important number to keep in mind is that the average balding male has between 5000 and 7000 FUs safely available for transplantation. The authors' guidelines are shown in Table 10-10.

In general, the authors first choice for the strip is centered at the level of the occipital protuberance.

One should avoid going into the neck (i.e. below the level of scalp at which the galea ceases). Additional harvesting in the temples can be used if necessary: (a) for large sessions requiring many FUs or in patients with lower density, and (b) to obtain hair that is possibly finer and will gray at the same pace as the original frontotemporal hair (Fig. 10-21).

Taking the strip: technique

The donor site is marked and clipped. It is recommended to leave the donor hair 3–4 mm long so that:

- the direction of the hair can be seen during excision/harvesting
- the visible hair sticking up will reduce the chance of inadvertently burying a graft while planting
- the hair gives the planters an atraumatic place to hold the graft while planting.

Anesthesia is next obtained and the area should be tumesced with saline or tumescent lidocaine until turgid (Fig. 10-22) (see section in chapter on anesthesia). Excision can be done with a multi-blade scalpel (Fig. 10-23) to speed up the dissection of the strip later as it is already partly divided. However, because of the documented significant increase in FU transection with this approach, most practitioners prefer to excise the strip as an undivided thin rectangle with tapered ends.

The excision should be carried out to a depth of 1–2 mm below the hair follicles. The direction of the blade should change to remain constantly parallel to the follicles, to reduce transection. Frequent inspection of the strip while cutting helps insure this is done with loupes while the assistant provides counter-traction with a hook or clamp of some kind. These steps are shown in Figure 10-24.

The strip is then handed to the technicians and bleeding cauterized (usually minimal).

Although some surgeons advocate undermining to facilitate closure, this is rarely necessary with appropriately wide donor strips, and is almost never done by the authors. The excision is then sutured closed. Most surgeons prefer layered closure and one of the authors uses a 4-0

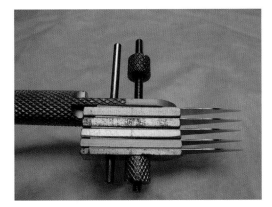

Figure 10-23 A multi-blade scalpel for donor site harvesting with adjustable spacers allowing the excision to be removed with four strips of variable width. There is increased transection of hair follicles with this approach

Vicryl buried suture followed by a meticulous running subcuticular suture with 3-0 polypropylene with small bites to minimize trauma to surrounding hairs. Choice of suture is as per surgeon preference.

The donor site should be immediately hidden by the remaining donor site hair. Some surgeons advocate a so-called trichophytic closure in which a 1-mm wide strip of the inferior wound margin is de-epithelialized and covered by the superior margin of the wound during closure. This may allow hair to grow through the scar, possibly increasing its camouflage. This technique is shown in Figure 10-25. An appropriately sized donor site can be expected to heal well and quickly in most cases, being easily camouflaged by existing hair immediately after the transplant as long as the hair is not too short (Fig. 10-26).

When harvesting a donor site in a patient who has had previous linear donor site excision, the authors prefer to incorporate the previous scar in the new excision, either in the middle or at the inferior border of the new strip. If this approach is taken, it will leave only one scar in the donor area. Because scar tissue may limit movement, it may be wise to err on the side of caution and take thinner strips on subsequent re-excisions.

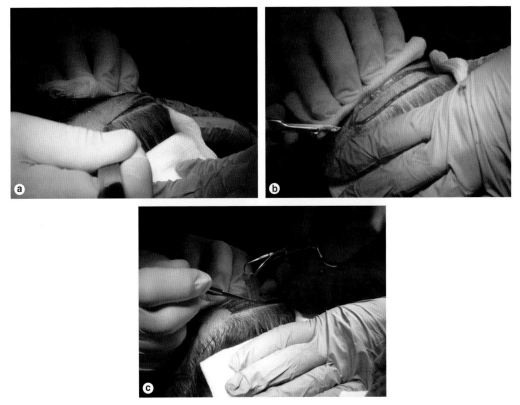

Figure 10-24 (A) The donor strip is first incised, making sure the blade is parallel to the hair follicles. (B) The donor strip is completely incised and ready for removal from scalp. (C) The strip is removed 1–2 mm below the level of the follicle bulb, taking care to avoid transection of the hair follicle or to cut too deeply and damage the occipital vessels or nerves

Follicular unit extraction

Traditional strip harvesting techniques usually result in a fine linear donor scar. Occasionally a less than ideal, wider than desired, scar will result. An alternative to strip harvesting employs a small traditional punch biopsy trephine, 0.7–1.0 mm in diameter, to excise 1- or 2-haired grafts directly as FUs from the donor area. The donor area can be the scalp or any other haired body part, as illustrated in Figure 10-27.

One technique involves using a standard 1-mm diameter sharp biopsy punch, incising approximately 2 mm into the dermis. The skin surrounding the graft is pressed down as the graft is grasped and pulled out with gentle traction. The resulting core is left to heal by secondary intention. The aim is to remove the graft without amputating the distal follicle. However, damage to the graft can occur with transection of the base of the follicle. A second step can be added to graft removal. Once the graft has been cored, the more distal portion of the graft can be dissected from the surrounding tissue, using a fine needle while gentle traction is exerted on the proximal end of the graft.

Owing to the high rate of follicular transection possible with this technique, a three-step technique has been developed. The epidermis is scored to a depth of 0.3–0.5 mm with a sharp 1-mm punch, and then, rather than cut through the entire full thickness to remove the graft, a dissecting, blunt punch is inserted over the initial scored graft gently to separate the graft from the surrounding dermal tissue. The intent of this approach is to avoid transection of the graft and allow for complete, easy, extraction of an intact FU.

Follicular unit extraction (FUE) has several disadvantages that have thus far precluded its routine use:

- FUE is technically more difficult to perform without transecting grafts or inadvertently burying donor portions of the donor hair follicle at the time of attempted harvest.
- It is slower, with fewer grafts typically harvested in a session.
- Donor scars may be problematic, especially if taken from areas of the body (e.g. keloid risk if taken from chest).

Nevertheless, FUE may have limited use in the following scenarios:

- Patients who wish to shave their heads in the future and do not want the linear scar.

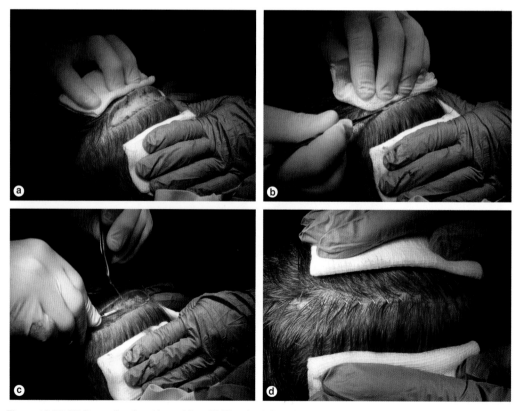

Figure 10-25 (A) Donor site after strip excision. (B) Trimming inferior border of wound at 45° angle to create a triangular strip, 1 × 1 mm, which will de-epithelialize one or two follicular units. (C) De-epithelializing the strip. (D) Following closure

- Patients with excessive donor scarring where there is difficulty in harvesting a strip.
- Patients with limited areas to transplant (e.g. scar, eyebrow).
- Patients who wish to use hair from other body areas (chest, back, arms, legs, feet, and beard), which may on occasion be a better match in character or in length of expected hair growth.

These indications and disadvantages are summarized in Table 10-11.

Graft preparation

Technique

Once the donor strip has been harvested, it is placed in chilled saline and handed to the technicians for dissection into FUs and MFUs. The ellipse is first cut into smaller strips under magnification in a process called "slivering" (Fig. 10-28). At all times, care is taken to cut between follicular units to avoid transaction.

The smaller slivers are then further dissected into FUs and MFUs by other technicians working in parallel (Fig. 10-29). Some technicians use scalpel blades (e.g. #10 or #11), whereas others prefer one-sided razor blades for this task. A small amount of surrounding adventitial tissue should be left around the follicles to maintain viability; some surgeons prefer more tissue ("chubby" grafts – Fig. 10-30), and others prefer less ("skinny" grafts). Chubby grafts may be more viable, although use of these grafts decreases the density of recipient sites that can be made, as skinny grafts can be placed in smaller sites.

Magnification is indispensable to avoid transaction of follicles and loss of viable hair. Backlighting of the strip is very helpful and commercially available backlighting platforms are sold by most instrument suppliers. Stereomicroscopes are now used routinely by some or all technicians in hair transplanting cases (Fig. 10-31). One published study showed a 17% greater yield of hair due to reduced transection rate when microscopes were used compared to loupes, and another showed a reduction of transection of 10% when using the

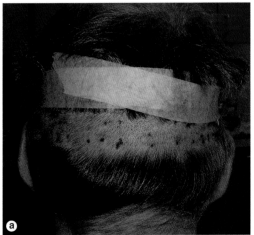
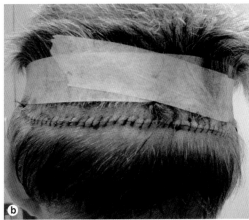
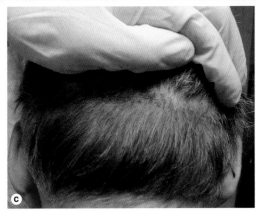

Figure 10-26 (A) Donor site shaved and ready for harvesting. (B) Donor site immediately after harvesting and suturing; can be covered by the hair above the site. (C) Donor site at suture removal 14 days after surgery

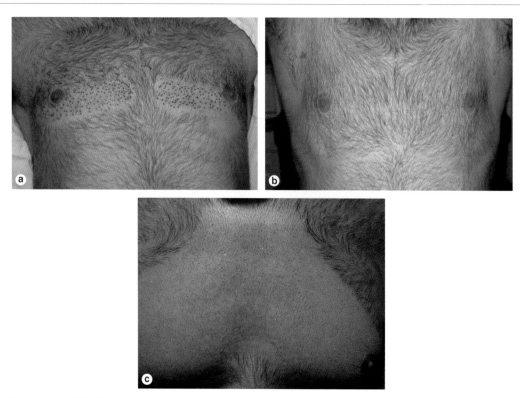

Figure 10-27 (A) Follicular unit extraction sites made at time of procedure using a 1.0-mm disposable punch trephine. (B) Ten days after surgery, showing sites healing by secondary intention. (C) Close-up of healed sites

Table 10-11 Follicular unit extraction	
Possible "indications" for FUE	Disadvantages of FUE
Avoid linear donor site scar	Technically difficult to do without transection and ingrown follicles
Excessive scarring at donor site precludes further excision	Time consuming
Patients with limited areas to transplant	Fewer grafts per session
Desire to harvest nonscalp hair	Possible problems with secondary intention healing of donor site

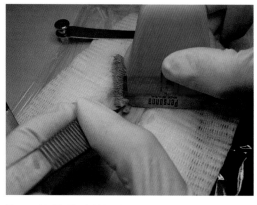

Figure 10-28 The initial strip is dissected into smaller "slivers" under magnification. These will then be further dissected into FU and MFU grafts

microscope compared with 20% without. Examples of commonly used microscopes include the Zeiss Stemi DV4, Mantis, Leica M Series (pick as quality varies), Nikon SMZ645, Olympus SZ40 Series, Motic K500P, K700HI, and the Mantis Stereomicroscope (Fig. 10-32). The reader is referred to the website www.microscopyu.com for further information relevant to choosing a microscope. It is likely that some experienced technicians can achieve excellent results with loupes alone. Because microscopes are ergonomically more uncomfortable, in some practices the initial slivering is done with a microscope and the subsequent preparation of FUs and MFUs is done with loupe magnification (Fig. 10-33).

As the grafts are prepared, the technicians should place them in continually chilled saline (Fig. 10-34). Grafts should be sorted by size, number of hairs, and quality so that they can be counted (allowing an estimate of how many different sized recipient sites will be needed) (Fig. 10-35). It is wise to keep the finest 1-haired FUs separate for the anterior hairline.

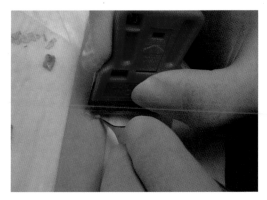

Figure 10-29 Follicular units are dissected from the initial slivers

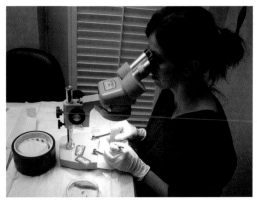

Figure 10-31 Technician using a stereomicroscope to sliver the initial donor strip

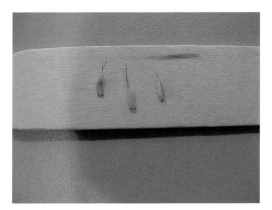

Figure 10-30 Examples of 1-, 2-, and 3-haired FU grafts. The fairly robust amount of adventitia and fat left on these grafts (particularly the 1-haired FU) would classify these as "chubby" grafts

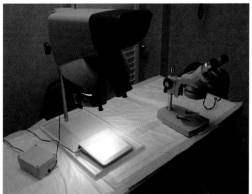

Figure 10-32 Examples of microscopes used in hair transplanting. *Left:* Mantis stereomicroscope with uplighter. *Right:* A Meiji microscope

Principles of graft care

Causes of reduced viability of grafts include:

- transection of follicles
- desiccation
- prolonged time at room temperature
- crushing.

Transection can occur at donor site harvesting, initial slivering of the donor strip, and graft cutting into FUs and MFUs. Studies have shown that a partially transected hair may still grow, but at a far reduced rate (and with lesser diameter) than an intact hair. For this reason transection should be avoided at each step in the transplant.

Desiccation is considered to be a major source of graft compromise, and grafts should be held until ready for planting in chilled saline at all times (e.g. Petri dish on top of ice packs). Once removed from the saline they should be planted quickly. Many believe that cooling the grafts prolongs viability. Care should be taken at all times not to crush the grafts, especially when planting.

Shaving or clipping the donor site, with attention paid to leaving 3–4 mm of hair sticking out of the donor skin before harvesting, will later allow the hair to be used to help safely grasp the FUs during handling. Likewise, leaving a small amount of fat below the hair bulb will reduce crush as the grafts are inserted.

Recipient site creation technique

Graft orientation in anterior and mid scalp: coronal versus sagittal

Sagittal, or parallel, angle grafting (SAG) has been the standard orientation for the incisions made when transplanting the frontal scalp. Natural hair direction is such that hair grows in a forward direction at the frontal scalp. Incisions, either with a blade or needle, are made to reflect this natural forward direction of hair growth and are oriented parallel to the intended direction of hair growth.

Coronal, or perpendicular, angle grafting (CAG) is a newer technique whereby incisions made when transplanting the frontal scalp are made perpendicular to the forward or anterior direction of hair growth. These orientations are illustrated in Figure 10-36. The rationale behind using CAG is that, on close inspection of the scalp, the FUs tend to orient not in an anterior/posterior pattern, but in a side-by-side pattern with the long axis arranged perpendicular to the direction of hair growth (Fig. 10-37).

Proponents of CAG note the following as advantages:

- FUs placed in a parallel incision will exit from the skin one behind another and, when viewed from the front or from above, they will line up this way leaving the appearance of less fullness, analogous to looking at a single row of people from the front. Additionally, the hair tends to stand up, with one hair lying against another. FUs placed in perpendicular incisions (CAG) will grow side by side at a

right angle to the hair direction. This allows for the hair to lie more flat against the skin and also give the appearance of more fullness when viewed from the front, analogous to a single row of people viewed from the side.
- Because a smaller chisel, rectangular, flat-edged blade is used to create CAG (0.6–1.2 mm in width), there is less penetration of the blade into the skin. This can lead to less injury to the local vasculature in the recipient site, which may allow for more dense packing of grafts without vascular compromise, as well as less bleeding. In the parallel incisions used in SAG, the depth created by incision of a needle or angled blade is not uniform and is deeper at the maximum point of entry.

Requirements for perpendicular angle grafting (CAG) include the following:

- As this technique is more inherently difficult, employing very small blades, higher densities, and numbers of grafts, it is strongly suggested that the surgeon have experience with SAG and dense packing first.
- Small 0.6–1.2-mm chisel blades.
- Recipient site tumescence (1 : 100 000 epinephrine).
- The use of "skinny" FUs (compared with "chubby" FUs).
- A greater possible need to shave the recipient area to assist in creating the very large number of small recipient sites.

Instruments

The decision of whether to choose needles or flat blades to create the recipient sites with FU grafting is physician dependent and based on the size of graft employed. Round and slot punches can

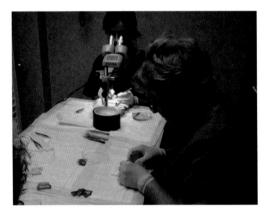

Figure 10-33 One technician slivering with a microscope while a second cuts grafts from the slivers using magnifying loupes

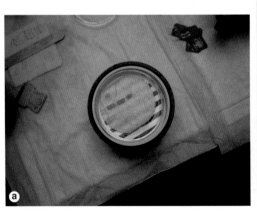
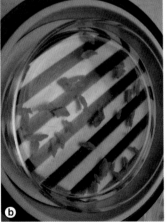

Figure 10-34 The initial slivers (A) and the subsequently cut grafts (B) should be kept in chilled saline at all times until just before transplantation

be used to make recipient sites that will accept MFUs and mini-grafts away from the hairline. Figure 10-38 illustrates the most common sizes and instruments used.

Needles

Needles are color coded and beveled. The commonly used sizes range from 18 to 22 gauge. Also available are color-coded solid needles with no central core. Owing to the lack of a central core there is no debris picked up in transfer during site creation, with concomitantly less risk of blood exposure from the accidental needlesticks.

The advantages of needles are:

- They are relatively inexpensive.
- The bevel aids in planting grafts.
- They can be useful for both perpendicular (CAG) and parallel (SAG) grafting.
- They provide dilatation when stick and place techniques are used.

Blades

Angled blades come to a point either in the midline (Spearpoint) or laterally (Minde, Sharpoint, Noker, custom-cut blades) (Fig. 10-39). They tend

to be sharper than needles, but do not offer much dilatation. Angled blades are used primarily for SAG when the cutting edge is angled such that the incision is made parallel to the intended direction of hair growth. Chisel blades are flat rectangular blades, which are primarily used for CAG when the cutting surface of the blade is angled perpendicular to the intended direction of hair growth. These blades are not suggested for SAG because, if used parallel to hair growth, when the incision is made, the leading edge can disturb blood vessels of the deeper supragaleal plexus.

The ability to control the depth of a recipient incision is important in order to minimize damage to the supragaleal vascular plexus. The Minde blades come with a handle that aids in depth control. Blade-holder handles (Fig. 10-40), or special handles designed to hold needles, can be used for blades or needles that come without handles. Figure 10-41 shows a needle driver being used as a blade holder. For blade holders or needle drive

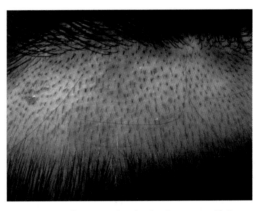

Figure 10-37 Close-up of scalp showing perpendicular orientation of FUs. Note that hair direction is superior–inferior, but hairs within the 2- and 3-haired FUs line up left to right (perpendicular to hair direction)

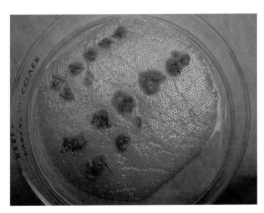

Figure 10-35 Grafts are counted, placed in uniform "piles" of a predetermined number, and kept sorted according to size and/or number of FUs

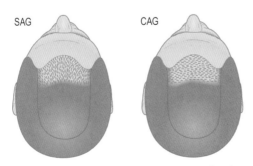

SAG CAG

Figure 10-36 Diagram showing the orientation of graft sites for traditional sagittal angle grafting (SAG) and the more recently described coronal angle grafting (CAG)

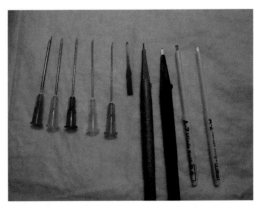

Figure 10-38 Examples of color-coded beveled needles (6, 18, 19, 20, and 21 G) commonly used to make recipient sites commonly used. Also shown are spear-tipped mini blades, flat-bladed chisels, and the Minde knife (1.8 and 3.0 mm)

| Angled blade | Angled blade | Chisel |
| midline point | lateral point | blade |

Figure 10-39 Examples of blades used to create recipient sites. (A) Angled blade with a central point. (B) Angled blade with a lateral point. (C) Chisel or flat blade

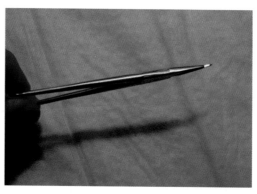

Figure 10-41 Needle driver being used as a graft holder that has been sized to the length of graft to be implanted

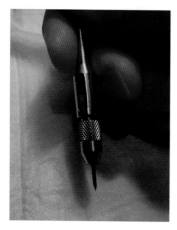

Figure 10-40 Example of a blade-holder

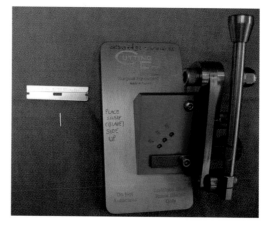

Figure 10-42 Example of a commercially available custom blade cutter, showing the device as well as the blade that is used to cut into smaller blades of custom widths

holders, maximal depth can be adjusted. A sample of a graft is used to estimate the required depth, and the blade is clamped onto the blade holder or needle driver at the appropriate depth.

A custom blade cutter (Fig. 10-42) is available that allows the surgeon to cut chisel-type and laterally angled blades to a variety of sizes ranging from 0.6 to 2.0 mm in 0.1-mm increments. These custom-made blades are thinner and possibly sharper than the usual pre-made blades, and are an inexpensive alternative once the cost of the blade cutter has been absorbed.

The forceps used for placing grafts (Fig. 10-43) need to have very fine tips so as to not injure or crush the graft. Jeweler's forceps are an example; they can be straight or curved. Owing to the fragile nature of their tips, which can be easily bent when cleaning, it is suggested that a rubber tip or plastic guard that can be sterilized be placed over the tip. Forceps with a disposable tip can also be obtained.

Some physicians advocate the use of multi-blade recipient devices as they can speed up the rate of making incisions and create a systematic grid work (Fig. 10-44). Because they can cut existing hair, these devices are limited in usefulness to areas that have virtually no preexisting hair.

The Choi implanter is an example of an automatic graft-placing instrument that is shaped like a pen. It is preloaded with one graft with each

use. An incision is made with the device and, as it is spring loaded, the graft is then injected into the site.

Transplanting a natural hairline zone

The actual creation of a natural hairline with grafts is best described as creating a zone of gradually increasing hair density, so as to mimic a natural hairline "zone." The observer's eye is drawn to abrupt lines and hairlines that are overall too symmetric or contrived. Natural irregularities need to be established, and with the use of 1- and 1–2-haired FUs this can be achieved. Macro and micro irregularities can be created to soften the hairline and avoid an abrupt transition to the more densely, posteriorly transplanted, grafts. The anterior hairline is thus seen as a zone, approximately 5–10 mm in width, starting as single, erratically placed, 1-haired FUs, blending into small peaks and valleys created using 3–6 single FUs (Fig. 10-45).

In a similar way, an anterior "transition" zone (0.5–1.0 cm) behind which lies a "defined" zone (2–3 cm in depth) can be defined for the

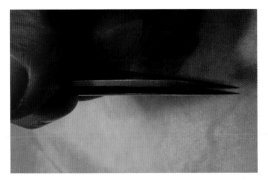

Figure 10-43 Placing a jeweler's forceps

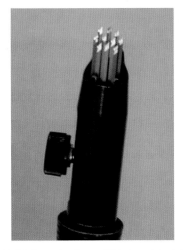

Figure 10-44 Example of a multi-blade recipient device. Courtesy of Sharon Keene MD

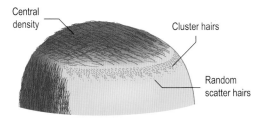

Figure 10-45 Creating a hairline zone. Anteriorly, groups of three to five 1-haired FUs are created in the shape of a triangle, placed irregularly in front of the increasingly more densely planted hairline zone posteriorly. As a last step, randomly placed, eccentric, 1-haired FUs are scattered

hairline. The central anterior scalp is termed the "frontal tuft" area. The transition zone is transplanted anteriorly with the finest 1-haired FUs, and posteriorly with 1–2-haired FUs. The defined zone receives 2–3-haired FUs anteriorly and multi-FUs more posteriorly, as indicated. Density is concentrated in the frontal tuft area. Figure 10-46 shows a hairline following incision placement illustrating these points.

Larger fluctuations in the hairline can be made by using a number of small FUs to create mounds,

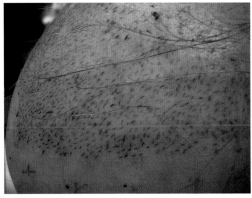

Figure 10-46 Bald frontal scalp following placement of recipient sites at first session of 1349 FUs and MFUs. Note the attempt to produce irregularities at the hairline, and that the recipient site sizes are smaller anteriorly and larger posteriorly. This helps to feather the hairline and allows placement posteriorly of larger MFUs for more hair density/graft

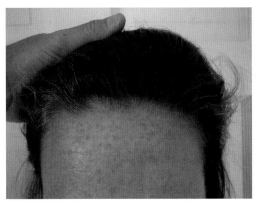

Figure 10-47 A natural hairline showing a widow's peak that adds irregularity to the hairline when seen at a distance

such as a widow's peak, that are more easily appreciated at a distance (Fig. 10-47).

Possible frontal scalp patterns

The following scenarios illustrate three possible patterns for the creation of the frontal recipient area.

SAG using a combination of FUs and MFUs

- This technique can be used by the physician who is a beginner or does not perform hair transplantation as a majority of their practice.
- Example: 1200 grafts – 600 1–3-haired FUs and 600 4–6-haired MFUs); approximately 4200 hairs.
- The least number of technicians is required.
- Can be completed in 3–4 h with well trained staff.

SAG using all FUs

- With the use of all single 1–3-haired FUs, there is a requirement for a greater number of grafts to fill an area and to achieve the illusion of density, by packing the grafts more densely.
- Example: 2100 grafts (all 1–3-haired FUs); approximately 4200 hairs. (Note: The same number of hairs transferred as with the above pattern).
- Requires more technicians to dissect donor tissue into all FUs.
- Longer operating time required to dissect tissue and plant grafts.
- Greater need for stick and place as graft numbers go up, and packing of grafts becomes tighter.

CAG

- Inherently the most difficult.
- Greater tendency for poor growth if not performed correctly.
- Greater need for tumescence.
- Need for all skinny FUs, made with flat-edged chisel blades.
- Requirement for higher numbers of technicians and longer operating time.

Reconstituting the whorl in the vertex

In a natural scalp there is a well defined whorl of hair direction change. If the entire vertex is to be transplanted, the center of the whorl needs to be identified. If there is any amount of even fine vellus hair present, a single whorl can be reconstituted based on the identified direction of the original hair. If the area is completely bald, an arbitrary whorl can be created.

The grafts are oriented in such a fashion as to radiate out in a 360° direction from the center (Fig. 10-48). Graft selection starts with 1-haired FUs at the eye of the whorl, followed by 2–3-haired FUs radiating outwards. Adequate coverage and density can usually be achieved with a single session. It is the authors' experience that patients often desire reasonable density to the frontal scalp and are happy with light coverage to the crown, avoiding a totally bald dome.

It should be noted that scalp reductions, extenders, and expanders are all techniques to minimize the alopecic area of the vertex with the intent of conserving donor scalp and achieving better overall scalp coverage. These techniques are beyond the scope of this chapter, and the reader is directed to other reference sources (Brandy 2002, Seery et al 2004).

Making the incisions

Once a decision on graft orientation (CAG versus SAG versus whorl) has been made for the area to be transplanted and anesthesia has been obtained, the surgeon may make the recipient sites.

General tips

Use of the tumescent technique in the recipient area may allow for more density as the tumescence stretches the skin, allowing incision placement. Once the incisions have been made and the tumescence has dissipated, the skin shrinks and the density of the sites increases. Loupes are indispensable, particularly when transplanting an area with still-existing hair.

Preparation with povidone–iodine (Betadine) will stiffen the existing hair, making it easier to move aside when looking for gaps in which to make incisions. It is helpful for the assistant continually to clean the field of any blood and judiciously brush aside any existing hair, so that the surgeon can see where to make the next incision.

The assistant should keep a running tally of the number and sizes of the sites made. This will allow the surgeon to make sure that the incision sites are appropriately distributed to match the actual or expected number of grafts for the planned areas to be treated.

Size of instrument

Blade or needle sizes used to make the incisions will vary depending on the size of the FUs and MFUs to be planted, and whether they have been cut skinny or chubby. As an example, the small 1–2-haired FUs that will be used in the anterior hairline in most transplants can be placed in holes made by a 19-G needle or comparable blade. Custom blade sizes of 0.7–0.9 mm may be used for grafts of this size.

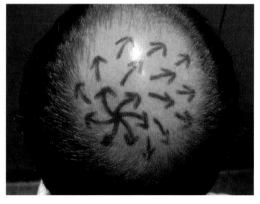

Figure 10-48 Arrows indicated direction of graft placement such that transplanted hairs will radiate out from center of newly created whorl

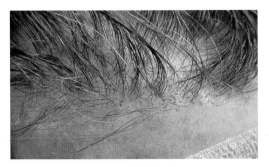

Figure 10-49 When transplanting hair-bearing skin, incisions are made parallel to and between the existing terminal hairs to avoid transection

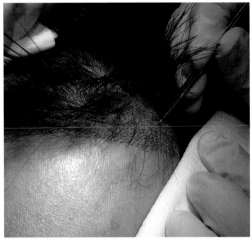

Figure 10-51 Planting the graft after all sites have been made. Two or three surgical assistants can plant at the same time. A jeweler's forceps is being used

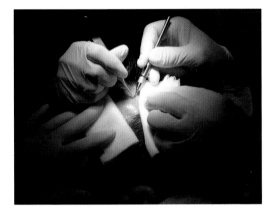

Figure 10-50 Planting the grafts using "stick and place." The physician or assistant makes the site and the graft is then implanted immediately

Angle of placement

This is a critical point. The angle of the incisions should always be made between and parallel to any existing terminal hairs to avoid transecting the existing follicles (Fig. 10-49). In situations where the recipient site hair is miniaturized and very fine, it may be reasonable to transplant through those hairs rather than around them on the assumption that they are contributing little cosmetically and are likely soon to be lost. The surgeon should be aware that these angles change depending on location (e.g. the hair emerges nearly flat at a very short angle in the temple or eyebrow). Even in a very bald patient there are usually some stray hairs to help in identifying the proper hair angle.

In areas where the existing hair is completely unavailable for guidance, it should be noted that the natural angle of hair in the frontal hairline is about 30–45°. As the incisions are made from the center towards the temporolateral angle, there should be a gradual transition in direction from pointing forward to pointing more down and posterior, along with a gradual decrease in angle to more acute.

"Stick and place"

In many practices the incisions are made first followed by graft placement. In some cases it is advantageous to use the "stick and place" method in which the physician or technician makes a site with a needle (18–27 G) or small blade and, as soon as the needle has been removed, the graft is immediately inserted (Fig. 10-50). This technique may be especially helpful at the end of a case when there are a few grafts left over without obvious recipient sites to place them.

Planting the grafts

Planting the grafts can be done by two or three technicians at one time, sitting on either side of the patient. The sites can then be planted (Fig. 10-51). Grafts should be kept moist or completely immersed in cooled saline. Dehydration during planting can lead to significant graft failure. Typically a few grafts are removed from the cooled Petri dish at a time and placed on the finger of the technician's nondominant surgical glove, from which they are individually and quickly removed for placement in the recipient site.

Grafts should not be allowed to sink below the surface of the skin. Otherwise, another graft may be inadvertently placed on top of the graft (called piggybacking), and an inclusion cyst may ensue. Existing hair in the recipient site should be combed aside frequently to make sure it has not been "trapped" in a recipient site under a planted graft. One larger recipient site may on occasion be filled with two small FU grafts (follicular pairing), taking care not to bury either graft. Figure 10-52 shows an anterior scalp transplant just completed in a man.

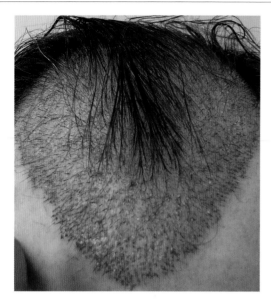

Figure 10-52 Appearance following completion of graft planting

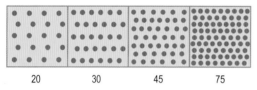

20   30   45   75

Figure 10-53 Representation of graft density. Dots have been placed at 20, 30, 45, and 70 FU/cm²

Table 10-12 Disadvantages of "megasessions" with dense packing

Disadvantage	Comment
More risk of vascular disruption and poor growth	Technically more difficult to perform without vascular disruption
Requires more time and/or technicians to complete the case	Works well in practice with many technicians, but otherwise prolonged time required may compromise graft survival
More difficult to plant	Large number of grafts in a small area may lead to more popping out of adjacent graft when new graft placed just next door
May require patient to shave recipient area	It is difficult to dense-pack between existing long hairs
Requires "skinny" grafts	Technically more difficult to obtain without compromising graft. Studies show possible decreased survival of skinny grafts
Longer day for patient	May require more anesthetic or sedatives and inactivity, theoretically increasing risk of safety issues (e.g. deep vein thrombosis)

"Dense packing"

The decision as to how many follicular units to plant and how densely to plant them can vary with the surgeon and patient. Certain areas of the recipient area (e.g. the mid-frontal forelock area) may be transplanted more densely than the rest of the hairline to mimic a natural pattern of hair growth and allow for good camouflage with combing. Densities greater than 30–35 FU/cm² in a single session are considered to be "dense packing."

Once the physician has gained sufficient experience, dense packing over 35 FU/cm² can be considered in certain areas, although it is important to keep in mind that consistently excellent results can also be obtained with sessions transplanted at densities of less than 30–35 FU/cm². Figure 10-53 gives a representation of creating recipient sites at 20, 30, 45, and 70 FU/cm². It is suggested that the novice physician gain experience in creating incisions at various densities.

Practices employing routine dense packing may typically transplant key areas in the 40–50 FU/cm² range, with some surgeons achieving 60 FU/cm² and higher. As the density of transplanted FUs increases, technical performance is more difficult, and a major concern with higher numbers of densely packed grafts is graft survival. This is attributed mainly to vascular compromise with the increased number of incisions in a confined area.

The major reason for incorporating dense packing into a practice is to maximize the density achievable in a single session, and possibly to increase the appearance of naturalness after a single session. The benefit of potentially reducing the number of sessions is clear, but for many surgeons excellent results can be routinely obtained with less density per session. It is important to remember that the recipient sites and graft sizes of necessity must be small in dense packing. Use of MFUs can give increased density with fewer recipient sites. Many of the difficulties or disadvantages that come with dense packing of large areas, and large or "megasessions," are primarily technical; however, these are not insignificant for most practices (Table 10-12).

PEARL

Technique for the novice

It is recommended that initially surgeons begin with a simpler technique, limited to the front one-third of the scalp.

It is recommended that the practitioner use a 19-G needle or comparably sized blade, creating recipient sites at moderate densities of 25–35 FU/cm².

Sessions should initially be limited to no more than 1500 FUs and MFUs.

Special considerations in women

In women, the sessions should be smaller (consider less than 1000 grafts/session) and grafts should be spaced further apart than might be done in a man, to minimize the risk of surgically induced telogen. In addition, in women, the selection of a higher proportion of 3–6-haired MFUs is preferred by the authors for transplanting behind the hairline. This serves the added benefit of allowing the physician more easily to identify and show to the patient the hair that has been transplanted.

Postoperative care

As is true of preoperative care, the use of topical and systemic antibiotics, postoperative corticosteroids to reduce swelling, or topical minoxidil to limit telogen is variable. The use of postoperative dressings is variable as well. Nevertheless, the authors offer the following postoperative suggestions, taken from their practice to deal with the usual postoperative sequelae. The Appendix contains the current postoperative instructions of one of the authors (D.B.).

General instructions

Patients are advised to rest on the evening of the surgery and to avoid aspirin products for a few days.

Bleeding

Significant bleeding is rare, and patients are instructed to apply pressure and call if they need to.

Swelling

Swelling on the forehead is common if the transplant involved the anterior scalp. It may be more noticeable beginning at day 2–3 after surgery, but usually resolves within 5–7 days. Eyelid swelling and even black eyes are uncommon but possible. Ice packs or packets of frozen peas applied over a towel (not directly over the grafts) may help with swelling. Some authors use postoperative oral steroids to try to reduce the swelling. Some have the patient use a sweat band at mid-forehead for 3 days so that the edema does not travel down to the eyelids. Some practitioners prescribe a short course of systemic steroids to reduce swelling.

To help decrease swelling, patients may sleep with the head elevated at a 45° angle for 1–3 nights following surgery.

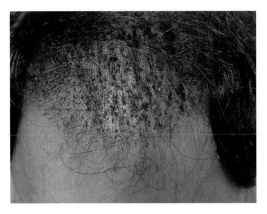

Figure 10-54 Crusting around grafts is inevitable and may last from 5 to 14 days, depending on both the individual patient and their postoperative care

Recipient site care

Bandages were commonly used in the early days of punch grafting, but are rarely employed today. Some practitioners ask the patients to use saline or proprietary graft solutions applied twice daily to keep the area moist in the first 2–3 days. Use of Aquaphor or antibiotic ointments may be soothing and reduce crust formation, but are greasy. Some authors advocate the use of hydrogel dressings for 1–3 nights, although these are difficult to use in patients with existing hair in the recipient area.

Grafts are well anchored almost immediately after surgery and are difficult to dislodge after 24–48 h. Nevertheless, patients are advised to touch gently and avoid picking or catching a fingernail or comb on the grafts or on the small crusts that inevitably form and last for 7–10 days (Fig. 10-54).

Donor site care

The donor site can be managed as for any surgical excision. It is likely that application of ointments (Aquaphor, Vaseline, antibiotic ointments) may decrease crusting, itching, or tenderness at the incision site.

Bathing

Patients may get the recipient site and donor site wet within the first 24 h in clean bath or shower water. They are advised to try not to let shower water beat at high pressure directly onto the recipient area until the crusts have gone. They may use a cup in the shower to help rinse the graft sites. They are advised that they can touch the grafts gently with the fingertips while washing in the shower, beginning 2–3 days after surgery.

Pain control

Most patients tolerate the procedure well and require minimal pain medication after the first 12–48 h. Typical prescriptions are for acetaminophen

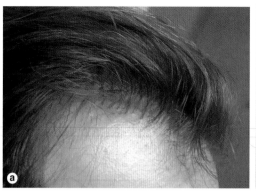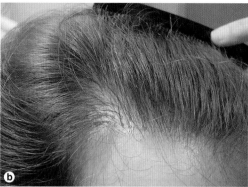

Figure 10-55 (A) Patient with previous large graft transplant and an abrupt slightly pluggy hairline. Hairline not too low. (B) Postoperative result after one session of small FUs and MFUs placed between and in front of old grafts

with codeine, acetaminophen with hydrocodone, or acetaminophen with oxycodone. Stronger medications are almost never needed.

Infection

Infection is rare. The graft sites and donor site should be kept clean and protected from dust and dirt.

Activity

Patients should refrain from heavy work or sports for 1 week to minimize bleeding or possible graft loss. They may return to work as early as the next day, and can wear a hat to cover the recipient site; however, because of the postoperative swelling and crusting at the recipient site, many prefer to avoid the public eye for a week or even longer.

Resuming hair care

Hairspray and mousse can be used 1 week after the transplant, but should be washed off daily. Patients should try to avoid hair dryers for 1–2 weeks to minimize the risk of burning the scalp. Hair coloring, perming, or cutting can be done once all the crusts have fallen off.

Suture removal

Sutures or staples can be removed in 10–14 days (longer if no absorbable sutures were used).

Special cases

Correcting previous work

The evolution of FU grafting away from the original procedures that utilized 3.25-mm and larger plugs, containing anywhere from 10 to 30 hairs and more, has led to a large group of patients hopeful that their results from previous techniques can be improved. A variety of techniques have been described to deal with various situations.

Some examples of how to "retrofit" previous transplants are:

- If a previously transplanted hairline is too dense or "pluggy," but has not been placed too low on the forehead, the use of multiple 1–2-haired FUs anterior to the old grafts can sometimes be enough to soften a hairline that initially appeared abrupt and linear, and make it look more irregular and natural (Figs 10-55 & 10-56).
- Patients who have had previous grafting with traditional 3.25–3.5-mm plugs may present with a corn row or "zebra pattern" effect. This can be handled in different ways. Some physicians use all FUs to fill in the vacant rows, whereas others may elect to employ MFUs (Fig. 10-57). Another technique is to punch out the alopecic scalp, in rows posterior to the hairline zone, using 1-mm trephines, and to place minigrafts.
- Hairlines that are too abrupt can be thinned by partial punch excision of existing large grafts and recycling of the newly reclaimed hair into FUs. This can be achieved by performing FU extraction in the middle of dense plugs. A 1-mm trephine can core out the centre of the offending hairline grafts; healing is by secondary intention, with the retrieved follicles to be used elsewhere. Alternatively, larger plugs can be more completely thinned using larger punches, with or without suturing.
- In patients in whom old, inappropriately placed, plugs need to be removed completely, these can be excised by utilizing a punch slightly larger in diameter than the plug to be removed. Once excised, the hole created is sutured closed. The excised graft can now be dissected into FUs and also recycled.

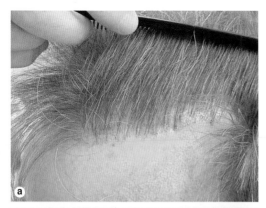

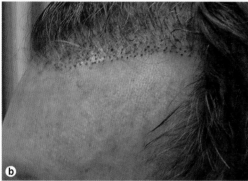

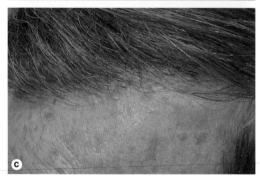

Figure 10-56 (A) Patient with previous large graft transplant and an abrupt, slightly pluggy, hairline. Hairline not too low. (B) Intraoperative photograph of session with small FUs and MFUs placed between and in front of old grafts. (C) Postoperative result

- Patients who have hairlines placed too low with larger traditional plugs can have an elliptical excision of a line of the frontal hairline grafts. This technique will raise the hairline and yield more reusable hair follicles to be used elsewhere. The resulting hairline scar can, at a later time, be camouflaged and softened with 1-haired FUs.

Transplanting other body sites

Other body areas that are amenable to transplants are the eyebrow, eyelash, moustache, and pubic areas.

When transplanting eyebrows it is important to follow the natural angle of the hair, keeping the hair oriented acutely to the face. There is a tendency for the transplanted hair to curl out or away from the natural direction of the eyebrows. Donor hair can be obtained from the lower occipital region or temporal region to try, as best as possible, to mimic the original eyebrow texture and color. It is important to warn the patient that consistent trimming of the hair every 5–6 days is needed because the transplanted hair will continue to grow at the same rate as from where it originated. In an attempt to minimize the need for frequent trimming, other potential donor areas can include the nape of the neck, chest, arm, and top of the foot.

Eyelash transplants are a technically more difficult hair restoration procedure, fraught with potential serious complications. Traditionally these procedures have been limited to adding hair owing to congenital absence, scarring due to burns, trauma, and trichotillomania.

Enthusiasm for transplantation for purely cosmetic enhancement of preexisting lashes should be tempered by remaining aware of the potential complications of entropion, ectropion, infections, and cyst formation.

Hair transplantation for absent or scant pubic hair is more commonly performed in Asian women where sparse pubic hair is considered more of an aesthetic concern. Single-haired FUs are utilized to reconstitute the area. Hair grafted to the pubic area can also be used to cover scars (Fig. 10-58).

Transplanting following rhytidectomy or burn scars

Hair transplantation can be used to correct hair loss and cover scars after facelifts. Women may present with the complaint of inability to pull their hair back behind their ears or to wear their hair up in a bun, due to the visibility of rhytidectomy scars.

A common principle to follow when transplanting scars is to leave adequate space between grafts and time between sessions to allow for revascularization. If this is done, transplanting into these areas works very well (Fig. 10-59).

Transplanting transgendered patients

Hair restoration is primarily useful for the male to female transgendered patient, seeking a more feminine, lower hairline and added fullness. Often other kinds of cosmetic changes are concurrently being made, such as hairline advancement and brow reconstruction, and as such the physician needs to plan accordingly. Hairline feminization entails lowering of the mid anterior hairline and rounding of the frontotemporal recessions (Fig. 10-60).

Specific to transgendered patients it is even more important than usual to assess for unrealistic expectations. If the degree of existing MPHL is too severe, a full wig may be the most appropriate solution. Often the patient wants to overemphasize their femininity and may want a lower hairline and fuller appearance compared with a typical genetic female patient.

Complications

Immediate postoperative swelling (particularly the forehead), crusting at the site of graft placement, and telogen/delayed growth of transplanted hairs are considered as expected outcomes of surgery and not as complications. Complications of hair transplantation have

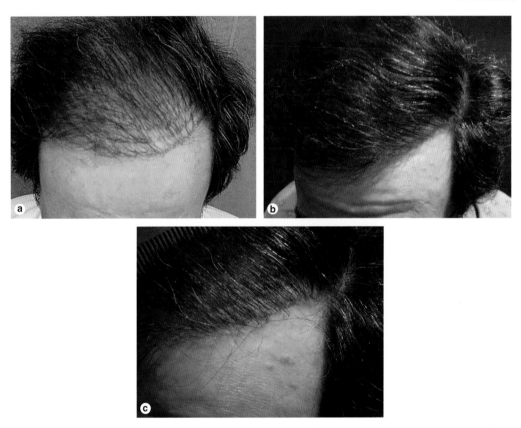

Figure 10-57 (A) Two sessions of traditional 3.25- and 3.5-mm punch grafts that presented years later to be updated. (B,C) One session of 1-haired FUs to soften the hairline, and 2–3- and 3–5-haired MFUs to in fill the 'zebra-like' rows behind the hairline

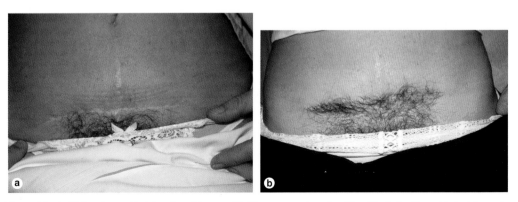

Figure 10-58 (A) Scarring and hair loss in pubic area. (B) After one session of grafting. The hair will need to be trimmed regularly

been subclassified into two categories: medical and aesthetic. Aesthetic complications are further subdivided into: (a) lower than expected density, and (b) unnatural appearance (Table 10-13).

Medical complications

Infection

Infection is very rare at either the donor or the recipient site (Fig. 10-61), occurring in less than 0.1% of patients. It can be diagnosed by clinical signs or culture, and may be expected to respond well to antibiotics.

Bleeding

Significant postoperative bleeding in the recipient area is unusual in a healthy patient and can be expected to respond to pressure. Donor site bleeding is also uncommon and usually responds to pressure. Rarely, bleeding may continue despite pressure, or a hematoma may develop, requiring the incision to be reopened and the bleeding vessel(s) cauterized or ligated.

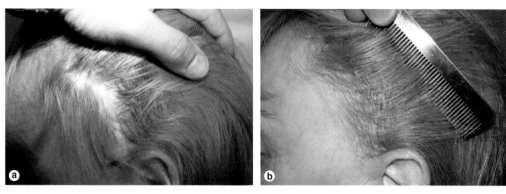

Figure 10-59 (A) Scarring to the temporoparietal scalp. (B) One session of grafting following the natural hair direction

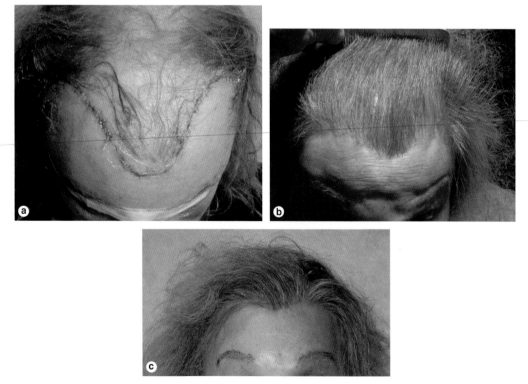

Figure 10-60 (A) Transgendered patient before hair transplant, showing recent scalp advancement and nasal/brow work. (B) After two sessions of grafting. (C) After two sessions of grafting showing hairline feminization as well as recent grafting to thicken eyebrows and cover incision scars

Table 10-13 Complications of hair transplant surgery

Medical complications	Aesthetic complications	
	Lower than desired density	Unnatural appearance
Infection	Poor growth of grafts:	Abnormal hair quality
Bleeding	• too much transection at harvesting	Plugginess
Dehiscence	• transection at graft preparation	Abnormal graft placement
Abnormal scar	• insufficient cooling of grafts	
Dysesthesia	• desiccation of grafts during transplant procedure	
Folliculitis	• trauma to grafts during insertion	
Necrosis	• patient factors (e.g. scar in recipient site, smokers) Transection of existing recipient hair during transplant Postsurgical effluvium Progression of underlying FPHL or MPHL	

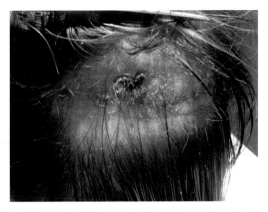

Figure 10-61 Donor site infection first noted 2 weeks after transplant and 1 week after uneventful suture removal. Extensive infection-induced telogen resolved with oral antibiotics and time, with an acceptable scar

Dehiscence

Donor site dehiscence is very rare with layered closure and as long as the strip is not too wide. If caught early and clean, dehiscence can be re-sutured. Otherwise, the wound can heal by secondary intention and the scar possibly re-excised later.

Abnormal scar

Keloid formation is very rare. Wide donor site scars are possible, especially with repeat sessions. Recipient site pitting or "cobble-stoning" can occur, although much less frequently with modern FU grafting. Pitting can be prevented by making sure that grafts do not sit below the surface of the skin.

Dysesthesia

Neuralgias from presumed surgical trauma to sensory nerves can rarely present after surgery. The patient can be reassured that these usually resolve quickly. Hypoesthesia of the scalp from transection of sensory nerves is much less common nowadays, with the use of tumescent technique, which allows the incisions to remain superficial to the larger sensory nerves.

Folliculitis and milia

These typically occur in the recipient site up to several months post-transplant and are related to ingrowing hairs or retained hair fragments, possibly due to inadvertent "burying" of a graft at the time of placement. Piggybacking of grafts occurs when one graft is inadvertently planted on top of another. An inclusion cyst may form, but should be uncommon with good technique. Solitary lesions can be incised, or even excised if they do not resolve.

Inflammatory papules along the donor site several weeks after surgery may represent suture granulomas from the absorbable suture, and will resolve.

Necrosis

Occasional but rare case reports of recipient site necrosis exist. Given the large numbers of grafts routinely transplanted in a modern case, this remains exceedingly rare.

Aesthetic complications: lower than desired density

An excellent transplant procedure can lead to a lower than desired density if the patient has excessive expectations about their likely hair growth. In addition to unrealistic expectations, lower than desired density can be caused by any combination of the following.

Poor growth of grafts

Most hair transplants should achieve greater than 90% successful growth of grafts. Possible causes of poor growth include technical considerations such as:

- too much transection at harvesting
- transection at graft preparation
- insufficient cooling of grafts

- desiccation of grafts during the transplant procedure
- trauma to grafts during insertion
- patient factors (e.g. scar in recipient site, smoker).

Even experienced hair transplant surgeons may have this complication on occasion, for unknown reasons, with one survey suggesting a prevalence of this phenomenon of as high as 6%.

Transection of existing recipient hair during transplant

Existing hairs may be transected by recipient site incisions that are not parallel to the existing hair. This should not be a factor if the surgeon uses both care and appropriate magnification.

Postsurgical effluvium

This may occur at the donor or recipient site and is secondary to the indirect trauma of the surgery near the follicles. This can lead to a devastating amount of thinning as the newly transplanted hairs take months to grow and the shedding may begin a few weeks after the transplant, leading to a thinned appearance compared with the preoperative state. Anagen effluvium refers to the sudden cessation of growth of the existing recipient hairs, beginning 2–3 weeks after surgery; this recovers quickly. Telogen effluvium occurs several weeks after surgery and may last for months, usually but not always with eventual regrowth of hair. Postoperative telogen effluvium is more common in women, and patients who are not prepared to take the risk of this phenomenon should not be transplanted. Perioperative minoxidil may help to reduce the risk.

Progression of underlying FPHL or MPHL

Pattern hair loss is unpredictable and the ongoing loss of hair over time may reduce the visible density/benefit of the transplant session. Patients should understand this possibility before surgery.

Delayed synchronized telogen

Some 2–3 years after the transplant, a large proportion of the transplanted hair can cycle into telogen at roughly the same time, leading to a noticeable thinning. This will resolve as the hairs cycle back to anagen.

Aesthetic complications: unnatural appearance

This complication may present in several ways.

Abnormal hair quality

In the first few months after the transplant, the growing hair may be finer or "kinkier" than in its original location (Fig. 10-62). This tends to improve with time. The occipital hair is the last to gray, and thus may lead to an unnatural color difference between the transplanted darker hair and the surrounding gray hair.

Plugginess

This is exclusively a complication of overly large grafts, mostly related to older transplants which used punch grafting techniques. It can usually be revised. Larger MFUs in patients with course hair may show a little bit of this, and should be avoided near the hairline.

Abnormal graft placement

Failure to plan hair transplantation adequately can lead to poor graft placement (e.g. too low or flat a hairline). The bad aesthetics of poor graft placement was compounded by the unnatural look of large round grafts in the earlier years of hair transplantation (Fig. 10-63). Sometimes grafts that were well placed originally become unnatural with the progressive loss of surrounding

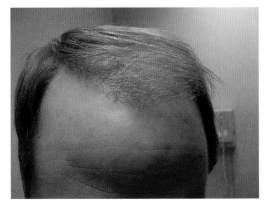

Figure 10-62 Six months after transplant of the anterior scalp and hairline, early growth of hair shows a finer "kinky" quality that can be expected to resolve largely or completely over the next few months (and did in this case)

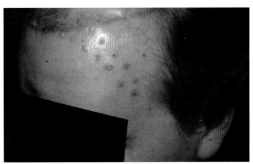

Figure 10-63 Thirty-five large punch grafts performed elsewhere, with unnatural and low placement of hairline compounding plugginess of large grafts. Punch excision and suturing, and then recycling of these grafts, was carried out, although laser hair removal could have been considered if the patient had wished no further transplantation

hair. To some degree this is not entirely preventable, but good planning can reduce the incidence or anticipate this problem. A wise surgeon leaves some donor hair to help later fill in cosmetically sensitive areas that may progressively lose more hair with time (e.g. frontotemporal angle).

Directions for the future

The field of hair restoration has evolved enormously since the first punch grafts for MPHL were performed over 50 years ago. Possible future horizons include the development of new medications for pattern hair loss or the study of existing medications such as dutasteride, currently not indicated for this purpose.

Development of improved graft storage may be on the horizon. Currently a chilled saline solution is used by most physicians temporarily to hold the grafts removed from the body until such time as they are planted back into the recipient sites. Injury can occur to the grafts during the period when the tissue has been removed from the body and is subjected to a reduction of oxygen, glucose, and other nutrients. Storage solutions aimed at reducing injury to harvested tissue are currently being studied. These include autologous platelet-rich gels and cell culture media as well as hypothermic storage solutions that lower the temperature of the storage solution in order to allow the tissue to be outside the body more safely for prolonged periods of time.

Low-level light laser therapy is being employed as an adjunct to the surgical and medical treatments available to treat MPHL and FPHL, and were recently given FDA approval as a safe device. More third-party studies need to be performed in order to assess the true efficacy of lasers and their subsequent place in hair restoration. At present, lasers have a limited role in hair transplantation, but this may change.

Hair restoration surgery is limited by the finite amount of donor tissue available in any one person. It has been shown that cultured human dermal papilla cells, when implanted back into the epidermis, can induce new hair growth. Several research centers are currently working at developing techniques that may one day aid the hair restoration surgeon.

Finally, the development of robotics holds promise in potential applications for hair transplantation.

Conclusions

Modern hair transplanting should allow the restoration of cosmetically pleasing and undetectable hair to a large number of balding individuals. This chapter has reviewed the key principles and practical points in both assessing patients, planning for, and performing hair transplantation.

Case examples of the results of modern hair transplantation are shown in Case Studies 10.1–10.7.

Case Study 10.1

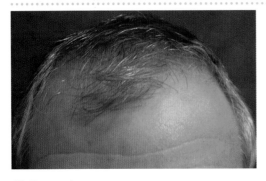

(A) Preoperative

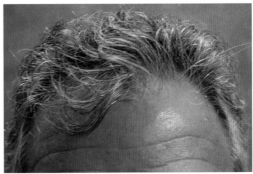

(B) At 10 months' follow-up after one session of 1395 FU and MFU grafts taken from a 20 × 1-cm strip

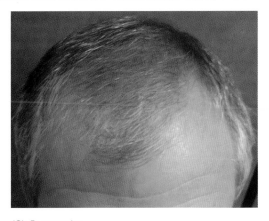

(C) Preoperative

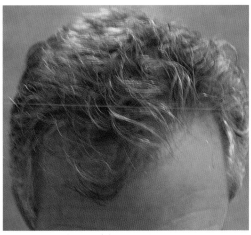

(D) At 10 months' follow-up after one session of 1395 FU and MFU grafts taken from a 20 × 1-cm strip

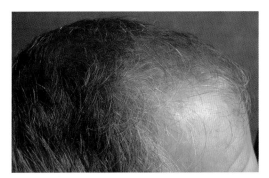

(E) Preoperative side view

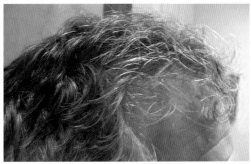

(F) Side view at 10 months' follow-up after one session of 1395 FU and MFU grafts taken from a 20 × 1-cm strip

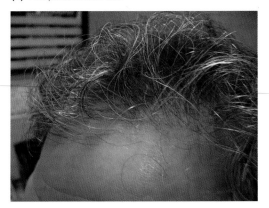

(G) At 10 months' follow-up after one session of 1395 FU and MFU grafts taken from a 20 × 1-cm strip. The photograph shows the natural appearance following modern grafting

Case Study 10.2

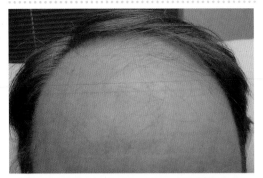

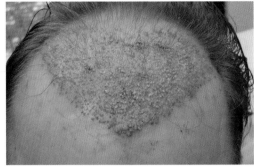

(D) Immediately after graft placement of recipient sites in session 1

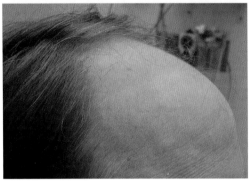

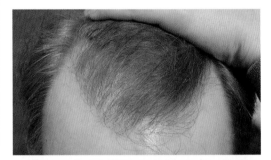

(A,B) Patient prior to hair transplantation to anterior scalp. He had an initial session (session 1) of 1349 FU and MFU grafts taken from a total 24 × 0.8-cm strip. This was followed 8 months later by a second session of 1531 grafts from a 19.5 × 1-cm strip

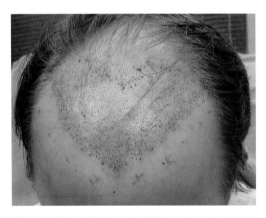

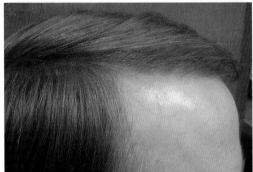

(E,F) Seven months after second session of 1531 grafts. Note natural appearance without "plugginess." Note also that final density is not the same as the original hair in that area, but still makes a dramatic aesthetic improvement

(C) Immediately after making 1349 recipient sites in session 1

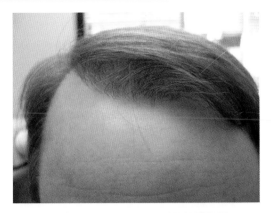

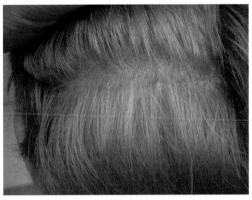

(K) Twenty-two months after second session of 1531 grafts. Note single donor scar, as second session excised original occipital scar

Case Study 10.3

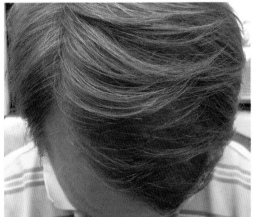

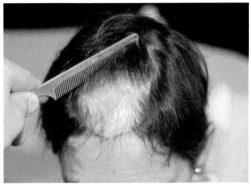

(A) Preoperative

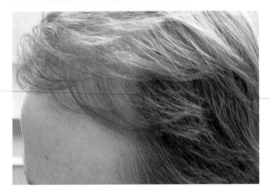

(G,H,I) Eleven months after second session of 1531 grafts

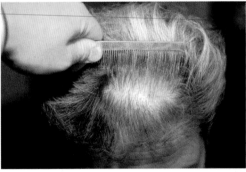

(B) After one session of approximately 900 FU and MFU grafts. Hair permed and colored lighter

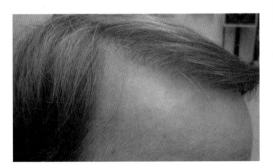

(J) Twenty-two months after second session of 1531 grafts

Case Study 10.4

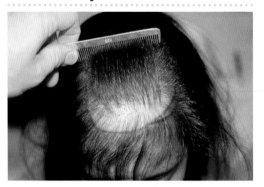

(A) Preoperative

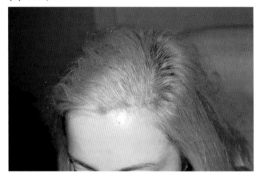

(B) After two sessions of approximately 1600 FU and MFU grafts. Hair dyed

Case Study 10.5

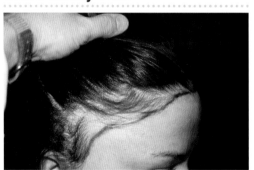

(A) Preoperative

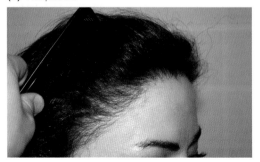

(B) After two sessions of approximately 2500 FU and MFU grafts in total

Case Study 10.6

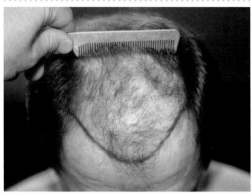

(A) Preoperative

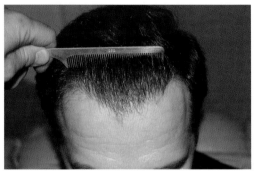

(B) After three sessions of approximately 4900 FU and MFU grafts in total

Case Study 10.7

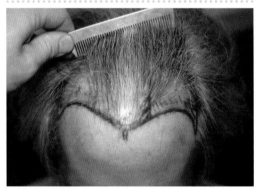

(A) Preoperative

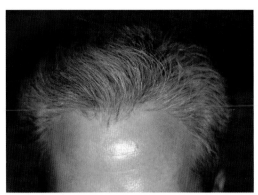

(B) After one session of approximately 1900 FU and MFU grafts in total

Appendix

Postoperative instructions for patients undergoing hair transplantation

General instructions

1 Immediately following surgery you should plan to go home and rest (minimal activity) until the next morning.
2 To help decrease swelling sleep with your head elevated at a 45° angle for 1–3 nights following surgery.
3 DO NOT use any aspirin-containing products or drink alcohol for 5 days following surgery.

What to do about …
Bleeding

1 Bleeding may occur the night after surgery or for up to a few days afterwards. This almost always stops if you apply firm, steady pressure over the area for 15 minutes (without lifting the gauze to "check" before the time is up). Press firmly but gently so as not to dislodge the surrounding grafts.
2 If you cannot control the bleeding with rest and pressure, you may reach the doctor or the resident on-call through the switchboard at
....
3 In the first 1–3 days, a graft may occasionally be knocked or combed out. Do not panic. This is uncommon and, even if it happens, it is rare to lose more than a few hair roots in this way.

Pain control

1 Many people require medication the first 1–2 nights following surgery. You should not have to suffer. The medication should control your discomfort.
2 You will have been given a prescription for Tylenol #3 or Percocet for pain control. Use these as directed.

Wound care

Immediately on discharge you will be provided with a kit to use as follows:

1 You will be given a spray bottle with sterile saline solution that you should use daily for the next 3 days after the surgery. Wet 2 to 3 pieces of gauze with saline solution and apply them on the transplanted area for 30 to 60 minutes twice daily. This will keep the transplanted area moist and will help speed the healing process.
2 For the donor site (in the back), please apply Polysporin, bacitracin, or Aquaphor ointment a couple of times a day to keep the site from drying out. Using ointment or K-Y water-soluble gel will help reduce crusting.
3 You will be given some sterile gauze to take with you. Use this to apply gentle pressure to any areas that may lightly bleed on the day of the surgery or in the next few days. If the bleeding is from the donor area, lift the hair before applying pressure to avoid the hair getting matted down.
4 We will speak by phone the next day to see if you need to be seen (many patients do not).

Swelling

1 Swelling may occur (especially after your first transplant), usually on the forehead and usually beginning around day 2–4 following surgery. This will not leave any permanent problems. As gravity works, the swelling may descend to the eyelids. *Rarely* black eyes may occur. This is uncommon, and though unsightly will not leave any permanent mark.
2 Swelling can be minimized by:
   a) Sleeping with your head elevated at 45° for 1–3 nights following surgery using a recliner or pillows.
   b) Apply icepacks (or bag of frozen peas) around the forehead and temples. DO NOT apply ice directly to the hair grafts.

Infection

Infection is rare. Avoid exposure to dirt in the air at work or at play for 2 weeks following surgery. Do not touch the donor area or the transplanted grafts, except with clean hands, to reduce the chance of an infection. Report any increasing tenderness or redness and swelling around the surgical site.

Exercise & work

1 Refrain from heavy work or sports for 1 week.
2 Refrain from weight lifting or heavy lifting, or swimming in chlorinated water, for 10–14 days.

3 Some people return to light work the day following surgery, although most people prefer to take at least 2–3 days off. Because of the possibility of swelling and some crusting following surgery, some people prefer to take 1 week off following surgery. This is especially true after your first procedure when everything is new for you. Crusting will be more visible if you have little hair to begin with. Crusts usually fall off 7–10 days following surgery.

Hair washing & hair care

1 Beginning on the day after surgery, you may begin to wash your hair gently in the shower. Try not to let the water beat directly onto the recipient area where the grafts are, until the crusts have gone. You may want to have a cup in the shower to help rinse the graft sites. Beginning 2–3 days after surgery you can gently touch the grafts with the fingertips while washing in the shower. Avoid catching the grafts with your fingernails.
2 Hairspray and mousse can be used 1 week after the transplant but should be washed off daily.
3 When combing, do so carefully to avoid dislodging the grafts.
4 Try to avoid hair dryers for 1–2 weeks, especially hot ones.
5 Hair coloring, perming, or cutting can be done once all the crusts have fallen off.

Sutures

1 Sutures will be removed from the donor area usually 14 days following the surgery.

Crusting

1 Crusts will usually fall off in 7–10 days, though this can last longer.
2 Applying ointment (Aquaphor or bacitracin or Polysporin) can be done (though not required) to try to soften the crusts if they are prominent. These preparations are greasy, however, and you can consider using K-Y gel (water soluble) instead.

Further reading

Andriole GL, Kirby R. Safety and tolerability of the dual 5α-reductase inhibitor dutasteride in the treatment of benign prostatic hyperplasia. Eur Urol 2003;44(1):82–88.

Avram MR. Hair transplantation in women. Semin Cutan Med Surg 1999;18(2):172–176.

Avram MR. Laser-assisted hair transplantation – a status report in the 21st century. J Cosmet Dermatol 2005;4(2):135–139.

Avram MR. Hair transplantation for men and women. Semin Cutan Med Surg 2006;25(1):60–64.

Avram MR, Leonard RT Jr, Epstein ES, et al. The current role of laser/light sources in the treatment of male and female pattern hair loss. J Cosmet Laser Ther 2007;9(1):27–28.

Beehner ML. A frontal forelock/central density framework for hair transplantation. Dermatol Surg 1997;23(9):807–815.

Bernstein RM, Rassman WR. Dissecting microscope versus magnifying loupes with transillumination in the preparation of follicular unit grafts. A bilateral controlled study. Dermatol Surg 1998;24(8): 875–880.

Bernstein RM, Rassman WR, Seager D, et al. Standardizing the classification and description of follicular unit transplantation and mini–micrografting techniques. The American Society for Dermatologic Surgery, Inc. Dermatol Surg 1998;24(9): 957–963.

Bernstein RM, Rassman WR, Rashid N, Shiell RC. The art of repair in surgical hair restoration – part II: the tactics of repair. Dermatol Surg 2002;28(10):873–893.

Bernstein RM, Rassman WR, Rashid N, Shiell RC. The art of repair in surgical hair restoration part I: basic repair strategies. Dermatol Surg 2002;28(9):783–794.

Brandy DA. An evaluation system to enhance patient selection for alopecia-reducing surgery. Dermatol Surg 2002;28(9):808–816.

Cooley JE. Complications of hair transplantation. In: Unger WP, Shapiro R, eds. Hair Transplantation. New York: Marcel Dekker, 2004:568–577.

Cooley JE, Vogel JE. Follicle trauma and the role of the dissecting microscope in hair transplantation. A multicenter study. Dermatol Clin 1999;17(2): 307–312.

D'Amico AV, Roehrborn CG. Effect of 1 mg/day finasteride on concentrations of serum prostate-specific antigen in men with androgenic alopecia: a randomised controlled trial. Lancet Oncol 2007;8(1):21–25.

Debruyne F, Barkin J, van Erps P, et al. Efficacy and safety of long-term treatment with the dual 5α-reductase inhibitor dutasteride in men with symptomatic benign prostatic hyperplasia. Eur Urol 2004;46(4):488–494.

Eaton JS, Grekin RC. Regional anesthesia of the face. Dermatol Surg 2001;27(12):1006–1009.

Finasteride Male Pattern Hair Loss Study Group. Long-term (5-year) multinational experience with finasteride 1 mg in the treatment of men with androgenetic alopecia. Eur J Dermatol 2002;12(1):38–49.

Frank EW. Scalp cyanosis during hair transplantation. Dermatol Surg 2000;26(4):402.

Gandelman M, Epstein JS. Hair transplantation to the eyebrow, eyelashes, and other parts of the body. Facial Plast Surg Clin North Am 2004;12(2):253–261.

Haber RS. Pharmacologic management of pattern hair loss. Facial Plast Surg Clin North Am 2004;12(2):181–189.

Hamilton JB. Patterned loss of hair in man; types and incidence. Ann N Y Acad Sci 1951;53(3):708–728.

Harris J. Follicular unit extraction: the SAFE system. Hair Transplant Forum International 2004;14(5):157, 163–164.

Headington JT. Transverse microscopic anatomy of the human scalp. A basis for a morphometric approach to disorders of the hair follicle. Arch Dermatol 1984;120(4):449–456.

Hordinsky MK. Medical treatment of noncicatricial alopecia. Semin Cutan Med Surg 2006;25(1):51–55.

Hunt N, McHale S. The psychological impact of alopecia. BMJ 2005;331:951–953.

Jimenez F, Ruifernandez JM. Distribution of human hair in follicular units. A mathematical model for estimating the donor size in follicular unit transplantation. Dermatol Surg 1999;25(4):294–298.

Kaufman KD, Olsen EA, Whiting D, et al. Finasteride in the treatment of men with androgenetic alopecia. Finasteride Male Pattern Hair Loss Study Group. J Am Acad Dermatol 1998;39(Pt 1):578–589.

Knudsen RG. The donor area. Facial Plast Surg Clin North Am 2004;12(2):233–240.

Langtry JA, Maddin WS, Carruthers JA, Rivers JK. Is there a rationale for the drugs used in hair transplantation surgery? Dermatol Surg 1998;24(9):967–971.

Leavitt M, Perez-Meza D, Rao NA, et al. Effects of finasteride (1 mg) on hair transplant. Dermatol Surg 2005;31(10):1268–1276.

Lee YR, Lee SJ, Kim JC, Ogawa H. Hair restoration surgery in patients with pubic atrichosis or hypotrichosis: review of technique and clinical consideration of 507 cases. Dermatol Surg 2006;32(11):1327–1335.

Limmer BL. Elliptical donor stereoscopically assisted micrografting as an approach to further refinement in hair transplantation. J Dermatol Surg Oncol 1994;20(12):789–793.

Lucky AW, Piacquadio DJ, Ditre CM, et al. A randomized, placebo-controlled trial of 5% and 2% topical minoxidil solutions in the treatment of female pattern hair loss. J Am Acad Dermatol 2004;50(4):541–553.

Ludwig E. Classification of the types of androgenetic alopecia (common baldness) occurring in the female sex. Br J Dermatol 1977;97(3):247–254.

Marritt E. Follimmerlicular transplantation. Giving credit where credit is due. Dermatol Surg 1998;24(8):925–929.

Motamed S, Davami B. Eyebrow reconstruction following burn injury. Burns 2005;31(4):495–499.

Nordstrom H, Stange K. Plasma lidocaine levels and risks after liposuction with tumescent anaesthesia. Acta Anaesthesiol Scand 2005;49(10):1487–1490.

Norwood OT. Male pattern baldness: classification and incidence. South Med J 1975;68(11):1359–1365.

Nusbaum BP. Techniques to reduce pain associated with hair transplantation: optimizing anesthesia and analgesia. Am J Clin Dermatol 2004;5(1):9–15.

Olsen EA, Dunlap FE, Funicella T, et al. A randomized clinical trial of 5% topical minoxidil versus 2% topical minoxidil and placebo in the treatment of androgenetic alopecia in men. J Am Acad Dermatol 2002;47(3):377–385.

Olsen EA, Messenger AG, Shapiro J, et al. Evaluation and treatment of male and female pattern hair loss. J Am Acad Dermatol 2005;52(2):301–311.

Olsen EA, Hordinsky M, Whiting D, et al. The importance of dual 5α-reductase inhibition in the treatment of male pattern hair loss: results of a randomized placebo-controlled study of dutasteride versus finasteride. J Am Acad Dermatol 2006;55(6):1014–1023.

Park SW, Wang HY. Survival of grafts in coup de sabre. Dermatol Surg 2002;28(8):763–766.

Parsley WM, Rose P. Science of hairline design. In: Haber RS, Stough DB, eds. Hair Transplantation. Philadelphia: Elsevier, 2006:55–71.

Rassman WR, Bernstein RM, McClellan R, et al. Follicular unit extraction: minimally invasive surgery for hair transplantation. Dermatol Surg 2002;28(8):720–728.

Ross EK, Shapiro J. Management of hair loss. Dermatol Clin 2005;23(2):227–243.

Ross EK, Tan E, Shapiro J. Update on primary cicatricial alopecias. J Am Acad Dermatol 2005;53(1):1–37.

Schulman C, Pommerville P, Höfner K, Wachs B. (2006). Long-term therapy with the dual 5α-reductase inhibitor dutasteride is well tolerated in men with symptomatic benign prostatic hyperplasia. BJU Int 2006;97(1):73–79.

Seager DJ, Simmons C. Local anesthesia in hair transplantation. Dermatol Surg 2002;28(4):320–328.

Seery GE, Unger MG, Marzola M, Cattani RV. Alopecia reduction procedures. In: Unger WP, Shapiro R, eds. Hair Transplantation. New York: Marcel Dekker, 2004:709–763.

Shapiro R. Follicular unit transplantation alone or follicular units with multi-FU grafts: why, when and how? In: Unger WP, Shapiro R, eds. Hair Transplantation. New York: Marcel Dekker, 2004:435–469.

Shapiro R. Principles and techniques used to create a natural hairline in surgical hair restoration. Facial Plast Surg Clin North Am 2004;12(2):201–217.

Shapiro R, Unger WP. Graft terminology, in planning and organization of the recipient area. In: Unger WP, Shapiro R, eds. Hair Transplantation. New York: Marcel Dekker, 2004:81–85.

Sinclair R, Wewerinke M, Jolley D. Treatment of female pattern hair loss with oral antiandrogens. Br J Dermatol 2005;152(3):466–473.

Stough D. Post-operative frontal central necrosis. Hair Transplant Forum International 1999;9:56–57.

Stough D. Dutasteride improves male pattern hair loss in a randomized study in identical twins. J Cosmet Dermatol 2007;6(1):9–13.

Swinehart JM. Local anesthesia in hair transplant surgery. Dermatol Surg 2002;28(12):1189.

Thompson IM, Goodman PJ, Tangen CM, et al. The influence of finasteride on the development of prostate cancer. N Engl J Med 2003;349(3):215–224.

Unger WP. The history of hair transplantation. Dermatol Surg 2000;26(3):181–189.

Unger WP. The incidence and degree of androgenetic alopecia at various ages in men and women. In: Unger WP, Shapiro R, eds. Hair Transplantation. New York: Marcel Dekker, 2004:51–56.

Unger WP, Beehner ML. Studies of hair survival in grafts of different sizes with additional hair survival studies and conclusions. In: Unger WP, Shapiro R, eds. Hair Transplantation. New York: Marcel Dekker, 2004:261–279.

Unger WP, Cole J. Donor harvesting. In: Unger WP, Shapiro R, eds. Hair Transplantation. New York: Marcel Dekker, 2004:301–337.

Unger WP, Shapiro R, Knudson R, Parsley WM. Basic principles and organization. In: Unger WP, Shapiro R, eds. Hair Transplantation. New York: Marcel Dekker, 2004:81–164.

Unger WP, Unger RH. Hair transplanting: an important but often forgotten treatment for female pattern hair loss. J Am Acad Dermatol 2003;49(5):853–860.

Vogel JE. Correcting problems in hair restoration surgery: an update. Facial Plast Surg Clin North Am 2004;12(2):263–278.

Wang J, Fan J. Cicatricial eyebrow reconstruction with a dense-packing one- to two-hair grafting technique. Plast Reconstr Surg 2004;114(6):1420–1426.

Ziering C, Krenitsky G. The Ziering whorl classification of scalp hair. Dermatol Surg 2003;29(8):817–821.

Liposuction

Murad Alam

Introduction, definition, and history

Liposuction, also referred to as "liposculpture," is a form of surgical "body contouring" that aims to reduce focal subcutaneous, suprafascial fat accumulation at various sites by transcutaneous vacuum-assisted extraction of fat particles through small punctures in the skin.

Liposuction was introduced to medicine in 1976 by Fischer, an otolaryngologist who pioneered the use of the hollow cannula. In France, Illouz and Fournier refined the process of liposuction, and their contributions included the "wet technique," or injection of hypotonic saline and hyaluronic acid prior to fat removal (Illouz); and the criss-cross motion of cannulas for smooth contouring and syringe removal (Fournier).

Although the first liposuction in the USA was performed in 1982, a sea change occurred in 1987 with Jeffrey Klein's report that liposuction with local anesthesia alone could be safe and effective. The advent of so-called tumescent liposuction eliminated the need for pain control through general anesthesia or conscious sedation. Additionally, as tumescent anesthesia entailed intralesional infusion of an extremely dilute anesthetic solution of lidocaine with epinephrine (Table 11-1), the resulting vasoconstriction markedly reduced intraoperative blood loss, which was one of the major causes of complications during nontumescent liposuction. This refined procedure enjoyed growing popularity, and authoritative reviews of tens of thousands of cases confirmed the safety of the procedure.

In recent years, concerns have been raised by some that liposuction may not be as safe as believed, and this has led to a move to restrict liposuction to physicians licenced to perform this procedure in hospital operating rooms. However, these fears have not been borne out, and tumescent liposuction continues to enjoy an unparalleled safety record when performed according to accepted protocols. Paradoxically, reports of deaths associated with liposuction have been associated exclusively with liposuction performed under general anesthesia or conscious sedation by nondermatologists.

In an era of minimally invasive, extremely safe, low-downtime cosmetic procedures, liposuction remains a timely and appropriate procedure. Unlike some minimally invasive procedures, however, liposuction is associated not with mild efficacy, but rather with dramatic cosmetic improvement. Up to several liters of fat aspirate can be removed in a single procedure. The cost–benefit trade-off associated with liposuction is thus exceptionally favorable.

Literature review/ evidence-based summary

As the cosmetic efficacy of liposuction is both clinically obvious and difficult to measure by objective techniques, few high-quality studies on clinical efficacy and persistence are available. In general, appropriate patient selection is associated with maximal efficacy. Efficacy appears to be diminished when liposuction is performed on obese patients; patients with significant excess or thin skin; patients with little or no excess fat; and elderly or deconditioned patients.

The largest body of studies pertains to establishing the parameters for safe liposuction, and assessing the benefits of these in protecting patients. The safety of tumescent liposuction was already well accepted in 1995, when a review of 15,336 patients who had undergone liposuction performed by members of the American Society for Dermatologic Surgery was carried out. Only minor complications, and no reports of death, pulmonary or fat embolism, hypovolemic shock, perforation of the peritoneum or thorax, or thrombophlebitis, were found. In 1996, a study of

Table 11-1 Recipe for commonly used tumescent anesthesia concentrations

Ingredient	Quantity	Final concentration or pH
Normal saline (0.9%)	1 L	–
Lidocaine 2% (select one)[a]	50 mL	0.1%
	37.5 mL	0.075%
	25 mL	0.05%
Epinephrine (1:1000)	1 mL	0.1%
Sodium bicarbonate (8.45%)	12.5 mL	pH 7.4
Triamcinolone acetonide (optional)	10 mg	–

[a]The different values for lidocaine dosage are alternatives; only one of these quantities should be infused in any given bag of saline

Table 11-2 Recommended maximum total tumescent anesthesia volumes (55 mg/kg total dose)

Bodyweight		Lidocaine solution (L)	
kg	lbs	0.1%	0.075%
40	88	2.2	2.9
50	110	2.7	3.7
60	132	3.3	4.4
70	154	3.8	5.1
80	176	4.4	5.9
90	198	4.9	6.6

a cohort of 60 patients showed that a mean lidocaine dose of 55 mg/kg bodyweight (Table 11-2) was not associated with lidocaine toxicity, whether assessed by subjective signs or by plasma lidocaine levels.

The low risk of liposuction under tumescent anesthesia was verified by a review of malpractice claims. Based on Physicians Insurance Association of America malpractice data from 1995 to 1997, hospital-based liposuction was found to be more than three times as likely to culminate in malpractice settlements compared with office-based liposuction. Fewer than 1% of liposuction claims settlements were found to be against dermatologists.

In 1999, a widely read article in the *New England Journal of Medicine* reported a series of so-called tumescent liposuction-related deaths over a 5-year period in New York. Notably, all four of the reported deaths were associated with so-called liposuction under general anesthesia or conscious sedation, and one was in a patient with severe coexisting morbidities and multiple interacting medications. As such, this case series did not provide any information regarding the safety of true tumescent liposuction technique under local anesthesia alone, as pioneered and perfected by dermatologists.

Following the sensational and poorly understood report from the *New England Journal of Medicine*, the dermatologic surgery community embarked on additional studies to assess the safety of true tumescent liposuction and to try to allay the concerns of patients and policymakers. In 2000, Florida mandated all adverse events occurring in physician's offices be reported, and a review was undertaken of all such reports from 2000 to 2004. Among these, there were seven complications and five deaths associated with the use of intravenous sedation or general anesthesia; liposuction and/or abdominoplasty under general anesthesia or intravenous sedation were the surgical procedures most commonly associated with complication and death. However, there were no adverse events associated with the use of dilute local (tumescent) anesthesia alone.

A study initiated by the Accreditation Association for Ambulatory Health Care Institute for Quality Improvement prospectively collected data from 688 patients undergoing tumescent liposuction at 39 centers between February 2001 and August 2002. Patients were followed for 6 months after surgery to track any delayed adverse events. Minor complications were found to occur at a rate of 0.57% and the major complication rate of 0.14% was accounted for by a single patient, who required hospitalization.

A mail survey of 517 dermatologic surgeons who were members of the American Society for Dermatologic Surgery in August 2001 elicited retrospective information on numbers of patients receiving liposuction, the operative setting, and associated complications for the period from 1994 to 2000. The overall response rate was 89%, of whom 78% had performed liposuction procedures during the interval of interest. Based on a total of 66 570 reported cases, the overall serious adverse event rate was 0.68 per 1000 cases. Complication rates were higher when intramuscular or intravenous sedation was used, versus no or oral sedation. No deaths were reported. Detailed information was obtained for each reported complication.

Experienced physicians have adapted liposuction to their practices, and minor differences in technique abound. However, certain studies describe elements of technique that are widely accepted. Many of these are described in the American Society for Dermatologic Surgery's recently updated guidelines of care for tumescent liposuction.

Other studies have indicated the utility of other technique modifications. Kaplan and Moy's double-blind randomized cross-over study in 1996 demonstrated that, upon infusion into subcutaneous fat, local anesthetic warmed to 40°C elicited reduced pain compared with anesthetic solution at room temperature. Similar work by Yang and colleagues in 2006 confirmed these results and also indicated a similar pain reduction benefit for neutral tumescent anesthesia with added sodium bicarbonate versus nonneutralized solution.

Although tumescent liposuction is most often performed with syringe suction or a mechanical aspirator, other approaches have met with variable success. Ultrasound-assisted liposuction, which was purported to be an improvement over standard mechanical suction, was one of the earliest such variations and has not been widely adopted by US dermatologists. A randomized controlled trial in 2000, comparing the efficacy and safety of liposuction with such high-intensity continuous-wave ultrasound with a placebo control of extremely low-intensity ultrasound, found no benefit of the therapeutic high-intensity ultrasound. More recently, power-assisted liposuction has been compared with traditional liposuction, with the former found to be associated with briefer procedure times, less intraoperative and postoperative pain, diminished surgeon fatigue, increased rate of fat aspiration per minute, and reduced recovery time with lower incidence of ecchymoses and edema. Laser-assisted lipolysis is a new technique in which a neodymium : yttrium–aluminum–garnet (Nd:YAG) or similar laser probe is introduced into the subcutis and used to melt fat. Laser lipolysis may be effective for the treatment of small pockets of fat or in combination with traditional suction liposuction for larger volume procedures.

The metabolic effects of tumescent technique and of liposuction continue to be studied. High-pressure injection of anesthetic solution does not appear to increase plasma levels or metabolic rate. On the other hand, the introduction of dilute epinephrine slows redistribution of lidocaine into the systemic circulation and delays the peak plasma concentration of lidocaine by more than 7 h. This effect may be partly responsible for the exceptional safety of tumescent anesthesia. Specifically, the delay in absorption may permit some lidocaine to be pre-emptively removed from the subcutis by liposuction; moreover, the gradual rise to peak plasma levels may enable the development of systemic tolerance to high lidocaine plasma levels. Interestingly, when tumescent anesthesia is injected into the head and neck, some of this benefit may be lost. Peak plasma lidocaine concentration after neck injection occurs in approximately 6 h, compared with 12 h after thigh injection.

Table 11-3 Patient selection criteria for liposuction[a]

Category	Specific criteria
Medical fitness	Not pregnant or seeking to be pregnant
	Good general health
	Medications do not interact with tumescent anesthesia
	Absence of serious bleeding disorders or abnormalities
	Liver function within normal limits
	Immune status consistent with low risk of infection
Medical indication	Patient not obese
	Focal areas of fat excess
	Either satisfactory "snap test" or patient amenable to postoperative skin excess or subsequent skin resection
	Targeted fat is not visceral fat
Emotional readiness	Reasonable expectations
	Patient accepts that perfect symmetry is not attainable
	Patient accepts that not all fat can or should be removed
	Patient accepts risks of mild, and rarely serious, adverse events

[a]Contraindications are rarely absolute, and must be assessed in the context of the patient's overall welfare and safety

Patient evaluation: examination and history

Prior to liposuction, the following must be assessed:

- The patient's medical suitability for safe liposuction
- The likelihood that the cosmetic deficit of concern will be addressed by the procedure envisioned
- The patient's mental state and expectations of the surgery.

Liposuction under tumescent anesthesia can be safely accomplished in most patients (Table 11-3), but there are some contraindications to treatment. Pregnancy is an absolute contraindication, and history and pregnancy tests should be obtained before surgery on women of childbearing age. Other relative contraindications include significant concurrent illness, including systemic immunosuppression, significant cardiovascular or neurovascular illness, bleeding disorders, hepatic disease, and wound healing diatheses. Numerous prior surgeries to the target site, such as multiple abdominal surgeries in a patient desiring abdominal liposuction or currently placed catheters or gastrointestinal devices, may also be contraindications, or at least strongly suggestive of a need to reduce the scope and intensity of any liposuction. Many but not all surgeons may request a preoperative complete blood count with differential and a comprehensive chemistry panel to confirm good general health. Coagulation parameters, hepatitis panels, liver function tests, and human immunodeficiency virus (HIV) tests may also be obtained.

Regarding the cosmetic deficit of interest, it is important that it be not only amenable to correction by liposuction, but also of salience to the patient. This distinction can be easily overlooked by an enthusiastic physician who is a novice at cosmetic dermatology. If there is an objectively obvious cosmetic deficit, such as bulging hips in an otherwise healthy young person of normal weight and with good skin tone, the patient may be an excellent candidate for liposuction, but if the patient does not perceive this deficit as problematic, even the most technically skilled procedure will not meet with the patient's approval. As cosmetic procedures are inherently optional and designed to please and not save the patient, it is imperative to focus on correcting problems that the patient considers major and to relegate areas of secondary interest to subordinate status.

Although liposuction is a safe procedure, there are associated risks and downtime that should be communicated to the patient. The procedure can last from an hour to several hours, and requires lidocaine and epinephrine injections followed by puncture incisions to permit entry of cannulas. As such, the area undergoing liposuction will eventually display several small dot-like atrophic scars which may be hypopigmented or hyperpigmented. Immediately after liposuction, significant swelling will result, with copious watery and serosanguinous drainage for at least 1 day. Widespread bruising to the treated site is inevitable, and may resolve gradually over 1–3 weeks. In the immediate aftermath of a liposuction procedure, reduction in apparent contour or girth is not evident, and the area may even seem thicker or fuller. Only after several weeks will the contour improve, as fluid is resorbed, edema diminishes, and the subcutis contracts and re-adheres to the fascial layer.

The evening after a liposuction procedure, patients should have a friend or family member staying with them, or at least checking to make sure they are doing well. Finally, patients who are unwilling to wear a support and compression garment to the treated site for several weeks after the procedure should be advised that this reluctance will diminish the efficacy of the procedure. It is often useful to provide patients contemplating a liposuction procedure with written material about liposuction, as well as a consent form. These documents should also encourage patients to avoid the preoperative use of unnecessary anticoagulants, such as alcohol, certain herbal medications, vitamin E, and self-prescribed nonsteroidal anti-inflammatory drugs. Patients who are unwilling to prepare appropriately for the liposuction procedure, or who cannot accede to undergoing some of the key steps, should be dissuaded from continuing. In some cases, other procedures may be suggested as an alternative option.

Index of devices or treatments available

Tumescent anesthesia is probably the most significant "device" for liposuction performed by dermatologists. Although technically tumescent anesthesia is neither a drug nor a device, it is a mixture of safe, separately approved, drugs that collectively enable liposuction under local anesthesia. The primary benefits of tumescent anesthesia are pain control, hemostasis, and hydrodissection of fat lobules (Fig. 11-1).

Hydrodissection is induced when the large volume of injected fluid separates subcutaneous fat into smaller particles to facilitate extraction by suction and reduce trauma; the infusion of up to several liters of aqueous solution also creates a cushion between the dermis and the underlying muscular fascia that further reduces the low risk of injury to underlying viscera. As serious adverse events associated with nontumescent liposuction are overwhelmingly associated with blood loss, the hemostatic benefits of tumescent anesthesia are arguably the most important. Liposuction aspirate collected after tumescent anesthesia is approximately 1–3% whole blood, compared with 40% for general anesthesia alone. Other benefits of tumescent anesthesia are intraoperative hydration and prolonged pain control for several hours after the procedure. Hence there is a reduced need for intraoperative intravenous fluid or additional postoperative pain medications. Epinephrine is responsible for the hemostatic benefits of tumescent anesthesia, as well as for increasing the duration of anesthesia. Epinephrine also slows the rate of systemic lidocaine absorption, thus ensuring slow mobilization of saline into the microvasculature and avoiding fluid overload. Peak plasma lidocaine levels are achieved for 6–24 h after surgery, with the gradual uptake and continuous metabolism of lidocaine protecting the patient from sharp peaks that could theoretically be associated with lidocaine toxicity if tumescent anesthesia were not employed.

The formulas for tumescent anesthesia are well established, with slightly more or less concentrated versions in use. Saline is the backbone

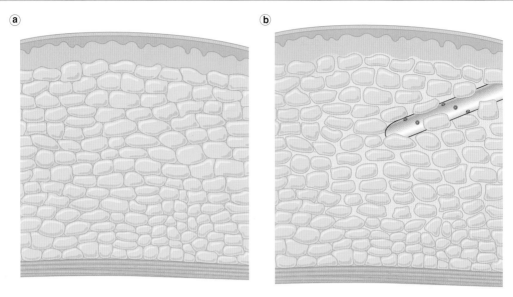

Figure 11-1 Infusion of tumescent fluid hydrodissects the fat, facilitating its removal, and also inflates the fat layer, which further cushions and protects underlying structures

of tumescent fluid. Lidocaine is the primary anesthetic agent. Significantly, even in concentrations as low as 0.05%, lidocaine has been shown to be bacteriostatic for *Staphylococcus aureus*. Although total lidocaine doses of 70–80 mg/kg have been used without inducing symptoms or signs of lidocaine toxicity, many liposuction surgeons adhere to the 55-mg/kg value shown to be safe by Moy and colleagues. Epinephrine is often used in a concentration of 1 : 1000 by volume, or 1 mL per liter of tumescent fluid. However, total epinephrine doses as high as 10 mg have been used without complications. Epinephrine toxicity, although extremely rare during liposuction, manifests initially as anxiety, agitation, and palpitations. Very high levels of epinephrine may be associated with hypertension, tachycardia, and arrhythmias. The addition of epinephrine makes the tumescent solution acidic, and burning may be felt during infusion. To avoid this, tumescent solution is buffered with sodium bicarbonate. Bicarbonate may also augment the antibacterial activity of lidocaine.

Lidocaine concentrations of 0.05–0.1% are commonly used in tumescent anesthesia. Higher concentrations (0.1%) are preferred for sensitive areas, such as the abdomen, lateral thighs, knees, inner thighs, periumbilical area, neck, and flanks. It has been suggested that, although the lower concentration may decrease the total lidocaine dose or enable treatment of greater body volume, this concentration may be inadequate to achieve prolonged anesthesia without supplementation with oral sedation. A compromise may be use of 0.075% solution, which is sufficient for anesthesia and yet reduces lidocaine load per liter of tumescent fluid. To estimate the total amount of tumescent fluid that may be infused at one time, it is necessary to know the patient's preoperative weight. For the prototypical 70-kg patient, approximately 4 liters of 0.1% tumescent fluid are acceptable, based on the Moy guidelines. Some surgeons choose to add triamcinolone to the infusion solution. Warming the solution has been shown to increase comfort, but hot solution is not recommended because of the risk of burns.

Infusion and aspiration equipment is used to inject tumescent fluid into the treatment area and then to remove aspirate containing fat. Infusion can be via a syringe attached to an infusion cannula (Fig. 11-2). A 60-mL syringe used in this manner may be appropriate for liposuction of small areas, such as the neck. For large areas, infusion is usually power assisted, either with a pressure cuff fitted over the intravenous fluid bag or, more commonly, with a motorized peristaltic pump. Pumps can be adjusted for speed of infusion, can be turned off and on manually or by foot switch, and require disposable tubing to deliver solution to the patient. The infusion tip can be a spinal needle or a specifically designed multiholed infusion cannula, with the latter being able to deliver more volume per unit time (75 mL/min for spinal needle versus 200 mL/min or more for infusion cannulas). In general, wider bore (2–3 mm), longer stem infusion cannulas are used for filling abdomen, thigh and hips, and shorter, finer cannulas for areas with small fat deposits, such as the neck.

Aspiration equipment resembles infusion equipment, but tends to be larger and more powerful. Syringe liposuction with a 60-mL syringe can be done, but is usually reserved for small areas.

Infusion cannula

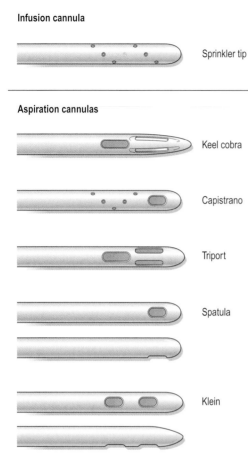

Sprinkler tip

Aspiration cannulas

Keel cobra

Capistrano

Triport

Spatula

Klein

Figure 11-2 Frequently used infusion and aspiration cannulas. Note that the more aggressive aspiration cannulas have multiple holes, often placed laterally or near the tip

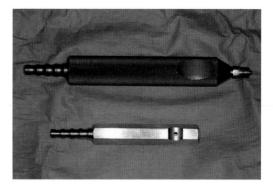

Figure 11-3 Cannula handles are available in various sizes and shapes. Thicker handles with thumb indentations are more comfortable for some

Toomey-type syringes have larger tip openings than standard Luer lock syringes, and syringes are available that either come with or can be fitted with special locks that maintain negative pressure during suction. Holding a 60-mL syringe for a protracted period with a single hand is fatiguing and has been noted by the author to cause transient compression injury to the thumb. Most surgeons use mechanical aspirators in lieu of syringe aspiration. Powerful piston-driven aspirators can be fitted with 1–3-L disposable bags for collection of aspirate and semirigid disposable tubing that will not collapse shut when vacuum is applied. Foot pedals and hand controls are available for starting and stopping suction, and some machines offer variable suction pressure for different body sites. Suction machines or syringes are used with aspiration cannulas, which are produced in many more varieties than infusion cannulas.

Ranging in length from about 3 to 14 inches, aspiration cannulas (Figs 11-2–11-5) are also distinguished by their bore, which can be measured in millimeters or gauge (Table 11-4), and by the

pattern, location, number, sharpness, and size of holes at the suction tip. Tip architecture, in turn, determines the degree of cannula aggressiveness (Table 11-5). The most aggressive cannulas remove fat the fastest and are useful for debulking relatively large volumes in areas of significant fat accumulation, such as the abdomen and hips. Medium to less aggressive cannulas are useful for areas of smaller fat deposits or for fine sculpting near the end of a liposuction procedure, when precision and small-volume correction are necessary to avoid skin dimpling or unevenness associated with excessive removal of fat. The most aggressive cannulas are no longer favored by most surgeons, as the risks of asymmetry, skin dimpling, and other adverse events appear to outweigh the benefit of a speedy procedure. As a rule of thumb, more aggressive cannulas are thicker (10–12 G, or 2.7–3.4-mm bore), more pointy, and have multiple, large holes near the tip of the cannula. Conservative cannulas are thinner (12–16 G, or 1.5–2.7-mm bore), blunt, and have one or two smaller holes, which are set back further from the tip. Smaller fat deposits may also benefit from shorter cannulas, which reduce the risk of skin tenting and consequent superficial suctioning when the cannula is fully inserted.

Cannulas are usually attached to the distal end of the suction tubing with a cannula handle. Ergonomic cannula handles are available that reduce fatigue by providing a big grip surface and an indented area to rest the thumb. Some liposuction cannulas are manufactured with handles attached.

Adjuvant equipment is sometimes used to speed liposuction or to increase its effectiveness. Powered liposuction, laser lipolysis, and external ultrasound are some of these additional technologies. External ultrasound is based on the theory that energy-actuated microcavitations in the subcutis might help destroy fat and also separate fat into minute particles more amenable to easy removal. Reports of seromas and skin burns,

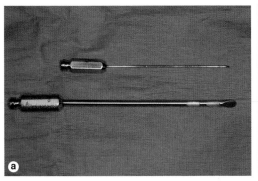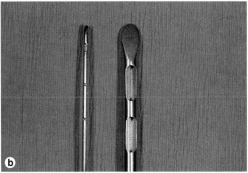

Figure 11-4 There are dramatic differences in the bore sizes of aspiration cannulas. Here 8-G Klein and 18-G Capistrano cannulas are placed (A) side by side and (B) in close-up

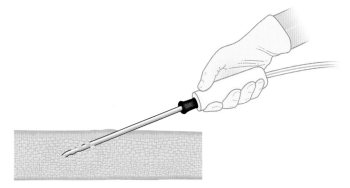

Figure 11-5 In general, the handle and cannula apparatus is held so that the suction holes are pointed downwards, away from the skin surface.

Table 11-4 Liposuction cannula diameters by gauge	
Gauge	Diameter (mm)
6	5.0
8	4.2
10	3.4
12	2.8
14	2.2
16	1.6
18	1.2

Table 11-5 Aspiration cannulas grouped by degree of aggressiveness		
Degree of aggressiveness	Type	Gauge or diameter
High	Keel Cobra	3 or 3.7 mm
	Capistrano	10 or 12 G
	Mercedes	10 or 12 G
	Pinto	10 or 12 G
	Toledo	10 or 12 G
Medium	Accelerator/Triport	3 mm
	Klein	12 G
	Capistrano	14 G
	Keel Cobra	2.5 mm
	Texas	2.5 mm
	Dual Port	2.5 mm
	Fournier	2.5 mm
Low	Capistrano	16 G
	Klein	14–18 G
	Spatula	2–3 mm

as well as studies indicating minimal intraoperative benefits, have resulted in this procedure not being widely adopted. Powered liposuction cannulas, on the other hand, are used by many busy liposuction surgeons to reduce operator fatigue and increase the efficiency of fat removal. Reciprocating action in powered liposuction moves the cannula tip back and forth at a rate of 3000 to 6000 strokes per minute, with this motion making it easier to move the cannula through the fat compartment. More recently, several laser devices have been developed that can be inserted into tumesced fat like liposuction cannulas. Laser lipolysis is achieved when the live laser tip melts proximal fat. The most commonly used laser lipolysis device is the 1064-nm Nd:YAG laser; as these lasers can injure the retina, eye protection must be used. Care should also be taken to avoid aiming the laser tip up into the dermis. Just as traditional liposuction cannulas can injure the dermis through oversuction, laser lipolysis tips can cause thermal injury and burns if applied too superficially. For small areas, like the neck, laser lipolysis may be sufficient for cosmetic correction, and no suction or fat removal may be required. Traditional liposuction may be performed in combination with laser lipolysis for treatment of bulkier areas. These innovations notwithstanding, traditional liposuction with syringe or machine suction remains favored by many experts and continues to provide excellent safety and efficacy.

Other equipment required for liposuction includes sterile gowns and gloves for the surgeon and assistants. Liposuction is best performed in sterile conditions to minimize further the low risk of infection. After the procedure, the patient is asked to wear compression garments to the body areas that were treated. These may be applied for a period of days to weeks, and arrangements to acquire one or two pairs of such washable garments that fit the patient should be concluded well before the procedure. Some surgeons provide patients with the relevant information and have them buy their own garments; other practices may order these and keep them onsite to dispense after the procedure (Fig. 11-6).

Device or treatment selection

As implied above, much of the variation in equipment used in liposuction is a function of surgeon preference rather than patient need. This may seem capricious, but it is not, as it is impractical for a liposuction surgeon to be equally familiar and facile with each of the plethora of available devices and cannulas. To ensure operator expertise and thus patient safety, it is preferable for a surgeon to master the operation of a modest array of devices that cumulatively permit the surgeon safely to treat fatty accumulations of different types and sizes in patients with various body habitus and skin elasticity.

The basic equipment used by liposuction surgeons often includes the following (Table 11-6):

- An infusion pump
- A mechanical aspirator
- One or two infusion cannulas
- A set of conservative, intermediate, and aggressive cannulas

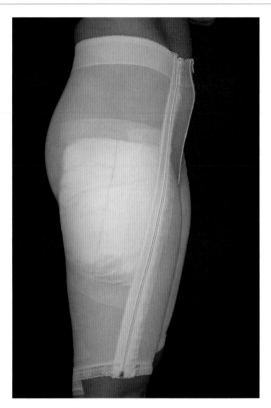

Figure 11-6 Binders and garments are applied after the procedure. Initially, these are worn over absorbent dressings designed to wick away the tumescent fluid, which may continue to drain from entry sites for hours. Several assistants may be required to apply compression garments properly to a sedated patient

- Disposable tubing (for the aspirator and infusers)
- One or two comfortable cannula handles.

Adequate supplies of epinephrine, lidocaine, and bicarbonate, as well as bags of intravenous solution, are also needed to make fresh tumescent solution. Postprocedure compression garments in routine sizes are also often stocked. Surgeons who perform only low-volume liposuction, such as neck or jowl procedures, may omit the infusion pumps and aspirators, and replace them with a set of self-locking 30- and 60-mL syringes for infusion and aspiration of fluid.

Whether or not a patient should undergo liposuction is an important determination that must be made after careful consideration of medical history, laboratory values, physical examination, and patient expectations. Medical history should be reviewed to rule out conditions that may exacerbate risk of bleeding, infection, emboli, thrombophlebitis, edema, and previous surgeries in the area of interest, particularly abdominal surgeries, which may increase the risks associated with

Table 11-6 Equipment and supplies routinely used for tumescent liposuction

Type of equipment or supply	Disposable	Alternative
Infusion pump	No	Large syringes
Infusion tubing	Yes	Large syringes
Mechanical aspirator	No	Large syringes
Suction tubing	Yes	Large syringes
Self-locking 60-mL syringes	Yes	Mechanical pumps
Infusion sprinkler cannula	No	Spinal needle
Aspiration cannulas (several)	No	–
Cannula handles	No	Large syringes
Sterile gowns and fields	No	–
Tumescent solution	Yes	–
Microwave oven	No	Unwarmed fluid
Pole for hanging tumescent fluid	No	Large syringes
Compression garments	Yes	–
Powered liposuction device	No	Unpowered

liposuction. Metabolism of lidocaine is via the liver, and specifically cytochrome P-450 enzyme CYP3A4, so patients on medications that inhibit P-450 function may not be optimal candidates. Concomitant use of selective serotonin reuptake inhibitors has been associated with lidocaine toxicity during liposuction, and other similarly metabolized drugs such as erythromycin or ketoconazole may pose similar theoretic risks. Hepatic disease, including a history of hepatitis or hepatotoxic chemotherapy, may also be contraindications to liposuction.

Laboratory values commonly checked prior to liposuction include liver function tests, hepatitis panel, chemistries and electrolytes, complete blood count with differential, prothrombin time, partial thromboplastin time, and a serum pregnancy test for premenopausal women. If appropriate, other infections may be assessed by urinalysis or other HIV testing.

Physical examination of the patient is commonly performed with the patient standing up, although sitting and supine examinations may be preferred by some surgeons. The purpose of the examination is to assess general health and, more specifically, suitability for liposuction. Key attributes are the outline of the subcutaneous

fat compartment, including its size and distribution, and the character of the overlying dermis. Regarding fat distribution, patients with overall obesity are poor candidates for liposuction, but those with focal, well demarcated, adipose depositions resistant to diet and exercise are good candidates. Fat pads deeper than the subcutis, such as visceral abdominal fat, are not accessible to liposuction. Dermal flaws that may contribute to unsuccessful liposuction are poor skin elasticity, skin laxity, and underlying muscle flaccidity. Liposuction does not reduce skin surface area directly, so to obtain a smooth postoperative contour the skin must be able to shrink smoothly and evenly. Excessively loose skin will not do this, and excess hanging skin may remain after surgery. Visible dimpling of skin, or cellulite, will not be corrected by liposuction. Kaminer's concept of "soft skin" refers to patients with loose, inelastic skin that does not rebound quickly to rest position when pinched (e.g. via the "snap test") or has widespread preoperative dimpling. Patients with soft skin should be apprised of the risk of skin excess, or even worsening of cellulite with aggressive suction. They may also be candidates for skin excision and muscle tightening procedures, such as abdominoplasty, or rhytidectomy (facelift).

Reasonable patient expectations include the understanding that liposuction can reduce localized fatty deposits and improve contour, but cannot perfectly correct either. Some patients believe that skin will contract markedly after liposuction, and they must be disabused of this notion. It must be made clear that cellulite is not improved and may be worsened by liposuction. Liposuction is also not a substitute for a diet and exercise regimen, which should be used in combination with the surgical correction. Patients with eating disorders, or apparent body dysmorphic disorder, as manifested by numerous prior surgeries for the same problem or excessive self-criticism, should be referred for psychologic consultation. Liposuction frequently does enable clothes to fit better in patients who previously had focal fatty deposits. For those who have an efficient exercise regimen and an appropriate calorie-limited diet, liposuction can be an effective and minimally invasive procedure for removal of resistant fat pockets.

In conclusion, liposuction is appropriate for healthy people without bleeding disorders, liver injury, or other significant complicating medical disorders. Patients with localized fat deposits but elastic, nonredundant, overlying skin, will have the best outcomes. Liposuction is inappropriate for the treatment of obesity, and patients with excess and soft skin may require either an alternative or concurrent skin resection procedure. Patients should understand that, although they are likely to have a permanent local improvement in body contour after liposuction, subsequent weight gain may negate this or cause fat accumulation elsewhere on the body.

Alternatives to liposuction do exist. Apart from skin resection procedures, patients may also select minimally invasive fat melting and tightening procedures. One of these is so-called "fat mesotherapy" (e.g. Lipodissolve), and entails injection of a mixture of phosphatidylcholine, deoxycholate, and sometimes other chemicals into the subcutis to dissolve fat. Current work is indicating that side-effects may be minimized by employing formulations that consist exclusively of deoxycholate, a detergent, eliminating other constituents in this mixture. There have been reports of peripheral neuropathy and infections associated with this procedure, and it is currently (2007) regarded with caution by major dermatologic surgery professional organizations in the USA. Further work on safety and efficacy is needed to assess the utility of this procedure. Potential benefits include fat loss without surgery, and potential risks include contamination of the injectable solution, minimal fat loss not comparable to that from a liposuction procedure, and other potential adverse events.

Laser, radiofrequency, and ultrasound devices are also becoming available that purport to shrink fat by delivering energy into the subcutis. The major challenge that remains is how to melt fat efficaciously without injuring overlying skin or deep structures, or inducing significant pain. There remains disagreement as to the degree of fat melting possible by such procedures, and, like mesotherapy, they do not at present offer a degree of improvement comparable to liposuction. As with mesotherapy, there remains the benefit of not requiring surgery and the promise of increased efficacy and safety in the future. Ultrasound may be the most promising modality for fat melting because it permits very deep heat deposition with relatively little dermal injury. If nonablative energy fat melting were to become markedly more efficacious, one residual challenge would be how to remove the copious quantities of necrosed fat from the subcutis, or whether to allow this to be metabolized at site.

Radiofrequency and light-based devices may also have utility for treatment of cellulite, which is not responsive to and may be worsened by liposuction. Some such devices are approved by the Food and Drug Administration for temporary reduction of the appearance of cellulite. Subcision, a procedure that entails insertion of a sharp needle into the superficial fat and abrasion of the subdermal area with back and forth movements of the same, may also help release fibrous attachments that may be responsible for cellulite.

Method of device or treatment application

Key Points

- Inject no more than recommended dose per weight of lidocaine.
- Minimize size and number of entry sites, and conceal locations.
- Avoid superficial suctioning to prevent dimpling and skin irregularity.
- Use prophylactic antibiotics.
- Encourage prolonged use (at least 6 weeks) of compression garments to minimize the risk of seroma and achieve an optimal contour.

Dose setting/selection

Liposuction is performed similarly at various body sites. Concentrated (0.1%) tumescent fluid may be used at more sensitive body sites, and dilute fluid (0.05–0.075%) at less sensitive sites. Total dose of lidocaine is usually adjusted in accordance with patient bodyweight to conform to a level of 55 mg/kg. Patients with skin of color may be more prone to hyperpigment or develop hypertrophic scars at puncture sites where cannulas are inserted. This risk is not mitigated by reducing the overall dose of lidocaine, but may be addressed by minimizing the number of entry sites, concealing these in skinfolds or other anatomic areas, and reducing skin trauma during liposuction to avoid spreading or tearing of skin apertures. Men may have more fibrous subdermal fat and also more total suprafascial fat thickness; this may require more aggressive infusion of anesthetic solution to prevent discomfort during suctioning, and also more aggressive suctioning during removal.

Treatment technique (Box 11-1)

Prior to treatment, a detailed patient consultation should be conducted, as described above. At this point, it is appropriate to provide prescriptions for preoperative, intraoperative, and postoperative medications (Table 11-7). Drugs may include oral antibiotics, which are usually started several days or at least an hour before surgery; sedatives or analgesics to be used intraoperatively; and post-treatment pain medications.

Preoperative photographs, often front and side views, are obtained. Informed consent is obtained, and, if so desired, the patient is premedicated with sedatives or analgesics, often oral diazepam. After discussion with the patient, and appreciation of which exact areas the patient is concerned about and which are feasible to treat, the sites to be treated are marked. A medium-tip black permanent marker (e.g. Sharpie) can be used to demarcate areas that require active suctioning; areas that require light suctioning, or feathering or blending with the surrounding areas; and areas that should not be suctioned (Fig. 11-7). Markers are also used to pinpoint entry sites, which are usually placed symmetrically on either side of the body, and in such a manner as to enable easy suctioning, triangulation during suctioning,

---

BOX 11-1

Major procedural steps in tumescent liposuction

Obtain consent and prepare patient

- Review consent form and answer questions
- Provide patient with opportunity to decline procedure
- Mark patient skin, and have patient review examine markings in mirror
- Provide oral sedation, if any

Sterile prep and drape

Infuse tumescent solution

- Anesthetize and perforate entry sites
- Infuse tumescent solution 1–2 cm beyond feathering borders at multiple levels
- Reposition patient and repeat infusion from other entry sites

Aspirate fat

- Optional re-preparation and drape
- Remove fat via criss-cross technique
- Observe and avoid danger zones
- Periodically pinch and palpate skin to ensure even and complete suctioning
- Usually, one side is suctioned, then the other; the process is repeated as needed

Prepare patient for discharge

- Clean patient skin and apply dressings to entry sites
- Apply compression garments
- Review postoperative instructions
- Schedule follow-up appointment

---

and optimal concealment of such sites after the procedure.

Thereafter, the patient is sterilely prepped and draped, and placed in a supine or prone position. A short, fine (e.g. 30-G, ½ inch) needle attached to a small (e.g. 3 mL) syringe containing 0.1–2% lidocaine solution is then used to raise blebs at the sites of cannula entry. A no. 11 blade or other similar device (e.g. 1.5–2-mm punch biopsy instrument) is then used at each potential entry location to make a shallow stab incision 3–4 mm in length, oriented along the relaxed skin tension lines (Fig. 11-8). A spinal needle or blunt-tipped infusion cannula is inserted and infusion of tumescent fluid is begun. The fluid flows from the peristaltic pump, passive pressure cuff, or large syringe into the subcutis.

To protect underlying structures, the insertion of the infusion cannula is initially vertical but then angled laterally as it is advanced. The cannula is advanced and retracted with full motions that ensure that the tip disgorging anesthetic covers the maximum radius and hence provides anesthetic to the largest possible area. Movement of the cannula should be gradual to allow adequate filling at each site. When the cannula is nearly withdrawn, it can then be redirected in a slightly different direction; in this manner, a round area around the cannula is infused. Redirection of the cannula should be performed only when the cannula is pulled back because intrastroke redirection puts stress on the entry site, with the attendant risk of friction trauma, and also causes tenting and dimpling of the skin that may result in subsequent uneven suctioning (Fig. 11-9).

Several layers of fat, including immediately subdermal, mid-fat, and deeper fat should all be infused, because each of these will ultimately be suctioned. Rates of tumescent fluid delivery vary, but very high flow speeds may be antithetical to even and complete anesthesia, patient comfort, and conservation of anesthetic fluid. Common infusion rates are less than 100 mL/min, with higher rates tolerable if the patient is relatively

---

Table 11-7 Oral medications frequently used in conjunction with tumescent liposuction

Medication category	Specific types	Indication	When dosed
Antibiotics	Broad spectrum (cephalosporins, other)	Infection prevention	Starting before procedure and usually for several days
Sedatives	Benzodiazepines (diazepam, lorazepam, other)	Intraoperative sedation, muscle relaxation	Immediately before procedure
Analgesics (if necessary)	Mild narcotics	Pain control	After surgery, usually for brief course
Antinausea agents (if necessary)	Nonsteroidal agents (prochlorperazine, ondansetron)	Nausea reduction	After surgery, if patient experiences significant nausea
Vitamins (less commonly)	C, K, multivitamins	Stress tolerance	Recommended before surgery by minority of surgeons

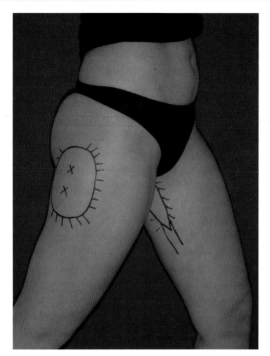

Figure 11-7 Marking of areas of excess fat should be done before infusion of tumescent fluid, which can distort anatomy. Notations should be used to distinguish between dense fat pockets, smaller areas of fat removal, and regions at the periphery that require light feathering only. Discussion with the patient can increase the likelihood that areas of particular aesthetic concern are targeted

more sedated. A small degree of burning sensation is to be expected immediately upon starting infusion at a particular site; this quickly diminishes. Especially when treating a larger area, it is important not to deplete prematurely the total allowable supply of tumescent fluid. After the fat has been infused adequately from one entry site, the cycle is repeated from the other sites. Horizontal and vertical criss-crossing of cannula paths from multiple sites is recommended to avoid missing areas that may then be painful during suctioning.

Delay required between infusion and suction varies according to anatomic site, and ranges from 15 to 45 min. Vasoconstriction may occur in as little as 15 min, but 30–45 min may be necessary for complete anesthesia, which enables precise and painstaking suctioning. Visible white blanch at the area to be treated is a good clinical indicator of adequacy of anesthesia.

If bilateral liposuction is being performed, fat removal commences on the side anesthetized first. Fat is removed from both areas of significant accumulation and from the edges of such areas. Feathering refers to the process of conservative fat removal from peripheral areas to create a smooth contour with the surrounding skin and

prevent a precipitous drop-off at the edge of the fat pocket of interest. As with infiltration, full back-and-forth cannula movements are needed to ensure even fat removal and to avoid oversuctioning at any one site (Fig. 11-10). Continual manipulation of the skin and subcutis is necessary to ensure that appropriate amounts of fat are being removed. Tactile feedback is provided by pinching, pressing, and moving the skin with the hand not holding the suction cannula (Fig. 11-11). In this manner, the surgeon ensures that the area is evenly defatted and that focal, asymmetric minipockets of fat do not elude treatment.

Compressing the skin with the nondominant hand also helps to guide the cannula to various depths, helping to remove not only mid-fat, but also superficial and deep fat (Fig. 11-12). For instance, if the skin and subcutis are pinched and then the cannula is used to push through the superficial pinched fat, fat just below the dermis may be gently removed; similarly, if a cannula is moved laterally below a handful of pinched skin, this may be preferentially target deeper fat.

Triangulation is a key concept in cannula movement (Fig. 11-13). To ensure a smooth, even decrease in the fat layer, localized fat deposits are suctioned from two or three sites located approximately 120° apart. If triangulation is not performed, there is a risk of oversuctioning in one or more grooves, thus creating an uneven topography of hills and valleys. Larger bore cannulas are used early in liposuction of a particular anatomic area (Fig. 11-14). At this point, anesthetic effect is at its peak, and the larger cannulas slide through the fat comfortably. As the volume of fat is decreased and much of the tumescent fluid is removed by suction, smaller bore cannulas come into use. Fine-diameter cannulas cause less trauma and hence less discomfort, and are also more effective for removing lesser amounts of residual fat without causing overlying textural abnormalities.

During the liposuction process, the surgeon needs to be aware of the evolving character of the liposuction aspirate. A pale yellow aspirate is ideal, but a degree of serosanguineous fluid is usually inevitably elicited as the procedure continues (Fig. 11-15). Frank blood is a sign of caution, and the aspiration cannula should be repositioned. Vigorous suctioning accompanied by very little fat removal indicates that a particular area or depth may have been fully suctioned. Lower or higher cannula elevation may result in further fat mobilization. Dimpling or worsened cellulite can be avoided by aiming the cannula holes downward. As the dermis on the trunk can be thick, the surgeon should understand that the first 0.5–1 inches pinched may be skin rather than subcutis. Suctioning should be discontinued at a point when sufficient fat remains to ensure a smooth postoperative contour.

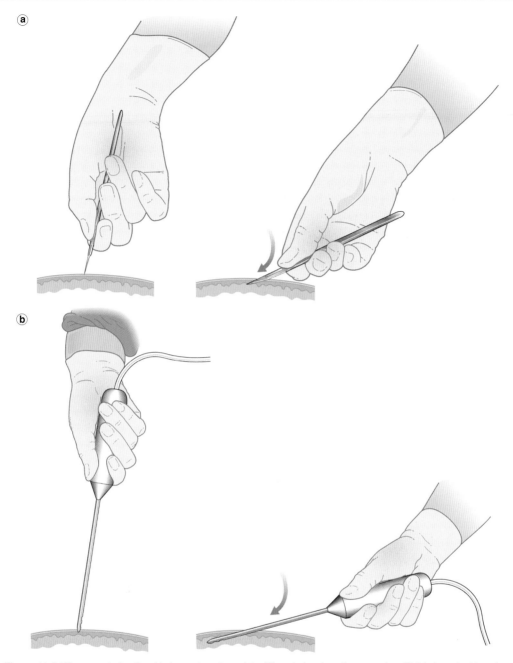

Figure 11-8 When puncturing the skin to create entry points, (A) and when inserting cannulas, (B) it is important to enter at a steep angle of 75-90 degrees and then quickly adjust to a more shallow angle (20-30 degrees) so as to avoid injury to deep structures

PEARLS

hUse warm tumescent fluid to enhance patient comfort.

Consider short-acting benzodiazepines (e.g. diazepam 5–10 mg) for anxious patients.

Assess patient medication list to verify that risk of intraoperative bleeding is minimal.

Discontinue nutritional supplements, vitamins, and herbal medications with anticoagulant properties prior to surgery.

Ensure before surgery that patient has transportation home.

Near the end of the procedure, stand patient up with support to assess bilateral symmetry.

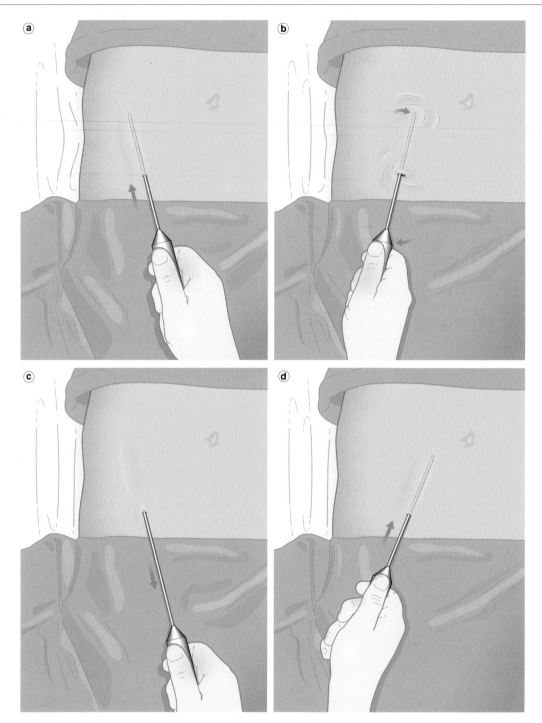

Figure 11-9 To redirect the suction cannula, first pull it back out nearly all the way, and then reinsert it in a new direction. Trying to turn the cannula tip sideways towards a new location while the cannula is still deeply inserted causes twisting of the skin and fat. This can result in suctioning of a different area than that intended, and it can tear or widen the aperture at the entry site

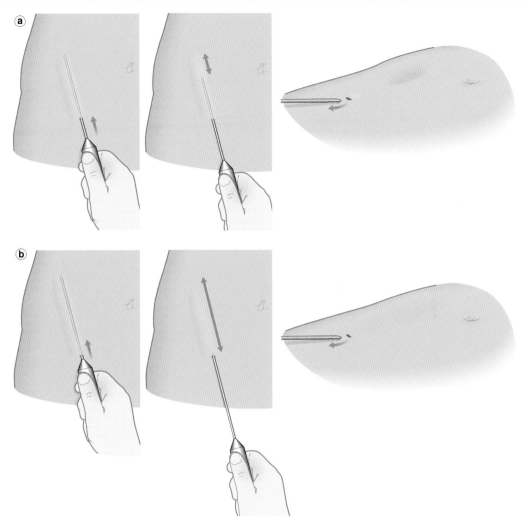

Figure 11-10 Suctioning requires long strokes that remove fat smoothly from a wide area, rather than short strokes that remove excess fat removal at one site

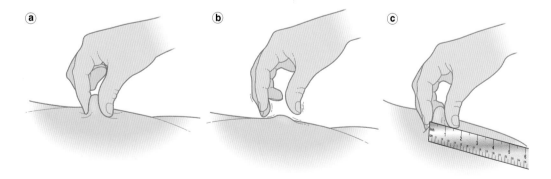

Figure 11-11 Tactile feedback can be used to assess (A) the "snap test," or whether skin elasticity is sufficient for eventual skin retraction after liposuction, and (B) the postprocedure endpoint, which occurs when a thumb and forefinger pinch of the abdomen collects less than half an inch (C) of tissue.

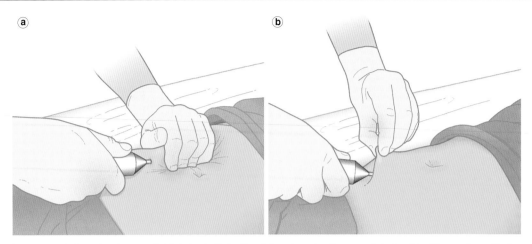

Figure 11-12 Grasping the superficial abdominal fat with a fist, and running the cannula below this, (A) permits suctioning of the deep fat. Similarly, pinching the upper fat and spearing the central core with the cannula enables complete removal of the mid to upper fat (B)

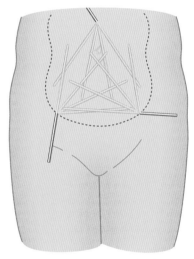

Figure 11-13 Triangulation, or suctioning from several entry sites in a series of overlapping fanning motions, allows even and smooth reduction of the fatty layer

Alternative treatment methods

Technique in liposuction is frequently anatomic site specific (Table 11-8), and distribution of fat can be gender specific (Fig. 11-16). Effective, speedy, and safe suctioning of different body areas requires minor, and sometimes major, adjustments.

Neck and jowls

Key Points

- Stay superficial to avoid injury to neurovascular structures.
- Hyperextend and support neck to avoid deep penetrance of cannula.
- Avoid excessive suctioning of jowls to stay away from marginal mandibular nerves.

The neck and jowls are perhaps the body region most commonly treated with liposuction. Neck youthfulness can be measured by the cervicomental angle (Fig. 11-17), which is the intersection of the vertical anterior facial plane and the submental plane. In young patients, ideal cervicomental angles are approximately 80–95°. Another important parameter is the submental–cervical angle, ideally relatively sharp, which is defined by the submental plane and the anterior border of the neck. As fat accumulates in the submental area and the skin becomes more lax, normal aging results in descent of the cervical point, the junction between the submental area of the face and the neck. Under the neck skin is the thin bilateral platysma muscle, the local continuation of the superficial musculo-aponeurotic system (SMAS), which may need to be resuspended in the aging neck. Subplatysmal fat that lies below the platysma may contribute to the appearance of a thickened anterior neck. Lateral jowl fat pads are accentuated as gravitational descent results in ptosis of the jowls. Depending on its position, the hyoid bone, a floating point within the anterior neck muscles that is important in swallowing, can make the anterior neck appear more or less full.

The optimal neck liposuction patient is a woman with excess submental fat. Lateral neck profile in such often mildly obese patients can be improved by liposuction alone. Elevation of the cervicomental point results in a better cervicomental angle. Jowls are treated more sparingly to avoid oversuction and consequent indentations.

Contraction of the skin can improve the overall outcomes of liposuction. Such contraction occurs as the dermis re-adheres to the underlying fascia postoperatively. Thinner patients with limited submental fat and excess skin may benefit from a concurrent skin resection procedure,

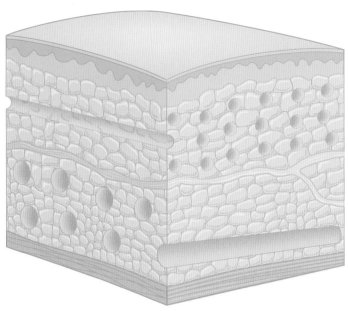

Figure 11-14 Finer cannulas are used for superficial suctioning after wider bore cannulas have debulked the deep fat

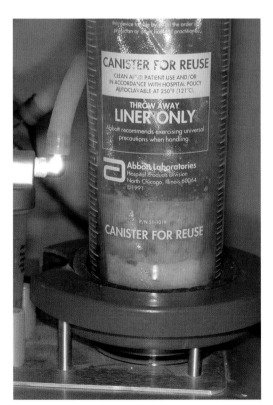

Figure 11-15 Aspirated fat is yellowish in color, but may be tinged with pink as the procedure progresses and additional suctioning is required to mobilize residual fat. Gradations on the canister attached to the mechanical aspirator facilitate measurement of the amount of fat and fluid removed

such as a rhytidectomy. Effects of skin removal may be enhanced by platysmaplasty, a procedure in which the platysma is tightened by suture plication (Fig. 11-18). Such a procedure can reduce platysmal bands, which may become evident once submental fat is removed. Subplatysmal fat can be removed by careful liposuction in patients with significant deep fat accumulation. Notably, an anteriorly displaced hyoid bone can complicate neck liposuction and reduce the enhancement associated with this procedure.

In the standard approach to neck liposuction, the patient is positioned with the neck hyperextended. Reduction of the anterior neck fat is commenced from one submental and two infralobular incisions. Jowls may be approached also from two infrajowl incisions. These three to five incisions may be suctioned by machine or syringe suction, with syringe suction alone often practical for less fatty necks.

Postliposuction, a pressure dressing and a compression garment resembling a chin-strap is worn by the patient day and night for several days. Thereafter this garment may be worn at night only.

Adverse events after neck liposuction include edema, swelling, and bruising, which are seen in most cases. Jowl swelling may remit more slowly than neck swelling and may be evident over a week later. Hematoma can occur, and is more common after platysmaplasty. Risk of seroma formation may be reduced by extended use of compression. In some cases of large-volume liposuction,

Table 11-8 Anatomic areas most commonly treated by liposuction (in descending order)

Men	Women
Flanks/love handles	Abdomen
Abdomen	Outer thighs
Neck/jowls	Hip/waist
Breast	Neck/jowls

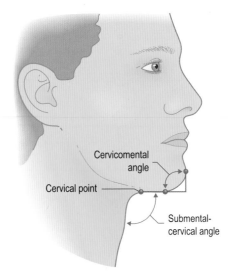

Figure 11-17 Angles associated with neck liposuction. Cervicomental angle is ideally 80–95°. Note the location of the cervical point (C), the junction between the submental area and the neck. Youthful appearance is also associated with a small submental–cervical angle

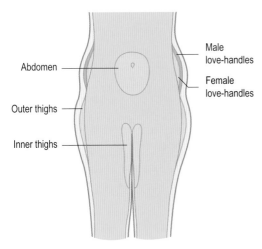

Figure 11-16 Men and women have predominant fat accumulation in different parts of the torso

a skinfold may emerge proximal to the submental incision; this may eventually involute or be treated with intralesional steroid injection. A potentially serious complication of neck and jowl liposuction is injury to the marginal mandibular nerve (Fig. 11-19). Liposuction cannulas do not usually sever the nerve, but may traumatize or stretch it, leading to temporary paresis of the ipsilateral lip depressors. Resolution within a few weeks to a month is routine.

Arms

Key Points

- Perform "snap test" to assess skin elasticity.
- Excess skin may need to be resected.

Fat accumulation in the arms tends to segregate in the lateral and posterior compartments. Staging is by having the patient extend the arm against resistance. Palpation reveals the component of excess tissue that is fat, rather than sagging skin. Women may be distressed by the size of their arms, which they view as disproportionately large compared with the rest of their body (Fig. 11-20). Patient goals may include wearing short-sleeved shirts or other revealing clothes

without embarrassment about the width of their arms.

During the preoperative evaluation, a "snap test" can be performed to see how rapidly the skin retracts to rest position after being pinched and released. A poor snap test result suggests that liposuction may have a suboptimal outcome. Combination of liposuction with brachioplasty, or skin resection, may improve this outcome. Some experienced practitioners also believe that a second liposuction procedure a year or more after the first may provide additional skin retraction.

As with liposuction at other anatomic sites, the presence of a discrete fat pocket increases the likelihood of a satisfactory result. Fat pockets are often localized to the lateral triceps or deltoid regions, with the medial upper arm being more excess skin than adipose. Younger patients with good skin tone and moderate fat excess tend to have better results than older patients with flaccid skin and large accumulations of fat.

Patients concerned about arm girth may also wish to address bulging at the far lateral chest, abutting the area inferior to the axilla. This area may include a tail of breast fat and may also protrude because of the manner of skin drape at this site. Given the thin overlying skin and possibility that genetic predisposition contributes to this appearance, experienced practitioners caution against aggressive suctioning, which may worsen the contour.

Insertion sites are often at the lateral epicondyle, the posterior axillary line, and the medial mid–upper arm. As the ulnar nerve passes

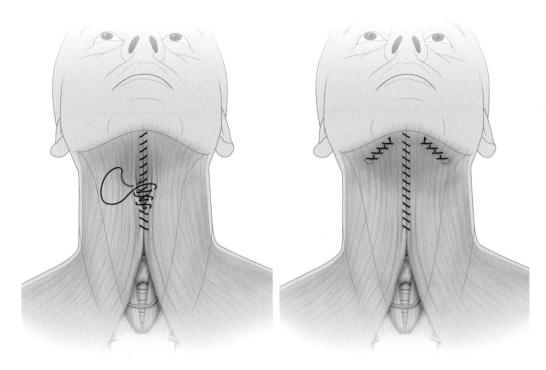

Figure 11-18 Plication of the platysma can improve the results of neck liposuction in patients with muscle laxity. However, meticulous surgical technique is required to minimize bleeding when suturing the nerve, and smooth reapproximation of the nerve is necessary to avoid subsequent bunching of the overlying skin

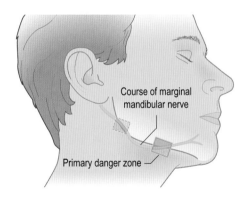

Course of marginal
mandibular nerve

Primary danger zone —

Figure 11-19 Neck and jowl liposuction should avoid the marginal mandibular nerve, which is most vulnerable when it crosses the jaw edge approximately midway between the point of the chin and the lateral jaw. Aspiration cannulas are relatively blunt and therefore unlikely to sever the nerve, but they can cause a temporary neuropraxia if used aggressively at this site

Upper arms may require 500 mL to more than 1500 mL of tumescent fluid. The initial patient position is lateral decubitus with the arm at the side and the elbow slightly bent; medial arm suctioning is performed with the patient supine, the elbow bent, and the hand raised and placed behind the head. Some conservative liposuction surgeons restrict themselves to longitudinal and oblique strokes, but others believe additional criss-cross technique is useful for adequate and smooth fat removal.

After liposuction, a compression garment is worn. Garments that cover the upper torso may be appropriate when axillary folds are treated as well. Otherwise, an arm garment connected by a band across the chest may be used. In either case, the garment should enclose the arm distal to the elbow. Heavy work and lifting should be avoided for several days after the procedure. Driving should be avoided for 1–3 days.

Common side-effects include those typical for liposuction at any site, including swelling, bruising, insertion site visibility and postinflammatory hyperpigmentation, and uneven final contour. Hematomas and seromas are less common, as are infections. Ulnar nerve neuropraxia is a rare, site-specific, adverse event.

superficially along the dorsum of the medial epicondyle, in order to prevent risk of neuropraxia an entry point should not be placed here. The radial nerve should also be avoided when it is high as it courses between the lateral and medial heads of the triceps on the mid–upper posterior arm.

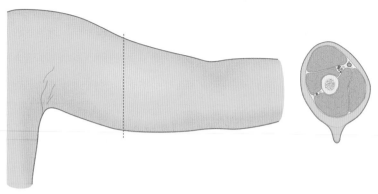

Figure 11-20 Arm liposuction is requested most often by women who regard their arms as disproportionately wide compared with the rest of their bodies. Fat removal may be insufficient in some cases as excess skin may only partially retract following the procedure

Female and male breast

* Fibrous tissue requires aggressive suctioning.
* Preoperative imaging desirable for female breast.
* Hide entry sites under breast.

Large female breasts can cause functional disability, including spine and gait abnormalities, and chronic back pain. Back and shoulder pain is reduced by removal of 30% or more of breast mass. Surgical excision remains a first-line procedure for breast reduction, but some patients may decline such a procedure because of the resulting visible linear scars, and need for general anesthesia and hospitalization. For patients with modestly enlarged breasts, breast reduction by liposuction is a reasonable option. A 1–2-inch reduction in bra size is likely, and the volume of the breast is usually reduced uniformly. Breast liposuction is not indicated as a treatment for nipple ptosis, as no skin resection or breast resuspension is performed to correct this. Rather, breast liposuction is appropriate for patients with slightly large but well shaped and positioned breasts in which the nipple–areolar complex is not displaced.

Preoperative assessment includes standard photography from front, oblique, and lateral views. Ptosis can be measured as the distance from the inframammary crease to the lowest point of the breast, and from the inframammary crease to the nipple. The volume of the breast before liposuction is measured by water displacement. A 4-L beaker is filled with water and then the entire breast is submerged, thus displacing an equivalent volume of water; to maximize precision, the procedure is repeated for each breast and the results are averaged.

Given the theoretic risk of altered breast stroma after liposuction, preoperative radiography and mammography are recommended by many.

Although breast liposuction has not been shown to increase the risk of breast cancer, to hasten its onset, or to induce calcifications or other abnormalities that may be confused with cancer on imaging or palpation, obtaining preoperative and postoperative studies simplifies future assessment of breast cancer risk by providing a baseline.

Tumescent fluid equal to 100–120% of the measured breast volume is typically infused initially. After 30 min, an approximately equivalent amount may again be infused to achieve more turgidity and anesthesia. Entry sites are created in the lateral and medial inframammary crease. A criss-cross technique is used, with aggressive, powered cannulas preferred because of the fibrous nature of breast fat. Larger fat deposits are deeper, but some superficial suctioning is necessary as well. Glandular tissue is preferentially concentrated around the nipple and in the upper lateral quadrant; these areas should be suctioned conservatively. Symmetric postoperative appearance of the breasts is crucial, so this must be assessed intraoperatively. If the breasts were of similar size prior to the procedure, a near equivalent amount of fat should be aspirated from each.

Breast contour must be aesthetically pleasing even as breast size is reduced. Large amounts of fat should not be removed from the superior breast to avoid textural irregularities. Too much suctioning under the nipple should be avoided as this can cause necrosis and loss of sensation. Subaxillary fat reduction will usually improve the overall result. If the breast stroma is very dense, smaller bore cannulas may be more effective in penetrating it and mobilizing fat.

After surgery, a pressure garment is worn for the first week to minimize the risk of seroma and edema. Subsequently, a sports bra may be sufficient compression. Vigorous physical activity must be postponed for several weeks as the breasts remain sensitive to motion. Firm masses become palpable in the breasts as edema recedes. Resolution of these masses can take many months, with masses in the inferior breast being the last to dissipate. Temporary loss of sensation around the nipple gradually recedes.

Significant adverse events are rare. Beyond the typical swelling and bruising associated with liposuction, common adverse events include self-resolving breast sensitivity and tenderness. Hematomas may develop more often than at other anatomic sites undergoing liposuction. Extraction of deep hematomas may require pretreatment infiltration with anesthesia.

In men, even modestly enlarged breasts may be socially unacceptable. Self-consciousness about breast size may preclude certain social activities or participation in sports. Exercise, particularly with weights, can worsen the problem by causing enlargement of the underlying pectoralis. As with female breast liposuction, liposuction of the male breast avoids unsightly scarring at the incision site. As male breasts tend to be less voluminous than female breasts, liposuction can be a definitive procedure for most male breast reduction, and surgical excision is seldom required for all but the most resistant cases.

Enlargement of male breasts is of two types, pseudogynecomastia and true gynecomastia. Pseudogynecomastia is an excess of breast fat that afflicts 50–60% of adult men. True gynecomastia, which is much less common, is an excess of glandular breast tissue. Fat is easier to remove by liposuction than fibrous breast stroma, so liposuction of pseudogynecomastia may be slightly easier and more successful.

Ideal candidates are young to middle-aged adults with near-normal weight and more soft fat accumulation than excess breast tissue. Presence of chest hair, nevi, and other benign skin lesions is desirable, as this can camouflage the small residual scars from cannula entry sites. Massive weight loss preceding breast liposuction is likely to have induced marked skin laxity, which may require resection. Patients younger than 21 years should be assessed carefully to ensure they are adequately mature to provide informed consent. Children younger than 18 years require even more complete preoperative evaluation to assess their mental state and motives; this may include discussion with parents and counselors.

Anabolic steroid use can predispose to recurrence after liposuction. A minority of male patients with very large breasts may require reduction mammaplasty rather than liposuction.

After surgery, a 50% size reduction can frequently be achieved. Clothes fit better. Even without clothes, most patients can expect markedly improved contour and, as the vestiges of the procedure are usually not visible, they may be less self-conscious.

At least three entry sites are typically used per breast. Inferolateral, medial, and superolateral access points allow removal of fat by triangulation. Small- and large-diameter cannulas are used to penetrate the often dense tissue and to remove both more and less fibrous particles. Grasping the breast allows the surgeon to direct the aspiration cannula efficiently to fat pockets at different depths. As with liposuction of the female breast, fat removal from the compartment anterior and inferior to the axilla can improve contour. The axilla itself should be avoided because of risk to neurovascular structures, including the brachial plexus. Significantly, there is less residual fat after male breast liposuction than after liposuction at most other body sites. That being said, as with female breast liposuction, periareolar and superficial suctioning should be limited to avoid the risk of necrosis. Postoperative care and adverse events after liposuction of the male breast are similar to those following female breast liposuction.

Back and abdomen

Key Points

* Suction upper and lower abdomen.
* Consider debulking with large-bore cannulas.

The torso is among the more common sites for liposuction, which can provide dramatic improvement of body contour in this area. Female and male body habitus differences require similarly diverse approaches to removal of fat. The ideal shape in women is an hourglass figure, with the minimal width at the hips contingent on the structure of the iliac crest. A "V" shape is more appropriate in men, in whom the chest tapers to the flatter hips. In both men and women, the ideal upper and lower abdomens, as well as the back, have little subcutaneous fat.

Stable pretreatment weight, and an ongoing diet and exercise regimen, are crucial preconditions for liposuction of the trunk. Personal trainers and nutritionists may be helpful consultants for those who have been unable to achieve physical fitness on their own. Resistant areas that persist despite attempts at modification by diet and exercise are optimal targets for liposuction. For instance, a patient in good physical shape and at near-optimal weight may have a lower abdominal bulge that no amount of exercise and only extreme weight loss can address. Focal treatment of this localized adiposity would be an indication for liposuction. Overall truncal obesity is not an indication for liposuction. Most patients undergoing truncal liposuction will be within 10–25 pounds of ideal bodyweight, and will have good skin tone that will allow the skin to contract postoperatively.

Although body contour may be abnormal, it may not be susceptible to improvement by liposuction. Skeletal abnormalities such as scoliosis or kyphosis must be excluded. Tactile assessment of the proposed treatment area with the "pinch test" will reveal the degree of subcutaneous adiposity. Intra-abdominal (i.e. "beer belly") and visceral fat is not amenable to liposuction. Such deep, sequestered fat may be relatively more copious in the male lower abdomen.

Silhouette in clothing is improved after truncal liposuction. Patients who are seeking this improvement will often be pleased with the results. Small corrections in patients with minor contour abnormalities may also improve appearance in more revealing clothing or bathing suits.

Truncal liposuction has the same anesthesia-associated risk as liposuction at other sites, but the greater volume of infused tumescent fluid potentially increases cumulative risk. Strictures on maximum total dose of lidocaine should be observed. If the area to undergo treatment would require more than the bodyweight-specific total dose, the liposuction must be divided into two or more procedures performed on different days.

Prior history of abdominal surgery must be elicited before abdominal liposuction. Scars and appliances will need to be avoided, or the areas around them treated exceptionally gently. Umbilical, ventral, and inguinal hernias should be noted on physical examination. Again, cautions should be observed intraoperatively, or the liposuction should be truncated or avoided. Severe laxity or redundancy of abdominal skin suggests that skin retraction after liposuction will be incomplete. Patients with such skin should be advised that skin resection or abdominoplasty may be necessary to treat excess skin, if removal of this is desired.

Within the trunk, there are several cosmetic units that may be separately approached. Women may be concerned about localized areas of the upper lateral mid-back. These so-called "bra bulges" are usually amenable to liposuction. At the hips, a double-bulge commonly observed in women can look unattractive in clothes. Suctioning the hips alone to reduce these protrusions and blend them better can be highly cosmetically effective. Both men and women frequently request reduction of the abdomen. Assuming the fat collection is not subrectus, and hence unreachable by liposuction, liposuction is often effective at reducing even relatively large accumulations. "Spare tire"-type circumferential fat coalescing into "love handles" at the lateral flanks is commonly seen in the lower abdomen of men. Liposuction of the lower abdomen and flanks is often effective at correcting this. In women, fat is frequently distributed in both the upper and lower abdomen. Although the fat accumulation in the lower area may be greater than that in the upper abdomen, adequate suctioning of both areas precedes good final contour. Temptation to concentrate on the lower abdomen can result in the undersuctioned upper abdomen pushing down on the lower and causing the umbilicus to be elongated horizontally, like an inverted crescent or an unhappy mouth.

Technically, a single supraumbilical entry site may be best for abdominal liposuction. Horizontal motion of the aspiration cannula at this site can create a well defined, cosmetically elegant midline sulcus between the upper and lower abdomen. This approach also permits use of fine cannulas to suction completely around the umbilicus. It is important to avoid "doughnut"-like residual fat around the umbilicus by adequate suctioning, and smaller cannulas can remove more of this fat while minimizing pain at this very sensitive area (Fig. 11-21).

Debulking of a large abdomen may require either large-bore, aggressive cannulas, or powered liposuction equipment. Transitioning to smaller cannulas after much of the fat has been removed permits even and smooth fat reduction. Scarpa's fascia divides the fat compartment, with some suctionable fat lying below this (Fig. 11-22). For optimal removal of abdominal fat, gentle mobilization and removal of fat below Scarpa's fascia is necessary. This should be done with great care to avoid injury to underlying muscle.

Given that abdominal and truncal liposuctions tend to be relatively extensive procedures compared with liposuction at other sites, several days of postoperative recovery may be required. Abdominal binders and garments should be worn to allow smooth contour emergence as swelling and bruising diminish. Pain control may require medication adjustment. Postoperative nausea may need to be treated with drugs. Occasional hematomas and seromas should be monitored for self-resolution, or drained if they are larger. Asymmetry or dimpling can occur, and usually at least 6–12 months is allowed to elapse before a touch-up procedure is considered. Uneven areas often spontaneously improve over this time window.

Legs

Key Points

- Lateral thighs respond well to liposuction.
- Suction carefully around Gasparotti's point.
- Anterior thighs and ankles should be suctioned sparingly.
- Inner thighs to knees to be suctioned continuously to avoid step-off.

Thighs are the part of the leg most commonly treated with liposuction. Contour improvement of the thighs can improve body silhouette and help clothes fit better.

Outer thigh adiposities may cause an unsightly bulge in clothes in patients with normal body

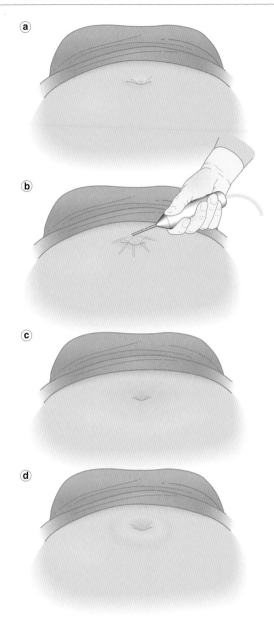

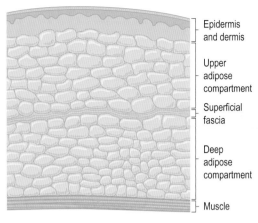

Figure 11-22 In the lower abdomen, suctionable fat is located above and below the superficial fascia. Mobilization of the infrafascial fat requires care so as to avoid injury to the underlying muscle

liposuction is challenging because much of the perceived cosmetic defect is flaccid skin rather than subcutaneous fat. Aggressive suctioning of fat at this area can also induce superficial skin irregularities, dimpling, and troughs. If only the upper inner thighs are treated, there can be a demarcation ridge or step-off separating the upper inner thigh from the lower inner thigh. Feathering of fat removal from the upper inner thigh down to the medial knee can reduce this problem. Before inner thigh liposuction it is important to convey to the patient that overall improvement at this site may be modest.

Treatment of the anterior and posterior thighs must be performed with great care to avoid dimpling and surface irregularities. Similarly, knee, calf, and ankle liposuction is a gentle procedure, designed to reduce very small pockets of fat. Significant venous disease and varicosities are relative contraindications. Some experienced liposuction surgeons attempt to dissuade patients from undergoing liposuction at these sites, given the limited improvement and risk of poor healing and asymmetry.

Anatomic features of the legs limit and guide liposuction. Much of the fat of the legs is below the muscular fascia, where it is inaccessible to aspiration cannulas. At the base of the buttocks, a fullness above the gluteal crease holds up the buttock and is contiguous with the fascial plane. Thinning this so-called "banana roll" with liposuction can result in buttock ptosis. Another danger zone is just posterior to the greater trochanter (Fig. 11-23). Known as "Gasparotti's point," this area can easily be oversuctioned to deep fat, thus creating a depression. Prior to liposuction in this region, abduction and internal rotation are useful for dropping the greater trochanter and preventing a point depression.

Figure 11-21 During abdominal liposuction, complete suctioning around the umbilicus with small-caliber cannulas ensures that residual periumbilical fat is not left behind to protrude

weight. Skin at the outer upper thighs tends to retract well after fat removal, making this area an attractive target for novice liposuction surgeons. Upper lateral thigh and distal lateral thigh suctioning should be conservative to avoid dimpling or contour irregularity at these sites.

Patients also frequently request treatment of the inner thighs. This may be to provide a diamond-shaped separation between the medial upper thighs, which may otherwise abut when standing erect with feet together. Inner thigh

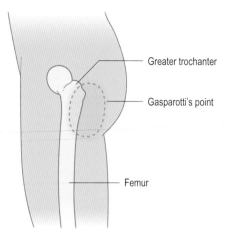

Figure 11-23 Soft tissue depression secondary to excessive suctioning can inadvertently occur at a point just posterior to the greater trochanter

Elevation of the legs and compression garments are important after leg liposuction, especially after calf and ankle liposuction. Ambulation will reduce the risk of deep vein thrombosis. Lower leg edema may persist for several weeks to months.

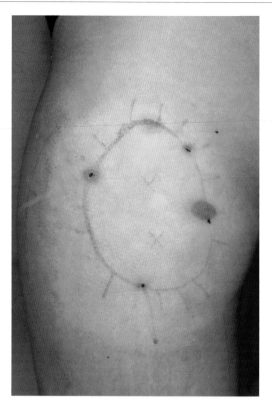

Figure 11-24 Immediately after liposuction of the outer thighs and hips, there are visible incision sites with slight peripheral erythema and minimal drainage. The baseline blanched color of the skin is an effect of tumescent anesthesia

PEARLS

Limit number of treatment areas to maximize safety and ensure adequate anesthesia.

See patient in follow-up 24–48 h post-procedure to identify concerns promptly and reassure.

Final results for liposuction will not be evident until 6–9 months later.

Contour irregularities can be corrected with fat augmentation or prepackaged fillers.

In some cases, large lipomas or congenital fat accumulations may be amenable to correction by liposuction.

Tumescent anesthesia has other applications: large Mohs surgery cases or reconstructions, hair transplants, endovenous laser/radiofrequency ablation.

Oral narcotic medications can be used for postoperative pain management.

Maintenance of stable weight and adequate exercise post-procedure will preserve aesthetic benefits.

Management of adverse events

Tumescent liposuction is a safe procedure, and following accepted practice reduces the risk of adverse events. Some adverse events are likely to be specific to the anatomic location, whereas others are seen more generally. Most adverse events are mild and self-limited.

Intraoperative concerns include infection risk, patient discomfort, and hypothermia. Sterile technique reduces risk of infection. Slow and gradual infusion of warmed tumescent fluid improves patient comfort. Hypothermia can be avoided by use of heating blankets and warming infusion fluid.

Common undesired effects after liposuction include diffuse erythema, edema, ecchymoses, drainage, focal erythema at cannula entry sites (Fig. 11-24), and mild tenderness. These conditions almost always resolve without intervention, with bruising and residual swelling lasting for several weeks. Eventually, small, pinpoint, hypopigmented or hyperpigmented scars may develop at the cannula entry sites.

Less common adverse events include hypertrophic scar or keloid developing at an entry site; this is more common in patients predisposed to poor wound healing, and may occur more often in darker skinned patients. Surface irregularities can be seen; these are sometimes persistent, and may be rectified by a touch-up procedure. Excessively superficial suctioning or too much fat removal from one entry site can cause skin unevenness, asymmetric depressions, or exacerbated cellulite.

Table 11-9 Toxicities associated with raised plasma lidocaine levels

Plasma lidocaine level (μg/mL)	Clinical signs and symptoms
<2	Mild to no effects
2–6	CNS: numbness of tongue, perioral tingling, metallic taste, tinnitus, visual disturbance, headache, lightheadedness, drowsiness, restlessness, muscular twitching, tremors, impaired concentration, dysarthria
	Cardiovascular (less common): hypotension by inducing both cardiac suppression and vascular smooth muscle relaxation
7–10	CNS: exacerbated
	Cardiovascular: exacerbated
11–30+	CNS: tonic–clonic seizures and, eventually, unconsciousness and coma
	Cardiovascular: respiratory and cardiovascular depression, and cardiovascular collapse

Seromas, skin necrosis, and necrotizing fasciitis have been reported rarely and may be associated with very vigorous superficial fat removal and excessive intraoperative trauma, such as that sometimes associated with internal ultrasonic cannulas. Prolonged use of compression garments improves final contour and skin smoothness in uncomplicated cases.

Infections are rare after liposuction. Preexisting immune compromise or severe wound healing diatheses may be contraindications for liposuction. Wound infections, when they have been noted, tend to be superficial infections around incision sites. Inadequate sterility and cleaning of surgical instruments have been implicated in atypical mycobacterial infections after liposuction.

Active bleeding is uncommon during liposuction. Congenital bleeding disorders, factor deficiencies, abnormal bleeding parameters, platelet dysfunction, severe liver disease, recent alcohol consumption, prescription or nonprescription anticoagulant agents, vitamin K deficiency, and other concerning conditions may be contraindications to liposuction. Significant bleeding and hematomas are more likely during treatment of large abdomens. Larger hematomas need to be aspirated for comfort and to ensure rapid wound healing.

Lidocaine toxicity is exceedingly rare when safety benchmarks for total dose per patient body weight are observed (Table 11-9). Staff and physician should be able to recognize early symptoms of lidocaine toxicity, including disorientation, tinnitus, nausea, gait abnormality, and perioral tingling.

Notably, serious side-effects associated with liposuction under general anesthesia have not been reported after tumescent liposuction under standard protocol. Perforation of the bowel or other internal organs, cardiorespiratory collapse, and pulmonary embolus are theoretical risks after standard tumescent liposuction, but these have developed in some cases after very high volume liposuction or nontumescent liposuction.

Directions for the future and conclusions

Liposuction continues to be the most commonly performed major cosmetic procedure. When performed according to generally accepted rules, tumescent liposuction is a highly effective, extremely safe, means for permanent body contour improvement. In the long run, noninvasive fat reduction techniques may displace liposuction, but these technologies remain in their infancy.

Dermatologists are uniquely qualified to refine tumescent liposuction, a procedure birthed in this specialty. Excellent references for further reading include: Hanke and Sattler's *Liposuction*, the chapter on liposuction in Kaminer's *Atlas of Cosmetic Surgery*, and Narins' *Safe Liposuction and Fat Transfer*.

Further reading

Ablon G, Rotunda AM. Treatment of lower eyelid fat pads using phosphatidylcholine: clinical trial and review. Dermatol Surg 2006;30:422–427.

Araco A, Gravante G, Araco F, et al. Comparison of power water-assisted and traditional liposuction: a prospective randomized trial of postoperative pain. Aesthetic Plast Surg 2007;31:259–265.

Butterwick K, Goldman M. Safety of lidocaine during tumescent anesthesia for liposuction. In: Hanke C, Sattler G, eds. Liposuction. Philadelphia: Elsevier, 2005: 34.

Coldiron B, Fisher AH, Adelman E, et al. Adverse event reporting: lessons learned from 4 years of Florida office data. Dermatol Surg 2005;31: 1079–1092.

Coleman IW, Hanke CW, Lillis P, et al. Does the location of the surgery or the specialty of the physician affect malpractice claims in liposuction? Dermatol Surg 1999;25:343–347.

Fournier PF. Why the syringe and not the suction machine? J Dermatol Surg Oncol 1988;14:1062–1071.

Fournier PF. Who should do syringe liposculpturing? J Dermatol Surg Oncol 1988;14:1055–1056.

Hanke C, Sattler G, eds. Liposuction. Philadelphia: Elsevier, 2005.

Hanke CW, Bernstein G, Bullock S. Safety of tumescent liposuction in 15 336 patients. National survey results. Dermatol Surg 1995;21:459–462.

Hanke W, Cox SE, Kuznets N, Coleman WP 3rd. Tumescent liposuction report performance measurement initiative: national survey results. Dermatol Surg 2004;30:967–977.

Housman TS, Lawrence N, Mellen BG, et al. The safety of liposuction: results of a national survey. Dermatol Surg 2002;28:971–978.

Illouz YG. Body contouring by lipolysis: a 5-year experience with over 3000 cases. Plast Reconstr Surg 1983;72:591–597.

Johnson D, Lillis P, Kaminer M. Liposuction. In: Kaminer M, Dover J, Arndt K, eds. Atlas of Cosmetic Surgery. Philadelphia: WB Saunders, 2002: 194–227.

Kaminer M, Dover J, Arndt K, eds. Atlas of Cosmetic Surgery. Philadelphia: WB Saunders, 2002.

Kaminer MS, Tan MH, Hsu TS, Alam M. Limited breast reduction by liposuction. Skin Ther Lett 2002;7:6–8.

Kaplan B, Moy RL. Comparison of room temperature and warmed local anesthetic solution for tumescent liposuction. A randomized double-blind study. Dermatol Surg 1996;22:707–709.

Katz BE, Bruck MC, Coleman WP 3rd. The benefits of powered liposuction versus traditional liposuction: a paired comparison analysis. Dermatol Surg 2001;27:863–867.

Katz BE, Bruck MC, Felsenfeld L, Frew KE. Power liposuction: a report on complications. Dermatol Surg 2003;29:925–927.

Kiak GA, Koontz FF, Chavez AJ. Lidocaine inhibits growth of Staphylococcus aureus in propofol. Anesthesiology 1992;77:A407.

Kim KH, Geronemus RG. Laser lipolysis using a novel 1064 nm Nd:YAG laser. Dermatol Surg 2006;32:241–248.

Lawrence N, Cox SE. The efficacy of external ultrasound-assisted liposuction: a randomized controlled trial. Dermatol Surg 2000;26:329–332.

Melton J, Hanke CW, Sattler G. Tumescent local anesthesia technique. In: Hanke C, Sattler G, eds. Liposuction. Philadelphia: Elsevier, 2005: 22.

Narins R. Safe Liposuction and Fat Transfer. New York: Marcel Dekker, 2003.

Ostad A, Kageyama N, Moy RL. Tumescent anesthesia with a lidocaine dose of 55 mg/kg is safe for liposuction. Dermatol Surg 1996;22:921–927.

Prado A, Andrades P, Danilla S, et al. A prospective, randomized, double-blind, controlled clinical trial comparing laser-assisted lipoplasty with suction-assisted lipoplasty. Plast Reconstr Surg 2006;118:1032–1045.

Rao RB, Ely SF, Hoffman RS. Deaths related to liposuction. N Engl J Med 1999;340:1471–1475.

Rotunda AM, Kolodney MS. Mesotherapy and phosphatidylcholine injections: historical classification and review. Dermatol Surg 2006;32:465–480.

Rotunda AM, Suzuki H, Moy RL, Kolodney MS. Detergent effects of sodium deoxycholate are a major feature of an injectable phosphatidylcholine formulation used for localized fat dissolution. Dermatol Surg 2004;30:1001–1008.

Rubin JP, Bierman C, Rosow CE, et al. The tumescent technique: the effect of high tissue pressure and dilute epinephrine on absorption of lidocaine. Plast Reconstr Surg 1999;103:990–996.

Rubin JP, Xie Z, Davidson C, et al. Rapid absorption of tumescent lidocaine above the clavicles: a prospective clinical study. Plast Reconstr Surg 2005;115:1744–1751.

Yang CH, Hsu HC, Shen SC, et al. Warm and neutral tumescent anesthetic solutions are essential factors for a less painful injection. Dermatol Surg 2006;32:1119–1122.

Advanced cosmetic surgical procedures **12**

Brian Somoano, Jeremy Kampp, and Hayes B. Gladstone

Key Points

- Tightening procedures are fundamental in addressing facial aging that results from loss of elasticity and a sagging envelope.
- The advent of tumescent anesthesia paved the way for these outpatient cosmetic surgeries, with decreased risks and postoperative downtime.
- Thorough understanding of cervicofacial anatomy is central to minimizing complications.
- Optimal cosmetic results are achieved when other elements of facial aging, such as actinic damage and volume loss, are also addressed.

Introduction

Cosmetic dermatologic surgery has advanced by leaps and bounds over the past 15 years. There are many reasons for this evolution. The formation of the American Society for Dermatologic Surgery (ASDS), composed of dermatologists interested primarily in surgery, particularly cosmetic procedures, laid the foundation for the discussion and dissemination of advanced techniques. Pioneers, such as Field, Alt, Asken, and Coleman, had a specific interest in cosmetic procedures, but the two most important steps in stimulating the development of advanced procedures in this field have been the increasingly complex reconstructions that Mohs surgeons were performing, and the invention of tumescent anesthesia by Jeffrey Klein. The latter has allowed advanced cosmetic procedures to be performed under local anesthesia and in an outpatient clinic setting.

Mohs and reconstructive surgeons such as Moy, Morganroth, Sengelmann, and Rotter have been able to apply their skills for cervicofacial rotation flaps and periorbital excisions to rhytidectomies and blepharoplasties. Other dermatologic surgeons, such as Eremia, Langdon, Brandy, Bisaccia, and Scarborough, have adapted techniques from plastic surgery colleagues, modifying these procedures for use in a less invasive outpatient setting.

Indeed, dermatologic surgeons have made major contributions to cosmetic surgery by emphasizing the less invasive aspects that reduce recovery time and risk of adverse effects, while still achieving reasonable results.

In this chapter, we discuss a select group of less invasive cosmetic procedures, including blepharoplasties, neck liposuction and platysmal plication, and facial lifting procedures. While facial aging is due to many components, including superficial photo-aging and volume loss, the decrease in elasticity results in a sagging envelope, which is still the most prominent marker (Fig. 12-1). Tightening procedures are the cornerstone for repairing this condition.

Blepharoplasty

Key Points

- Referral to ophthalmology is mandated prior to surgery if the preoperative evaluation suggests pathology, whether intrinsic or a result of a systemic condition such as Graves' disease.
- During upper blepharoplasty, lateral dissection increases the risk of lacrimal gland injury whereas medial extension predisposes to a visible scar or webbing.
- During lower blepharoplasty, aggressive fat removal increases the risk of a suboptimal hallowed appearance and damage to nearby structures, especially the inferior oblique muscle.
- It is important to recognize possible complications, especially retrobulbar hematoma, and how to initiate management immediately to avoid permanent loss of vision.

Relevant anatomy

Although it is important to recognize the anatomic variations that exist between the eyelids of different ethnic groups, such as among those individuals of Caucasian and Asian descent, knowledge of several fundamental anatomic structures common to all patients undergoing blepharoplasty

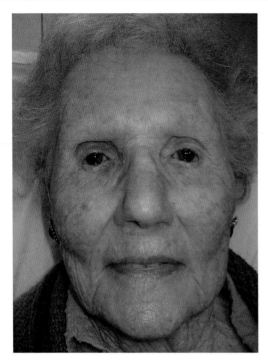

Figure 12-1 Facial aging

oblique muscle tendon and the trochlea can also be damaged during this procedure.

Patient selection and preoperative evaluation

Although the same principles apply for both upper and lower blepharoplasty, patient selection is different. Indications for an upper blepharoplasty include dermatochalasis (excess sagging skin) and fat herniation. In many patients there will be lateral hooding, which needs to be addressed. When addressing the upper eyelid, the brow must also be taken into account, particularly in women. Removing skin and muscle from the upper eyelid will often lower the eyebrow, and this can be problematic in women, where generally an arched eyebrow above the orbital rim is considered aesthetically desirable.

Patients with lower eyelid "bagginess" are candidates for a lower blepharoplasty. This puffiness is secondary to fat herniation from one of the three fat pads and needs to be distinguished from orbicularis oculi muscular hypertrophy, which appears more linear. Often there will also be dermatochalasis, which needs to be addressed.

In any patient undergoing eyelid procedures, an eye examination should be performed. This includes documenting not only vision, but also intraocular muscle function, tear production, lower lid laxity, and brow position. A patient with eyelid pathology, either intrinsic or secondary to a systemic condition such as Graves' disease, needs to be evaluated by an ophthalmologist.

Technique

Upper blepharoplasty

As with any technique, several methods are available. With the upper blepharoplasty (Fig. 12-2), the technical considerations include how much skin, muscle, and fat to remove, and marking is also critical. The amount of skin to be removed can be determined using calipers or simply by pinching the amount of skin with Adson forceps. Although markings should be tailored to the patient's anatomy, there are some general guidelines when using calipers. For the female upper eyelid, the marking for the lower incision, which is recreating the crease, should be 10 mm above the tarsal edge. The midpoint of the superior incision should be 12 mm below the eyebrow. The markings do not extend to the medial canthus, as this can result in webbing. Laterally, the inferior and superior incisions meet in an upward orientation and can go beyond the eyelid skin in order to reduce lateral hooding.

The incision can be performed with a no. 15 blade scalpel, a laser, or radiofrequency, but the authors prefer cold steel because of its tactile

is paramount. Below the eyelid skin is the orbicularis oculi, the primary muscle of lid closure. Deep to the orbicularis is the orbital septum, a thin fibrous membrane that serves as a key landmark because it must be penetrated during upper or lower blepharoplasty if access to the underlying orbital fat is to be gained.

Three distinct fat-containing compartments are found in the lower eyelid (referred to as the medial, central, and lateral fat pads), and injury to nearby extraocular muscles must be avoided during lower eyelid blepharoplasty. The inferior oblique is of chief importance, arising near the medial surface of the orbit and traveling posteriorly between the medial and central fat pads, where injury and resultant diplopia may occur if this muscle goes unrecognized.

In comparison, the upper eyelid has two recognized fat compartments: a larger and more yellow central fat pad, and the more medial nasal fat pad, which is paler in color. The term preaponeurotic fat is also often used to describe this superior orbital adipose tissue, given that the levator aponeurosis, the tendon of the levator palpebrae superioris (the main elevator of the upper eyelid), lies directly beneath these compartments of fat. Care must be taken to avoid injury to the levator or its tendon during fat removal in upper eyelid blepharoplasty, as this can result in ptosis. Furthermore, lateral dissection of the upper eyelid should not be pursued to avoid injuring the lacrimal gland found in this region. The superior

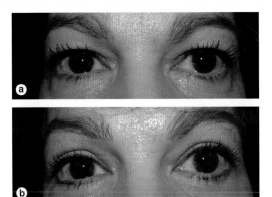

Figure 12-2 (A) Before and (B) after upper blepharoplasty

exposing the three fat pads. The fat needs to be handled delicately while being removed with the Colorado needle, as "pulling" on it can disrupt blood vessels and cause bleeding. Meticulous hemostasis with bipolar electrocautery is achieved. The conjunctiva does not need to be sutured. It is important not to remove too much fat as this will leave a hollowed appearance. For tear trough deformities, a fat pedicle can be developed from the medial fat pad and transposed into the concavity.

Infraorbital lasering is usually performed in conjunction with the lower blepharoplasty in order to tighten loose skin and ablate fine rhytides. A carbon dioxide laser can be used, although the authors prefer a long-pulsed erbium laser.

Postoperative care and complications

Postoperative care for upper blepharoplasties consists of gentle cleaning and use of an antibiotic ointment on the incision. For lower blepharoplasties, the incision does not need to be taken care of, although artificial tears during the first week may help to reduce irritation. Aquaphor is placed on the lasered site two to four times per day for the first week. The patient may perform normal activities but should refrain from bending or heavy lifting as this can promote bleeding. Ice packs or bags of frozen vegetables should be placed periorbitally to reduce swelling and the risk of bleeding.

The potential for complications in blepharoplasties is high, but, with careful patient selection and meticulous technique, they can be minimized. The retrobulbar hematoma is the most dreaded complication as it can cause blindness; however, it rarely occurs. If one does not recognize that the lacrimal gland sits in the lateral aspect of the upper eyelid, it can be injured. While performing the lower blepharoplasty, if one is too aggressive in teasing the fat pads out, the inferior oblique can be injured. An incision too low on the upper eyelid can lead to levator muscle injury and ptosis. Of course, overzealous removal of fat that skeletonizes the orbital region can be viewed as a complication, or at least a source of patient dissatisfaction, as can insufficient fat removal. Excessive removal of skin in the subciliary approach for the lower blepharoplasty can lead to ectropion. A patient may also develop conjunctival injection, conjunctivitis, or dry eyes. These usually subside, although eyedrops may be necessary. Gentle technique with eye shields is important to avoid corneal abrasions. As with any surgical procedure, infections can also occur. Although eyelid skin heals well, suture granulomas can occur, and, if the incision is extended onto glabrous skin, the scar may be noticeable. Because the infraorbital skin is thin, lasering should be judicious in order to avoid prolonged erythema and possible scarring (Table 12-1).

quality. When making the incision, it is important to incise sharply but superficially in one bold stroke as repetitive incisions may make multiple lines. Using tenotomy scissors, the skin and muscle is removed. Remaining thin strands of muscle should also be removed. In recent years, there has been a trend away from removing fat. However, if there is fat protrusion, particularly in the medial fat pad, it should be removed via buttonhole incisions through the septum. It is important to remember that there are only two fat pads in the upper eyelid. Laterally lies the lacrimal gland, which should not be violated. Meticulous hemostasis should be performed with bipolar electrocautery. Closure is performed in one layer and several methods exist, including interrupted, running, and subcuticular. The authors prefer an absorbable running suture with 6-0 fast-absorbing gut. As these sutures do not require removal, the healing blepharoplasty is not disturbed.

Lower blepharoplasty

The lower blepharoplasty (Fig. 12-3) can be performed via a ciliary or transconjunctival approach. Unless the patient has a significant amount of excess skin, the transconjunctival approach is preferred. Although exposure, particularly laterally, is more challenging with this method, there is less risk of lower eyelid malposition and no visible scar results.

Following the application of anesthetic drops, the lower eyelid is anesthetized via the conjunctiva with 1% lidocaine and 1:100000 epinephrine. The authors do not use eye shields for the upper blepharoplasty, but they do for the lower blepharoplasty. Similar to the upper blepharoplasty, the incision can be made with several devices. The authors prefer the Colorado needle because of its tactile feedback, small footprint, and coagulation capabilities. Incisions can be made pre- or post-septally. Generally, a linear incision is made midway through the conjunctiva. The lower lid retractors are bluntly dissected with tenotomy scissors,

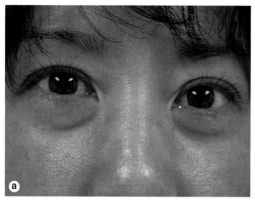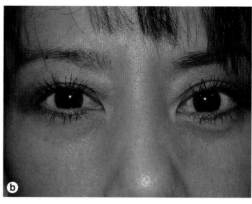

Figure 12-3 (A) Before and (B) after lower blepharoplasty

Table 12-1 Complications of blepharoplasty	
Adverse event	Procedural considerations
Blindness	Meticulous hemostasis important to avoid retrobulbar hematoma
Fat asymmetry	Evaluate location and degree of fat pad excision needed preoperatively
Hemorrhage	Avoid predisposing medications; meticulous intraoperative hemostasis
Bradycardia/dysrhythmia	Minimize ocular manipulation that may trigger oculocardiac reflex
Diplopia	May be due to edema, local anesthesia, or injury to inferior oblique muscle
Ptosis	Avoid trauma to tendon of levator muscle
Lid retraction (scleral show/ectropion)	Attempt conservative excision during transcutaneous lower blepharoplasty
Keratoconjunctivitis/ dry eyes	Lubrication and taping of lids may help
Lagophthalmos	Attempt conservative skin excision of upper eyelid
Medial canthal web	Avoid extending upper lid incision too medially
Hollowed appearance of upper eyelid	Seen with excessive removal of fat pads

Neck liposuction and platysmal plication

* When sculpting near the mandible, gentle technique and use of the smart hand can help avoid risk of marginal mandibular nerve injury.

* Overly aggressive fat removal may predispose to dermal scarring and skin dimpling.
* Compliance with the use of postoperative compression garments should be stressed to minimize ridging and puckering of the skin.

Background

Liposuction ranks among the most frequently performed aesthetic operations. A number of facial regions are amenable to lipoplasty, including the submentum, lateral neck, jowls, and buccal and nasolabial areas. Submental and neck lipoplasty is frequently requested because it offers the potential for remarkable improvement in the cervicomental angle with limited downtime. Restoring the aesthetic neck contour is an integral component of facial rejuvenation. The anterior neck is often the first region to capture the eye of an observer when viewing an aging face. Characteristic signs of the aging neck include lipodystrophy and platysmal bands, reducing the aesthetic quality of the lower face. These deformities are the result of skin laxity, platysmal ptosis and redundancy, ptosis of the submental fat pad, and prominent submandibular salivary glands or digastric muscles.

Relevant anatomy

The anatomic limits of the neck are the inferior border of the mandible superiorly, the supraclavicular area inferiorly, and the anterior borders of the trapezius muscles laterally. The platysma originates from the fascia overlying the pectoralis and deltoid muscles, and inserts in multiple points above the angle of the mandible. Posterior fibers intertwine with the depressor anguli oris, mentalis, risorius, and orbicularis oris before inserting at the level of the commissures. Central fibers insert directly into the periosteum of the mandible. Along its course, partial decussation of the muscle fibers is seen in approximately 61–75% of the population. When the muscle decussates from hyoid to chin, a supportive sling is fashioned for the submental area. Other variations include close approximation but no decussation (10%), and total muscular decussation from mandible to thyroid (15%). When the decussation of the platysma is absent, the free medial edges can be responsible for an anterior neck deformity, which appears as two vertical bands.

Patient selection and preoperative evaluation

Optimal candidates for neck liposuction include patients with full jowls but otherwise good skin elasticity, patients with high-set hyoid bones, and those with palpable submental fat pads. Patients with prominent platysmal banding should be given the option for platysmal repair at the time of neck liposuction in order to maximize the final results.

Patient evaluation should begin with an assessment of the degree of skin laxity and the amount of preplatysmal fat. The submental and submandibular fat deposits should be palpated, and the presence of malpositioned or ptotic submandibular glands noted. A fatty neck can obscure the ptotic glands, and patients must be aware of the possibility of unmasking this deformity with the neck rejuvenation.

Dynamic evaluation of the neck begins during the initial patient interview. The surgeon observes the neck during normal conversation for deformities that plague the patient during the majority of daily activities. The patient is then asked to animate in order to display potential medial or lateral platysmal banding. Jowls may be present, and the contribution of the skin, subcutaneous fat, platysma, and submandibular gland to this deformity is assessed and recorded.

A standard facial photographic series, including anterior, lateral, and oblique views, should be obtained. An additional view with the patient's neck flexed, as if reading, may also be helpful in revealing platysmal laxity. On the basis of the preoperative evaluation, the majority of patients can be subdivided into four categories:

- Type I – no skin laxity, excellent skin tone, and lipodystrophy
- Type II – mild skin laxity with or without narrow medial platysmal bands (<2 cm)
- Type III – moderate skin laxity with or without wide platysmal bands (>2 cm)
- Type IV – moderate to severe skin laxity and significant lipodystrophy.

Technique

Neck liposuction

There are several key points that will make the procedure go smoothly and result in a successful outcome. Following photography, the patient's neck is

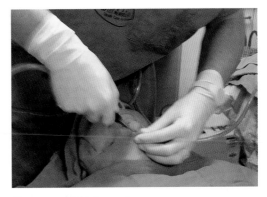

Figure 12-4 Neck liposuction

marked. This includes marking the border between face and submentum, submental and infra-auricular entry points, the thyroid cartilage and the border of the neck and chest. The neck is then tumesced with 0.1% lidocaine and 1:500000 epinephrine. It is important to warn the patient of the neck fullness that they will feel and to instruct them to tell the surgeon if they are having any difficulty breathing. After waiting 20min, the neck liposuction begins with a 16-gauge cannula using the smart hand to guide it in a criss-cross pattern (Fig. 12-4). The cannula is then changed to a 14 G for more defined sculpting. Liposuction is then performed from the bilateral infra-auricular entry points. When sculpting along and superior to the mandible to achieve a more acute cervical mental angle, it is important to be gentle and use the smart hand to lift the skin in order to avoid injuring the marginal mandibular nerve. Although it is important to be thorough, overzealous sculpting can lead to a concave submentum and unevenness, which is unflattering.

Platysmal plication

Platysmal plication follows liposuction and may be performed as an independent procedure or as part of a formal neck or face lift. A small fusiform incision is first made in the submental crease, after which neck liposuction is performed. The platysma is then dissected off of the skin and the remaining fat is cauterized. The separated platysmal bands, which should be apparent at this point, are then sewn together with 4-0 Prolene in an interrupted fashion. Although the authors prefer this method, because it leads to a smoother platysma, some prefer a corset technique, whereas others believe that trimming the platysmal bands will provide the best results.

Postoperative care and complications

Postoperative complications include hematoma, seroma, infection, anterior neck hypothesia, skin dimpling, and prominent jowls. The risk of hematoma formation can be reduced through meticulous surgical technique, hemostasis, and adequate compression bandages postoperatively. Infection can be minimized with the use of sterile technique and consideration of postoperative antibiotics. A certain amount of anterior neck hypothesia is expected with these procedures, with gradual recovery from weeks to months. To avoid dermal scaring and skin dimpling during neck liposuction, it is essential to leave several millimeters of fat on the skin flap to protect the dermis. Prominent jowling can appear when there is aggressive central submental fat removal without equal attention to peripheral liposuction.

Compression garments are worn for 23 h a day for the first postoperative week, then 8–10 h a day for the next month. Failure to compress and support the skin adequately during the first week after surgery can produce skin that shows signs of ridging and puckering.

Minimum-incision facelifts and suspension lifts

Background

Minimum-incision facelifts

Despite the multiple differences among the various facelift techniques, all share in common the elevation of ptotic facial tissue following the dissection of one or more anatomic planes. The traditional rhytidectomy, via more extensive undermining of larger flaps and often deeper tissue planes, has long been recognized as being capable of achieving extraordinary results in surgical facial rejuvenation. More recently, it has become evident that less invasive variations of this procedure are also able to achieve significant outcomes, an option increasingly sought by those desiring less dramatic results with shorter postsurgical recovery time. These more conservative procedures are often collectively called minimum-incision facelifts, or "mini-lifts," and numerous modifications to this somewhat simpler technique have been proposed over the years in regard to the exact plane and extent of dissection, tightening technique employed, and the anatomic site of fixation.

In the late 1970s and 1980s, Webster described a less radical facelift utilizing a smaller skin flap with shorter anterior and posterior incisions. The "Webster lift" utilized simple plication, tightening and elevating the superficial musculoaponeurotic system (SMAS)–platysma unit by suturing this tissue to itself. In 1999, Saylan popularized the Ansari modification of the original short scar facelift by Parisian cosmetic dermatologist Suzanne Noel in the early 20th century. This facelift is characterized by an even smaller incision localized mainly to the preauricular region, coining the term S-lift given the S shape of the incision, which began behind the ear lobule and terminated in the hair-bearing region of the temple. Although this approach limited the surgeon's ability to dissect and improve the lateral neck, good results were achieved with decreased downtime, and with the elimination of the classic retroauricular scar. Although the S-lift was often performed with simple plication of the SMAS–platysma unit, Baker argued that the vectors created with lateral SMAS-ectomy instead would better correct the nasolabial fold and lower face. Many other modifications have been reported, including a less conventional approach advocated by Hoefflin, which utilizes suspension of an extended supraplatysmal flap composed only of skin and subcutaneous fat, omitting tightening of the underlying SMAS altogether.

The final cosmetic results achieved by any of the above variations on rhytidectomy may be improved when used in conjunction with liposuction, chemical peels, laser resurfacing, or other adjunct cosmetic procedures. Regardless of the technique employed or the provider's surgical experience, optimal results can be achieved only when patient selection and expectations are appropriately addressed upfront, especially in light of the mini-lift's limitations in correcting severe cervical laxity.

Suspension lifts

Rhytidectomy can be used to correct sagging of the lower face and jowling, but significant improvement in mid-facial laxity can be variable. Suspension lifts, performed with one of several available modified sutures, represent a minimally invasive option for the purpose of elevating ptotic tissues of not only the midface, but also the neck, jowls, and brow.

Sulamanidze helped to popularize this technique in Russia in 2002, with the introduction of APTOS (anti-ptosis) threads. This procedure, which has been marketed as the FeatherLift®, utilizes specialized sutures comprised of polypropylene that are studded with small barbs along the shaft. These hook-like projections face in opposite directions, with barbs on each half of the suture angled inward so as to converge centrally; this bidirectional orientation allows the thread to anchor itself to and fix the surrounding facial soft tissue. Although the use of these threads has not yet been approved by the Food and Drug Administration (FDA), suspension lift procedures with Contour Threads™ were approved in 2004. Unlike the unsecured, free-floating APTOS threads, this suture has unidirectional barbs and, once deployed in the mid-subcutaneous tissue, must be secured to fascia by the curved needle at the proximal end. The term "thread lift" is now commonly used in reference to either of these procedures.

Some have suggested that the cuts placed along the shaft when creating barbed sutures may confer an inherent weakness to these threads, and alternative suspension lift options have been introduced. Eremia described a technique that utilizes an anchor suspension suture created by tying five to nine small suture bits (each piece about 7–9 mm in length) onto a longer, slowly absorbable, 2-0 monofilament suture. The suture bits, secured by basic square knots at about 1-cm intervals, anchor and elevate adjacent tissue once the 2-0 suture backbone is secured to fascia. In comparison, the Silhouette Mid-Face Suture™ (FDA approved in October 2006) utilizes clear, hollow, absorbable cones to engage and mobilize subcutaneous facial tissue. Endotine, a bioabsorbable implant shown to be effective in lifting the midface and brow tissue, is yet another available fixation device.

Common to these suspension lift techniques is the use of multiple supporting structures, permitting tension to be spread over a larger area of the soft tissue being elevated. Indeed, limited studies to date have demonstrated that this approach is capable of yielding excellent initial cosmetic results, clinically evident immediately after the procedure, and a relatively good safety profile has been documented. Although it has also been argued that sustained results may be feasible as a result of the fibrosis that develops around these modified sutures, preserving their ability to anchor and displace adjacent tissue, large long-term follow-up studies are limited and some available data have suggested that benefits may not be longlasting. Eremia recently reported that, among 14 individuals undergoing lifts with anchor suspension sutures, nearly all correction of the jowl and mid-face had been lost by 12 months.

Variations to the standard pure suspension lift have also been proposed, and some have advocated the use of a dual-plane thread lift, touting improved and longer lasting correction, especially for the brow. Although the suspension lift's popularity has stemmed largely from its role as an alternative to more invasive surgeries such as rhytidectomy, reports suggest that the use of threads in conjunction with minimum incision lifts may be a good option to address moderate facial aging. This combination has yielded impressive results with greater persistence over time, and the raised rhytidectomy flap makes accurate thread placement a relatively quick and easy undertaking.

Relevant anatomy

Minimum-incision facelifts

Key Points

- Patient selection and expectations are key in achieving optimal results, especially as prominent cervical laxity can be difficult to address with a purely preauricular incision.

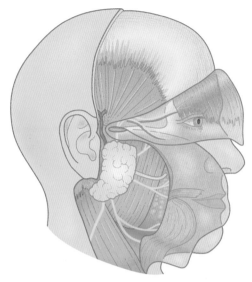

Figure 12-5 Cervicofacial anatomy

- Avoid aggressive undermining at sites of high risk for nerve injury, especially the zygomatic arch (temporal branch of facial nerve) and the lateral neck (greater auricular nerve).
- Excessive flap trimming should be avoided to prevent tension along incision lines and more prominent scars.
- The unnatural wind tunnel appearance can be avoided by ensuring that plication sutures and skin trimming is oriented to create a vertical vector.

A broad working knowledge of cervicofacial anatomy (Fig. 12-5) is central to achieving optimal results and avoiding complications when performing cosmetic surgical procedures. This is especially true of minimum-incision facelifts, for which a thorough understanding of the SMAS and the branches of the facial nerve is required.

The SMAS represents the fibromuscular superficial fascial layer of the face and neck. Its inferior margin is continuous with the superficial cervical fascia and platysma muscle, from which it extends superiorly across the mandible and facial muscles, approaching the zygomatic arch and eventually transitioning to galea and superficial temporalis fascia at its superior border. It lies superficial to the parotid gland at its lateral most position, where it inserts tightly to overlying parotid fascia, and advances medially where it nears the nasolabial fold. Most of the muscles of facial expression can be found within these defined boundaries, where they are enclosed by the SMAS. Given that numerous ligamentous extensions also attach the SMAS to the overlying subcutaneous fat and dermis, a complex network is formed which allows these muscles to transmit motion into appreciable facial expression. This concept is central in mini-lift procedures, as the exertion applied during SMAS–platysma tightening, as a result of plication or partial excision, thus allows for the correction of ptotic tissues overlying the lower face and neck.

The more limited dissection and undermining performed in mini-lifts may lessen the risk of surgical complications, but caution must still be exercised, especially to avoid injury to the temporal branch of the facial nerve. Although the temporal branch is fairly protected proximally where it lies deep to the parotid gland, it becomes more vulnerable to trauma as it traverses distally over the zygomatic arch, where the overlying SMAS can be especially thin. As the undermining required in mini-lifts utilizing plication is limited to the plane above the SMAS, the underlying motor nerves are generally shielded from injury. The greater auricular nerve, which ascends the neck along the sternocleidomastoid and branches near the parotid gland, is thought to be the most commonly injured sensory nerve during facelifts, and undermining of the neck should be superficial to the platysma to avoid trauma.

Suspension lifts

Providers utilizing suspension lifts for facial rejuvenation should be especially comfortable with subcutaneous tissue planes, as the ideal depth of their deployment can vary between threads. Contour and Aptos threads were designed for placement in the mid to superficial subcutaneous tissues, and inappropriately buried threads may predispose patients to developing an inflammatory response. Contour threads have been excellent for the midface and brow lift, although the duration is rarely longer than 1–2 years (Fig. 12-6). In comparison, anchor suspension sutures should be placed significantly deeper, ideally just above the SMAS, as this larger suture may result in a clinically palpable component if inserted more superficially. Although threads are minimally invasive, the risk of adverse effects, particularly thread migration, is not uncommon (Box 12-1).

Technique for minimum-incision facelifts

While the patient is in a sitting position, the incision path is marked. The superior aspect of the incision skin mark begins at the root of the helix and descends along the tragus, then around the earlobe, ascending postauricularly to the level of the external auditory canal and then turning 90° and going 5–6 cm posteriorly into the scalp. The patient is then tumesced with 0.1% lidocaine and 1:500 000 epinephrine. Neck liposuction is then performed, followed by platysmal plication if desired. The advantage of doing a platysmal

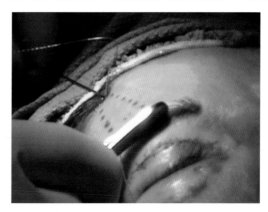

Figure 12-6 Suspension lift

BOX 12-1

Complications of thread lifts

Foreign body-induced reaction

Palpable or visible component:

- Thread breakage
- Thread migration/partial expulsion
- Aasymmetry
- Skin dimpling
- Infection
- Injury to local nerves

Dysesthesia

Fasciculations

Prolonged pain

plication in conjunction with a facelift is that it allows access to the neck so that undermining can be performed widely.

An incision is then made along the marked line and the flap is raised. The flap is initially raised sharply. A liposuction cannula can be used without suction in order to create supra-SMAS tunnels. The anterior and posterior aspects of the flap are completed with either Mayo, Gorney, or "baby" Metzenbaum scissors. The scissor dissection should alternate from a tips-up orientation and perpendicular to the SMAS. The flap should be thin and able to be transilluminated. Particular care should be taken in the posterior aspect where the greater auricular nerve lies superficially and where the skin is bound down. Meticulous hemostasis is obtained with cautery. SMAS plication sutures with either 4-0 Prolene or Vicryl are placed in a 60–90° vertical orientation. Excess skin is then trimmed, although no tension should result. The skin flap is then closed in two

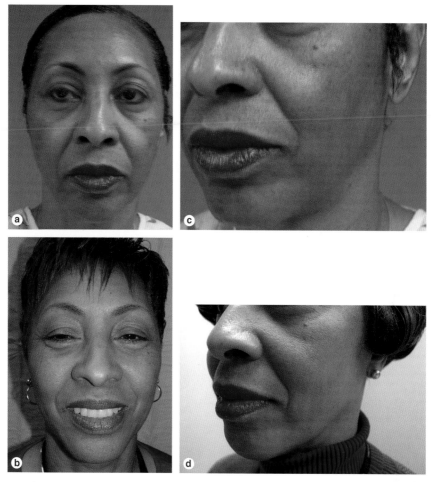

Figure 12-7 (A,C) Before and (B,D) after a minimum-incision facelift

layers with 4-0 Monocryl buried sutures and 6-0 fast-absorbing gut anteriorly and 5-0 fast-absorbing gut in the posterior aspect of the flap. Because there may be some tension in the posterior aspect, the buried sutures are anchored by taking deep initial bites. The authors do not place drains unless there has been an uncharacteristic amount of bleeding during the procedure (Fig. 12-7).

Postoperative care and complications

After a minimum-incision facelift, the patient is seen the next day for a bandage change, at which time a compression garment is fitted. The patient is instructed to wear this garment as much as possible for 2 weeks and is also shown how to change bandages. There is usually 1 week of recovery, although this is usually limited to mild swelling and bruising, as well as a sensation of facial tightness. Because the procedure is performed under local anesthesia, the patient has none of the sequelae

normally associated with general anesthesia. Nevertheless, they should be cautioned to reduce their activity during the first week to minimize risk of hematoma or dehiscence.

Hematoma is the most common major complication of facelifts (Table 12-2), and men are generally at higher risk. Infection is less likely given facial vascularity; however, this may result secondary to a hematoma or necrotic flap. Nerve injury is a major complication, but fortunately occurs rarely. Damage to the greater auricular, the most commonly injured nerve, can be particularly vexing because it leads to numbness of the earlobe, making putting on earrings difficult. The marginal mandibular branch of the facial nerve is less likely to be injured in the supra-SMAS approach, but it can be compromised by entrapment during plication. Wound dehiscence and skin necrosis can occur due to excessive tension. Buttonholing of the skin may occur, particularly in the posterior dissection, if care is not taken given the bound-down nature of the skin. Although there may be

Table 12-2 Complications of facelifts

Adverse event	Procedural considerations
Bleeding (ecchymosis, hematoma)	Avoid predisposing medications; meticulous intraoperative hemostasis
Swelling	Time will resolve
Injury to motor nerves (facial nerve)	Special care at high-risk anatomical sites, including:
• Temporal branch	• Area overlying the zygomatic arch
• Marginal mandibular branch	• Jawline, especially during liposuction
• Buccal branches	• Medial to the parotid gland
Injury to sensory nerves	Special care at high-risk anatomical sites, including:
• Greater auricular	• Neck, near the sternocleidomastoid muscle
Neuropraxia or dysesthesia	Usually temporary; minimize trauma to above nerves
Hairline distortion	Attention to retroauricular incision closure
Retroauricular dog ear	May require lengthening of retroauricular incision
Earlobe deformities (pixie ear)	Leave sufficient skin on redraped flap around lobe to minimize tension
Widened scars	Minimize tension of redraped skin flap
Skin flap necrosis	Predisposed by patient smoking and hematoma
Superficial slough	Minimize tension
Asymmetry	Similar number of plication sutures on each side and skin removed
Infection	Minimize tension; sterile technique
Dyspigmentation	Postoperative hyroquinone

hair displacement and alopecia with other types of facelift techniques, these complications are rare with this method because the incision does not extend into the scalp. Pixie ear deformity can occur if the earlobe is pulled downward due to excessive inferior trimming of the flap. The dreaded wind tunnel appearance can occur if the plication vector and skin trimming is in a horizontal rather than vertical direction.

Conclusion

Minimally invasive cosmetic surgery has become very popular given the public's demand for less downtime but effective results. These procedures can be performed under local anesthesia. They include traditional mainstays of surgical rejuvenation such as blepharoplasty. Other procedures such has rhytidectomies have been modified with varying results, while thread lifts are still evolving. Although these procedures are less invasive, there can still be complications from asymmetry to hematomas, and meticulous technique with its basis in the fundamentals in dermatologic surgery is obligatory.

Further reading

American Society for Dermatologic Surgery. Technology Report: Suspension Sutures. Available: http://www.asds.net/TechnologyReportSuspensionSutures.aspx

Baker DC. Minimal incision rhytidectomy (short scar face lift) with lateral SMASectomy: evolution and application. Aesthetic Surg J 2001;21:14–26.

Brennan H, Koch R. Management of aging neck. Facial Plast Surg 1996;12:241–255.

de Castro C. The anatomy of the platysma muscle. Plast Reconstr Surg 1980;66:680–683.

Doerr T. Lipoplasty of the face and neck. Curr Opin Otolaryngol Head Neck Surg 2007;15(4): 228–232.

Eremia S. Rhytidectomy. Dermatol Clin 2005;23(3):415–430.

Eremia S, Willoughby MA. Novel face-lift suspension suture and inserting instrument: use of large anchors knotted into a suture with attached needle and inserting device allowing for single entry point placement of suspension suture. Preliminary report of 20 cases with 6- to 12-month follow-up. Dermatol Surg 2006;32(3):335–345.

Fulton JE, Saylan Z, Helton P, et al. The S-lift featuring the U-suture and O-suture combined with skin resurfacing. Dermatol Surg 2001;27(1):18–22.

Hoefflin SM. The extended supraplatysmal plane (ESP) face lift. Plast Reconstr Surg 1998;101(2):494–503.

McCarty ML, Brackup AB. Minimal incision facelift surgery. Ophthalmol Clin North Am 2005;18(2):305–310.

Robinson J, Hanke W, Sengelmann R, et al. Surgery of the Skin. Philadelphia: Elsevier, 2005.

Rohrich R, Rios J, Smith P, et al. Neck rejuvenation revisited. Plast Reconstr Surg 2006;118(5): 1251–1263.

Saylan Z. The S-lift for facial rejuvenation. Int J Cosmet Surg 1999;7:18–23.

Souther S, Vistnes L. Medial approximation of the platysma muscle in the treatment of neck deformities. Plast Reconstr Surg 1981;67:607–613.

Sulamanidze MA, Fournier PF, Paikdze TG, et al. Removal of facial soft tissue ptosis with special threads. Dermatol Surg 2002;28(5):367–371.

Sulamanidze MA, Paikidze TG, Sulamanidze GM, et al. Facial lifting with "APTOS" threads: Feather-Lift. Otolaryngol Clin N Am 2005;38(5): 1109–1117.

Vistnes L, Souther S. The platysma muscle: anatomic considerations for aesthetic surgery of the anterior neck. Clin Plast Surg 1983;10:441–448.

Watson D. Submentoplasty. Facial Plast Surg Clin North Am 2005;13(3):459–467.

Webster GV, Davidson TM, White MF, et al. Conservative face lift surgery. Arch Otolaryngol 1976;102:657–662.